HIV AND AIDS

SOURCEBOOK

EIGHTH EDITION

Health Reference Series

HIV AND AIDS
SOURCEBOOK

EIGHTH EDITION

Provides Basic Consumer Health Information about Human Immunodeficiency Virus (HIV) and Acquired Immunodeficiency Syndrome (AIDS), Including Facts about Its Origins, Stages, Types, Transmission, Risk Factors, and Prevention, and Features Details about Diagnostic Testing, Treatments, and Co-occurring Infections, Such as Cytomegalovirus, *Mycobacterium avium* Complex, *Pneumocystis* Pneumonia, and Toxoplasmosis

Along with Tips for Living with HIV/AIDS, Reports on Current Research Initiatives, a Glossary of Related Terms, and a List of Resources for Additional Help and Information

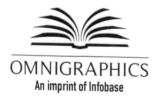

OMNIGRAPHICS
An imprint of Infobase

Bibliographic Note

Because this page cannot legibly accommodate all the copyright notices,
the Bibliographic Note portion of the Preface constitutes an extension
of the copyright notice.

* * *

OMNIGRAPHICS
An imprint of Infobase

132 W. 31st St.
New York, NY 10001
www.infobase.com
James Chambers, *Editorial Director*

* * *

Copyright © 2022 Infobase
ISBN 978-0-7808-1988-7
E-ISBN 978-0-7808-1989-4

Library of Congress Cataloging-in-Publication Data

Names: Hayes, Kevin (Editor of health information), editor.

Title: HIV and AIDS sourcebook / edited by Kevin Hayes. Other titles: AIDS sourcebook.

Description: Eighth edition. | Series: Health reference series | Revised edition of: AIDS sourcebook. Seventh edition. [2018]. | Summary: "Provides consumer health information about transmission, testing, stages, and treatment of human immunodeficiency virus (HIV), with facts about prevention, related complications, tips for living with HIV/AIDS, updated statistics, and reports on current research initiatives. Includes index, glossary of related terms, and other resources"-- Provided by publisher.

Identifiers: LCCN 2022000779 (print) | LCCN 2022000780 (ebook) | ISBN 9780780819887 (library binding) | ISBN 9780780819894 (epub)

Subjects: LCSH: AIDS (Disease)--Popular works. | HIV (Viruses)--Popular works. | Teenagers-- Health and hygiene.

Classification: LCC RC606.64.A337 2022 (print) | LCC RC606.64 (ebook) | DDC 616.97/92--dc23/ eng/20220111

LC record available at https://lccn.loc.gov/2022000779
LC ebook record available at https://lccn.loc.gov/2022000780

Table of Contents

Part 3. Receiving an HIV/AIDS Diagnosis

Preface

ABOUT THIS BOOK

Approximately 1.2 million people in the United States have human immunodeficiency virus (HIV). HIV continues to have a disproportionate impact on certain populations, particularly racial and ethnic minorities and gay, bisexual, and other men who have sex with men. In 2019, an estimated 34,800 new HIV infections occurred in the United States. In 2019, 36,801 people received an HIV diagnosis in the United States and 6 dependent areas – an overall 9 percent decrease compared with 2015. This devastating disease attacks the immune system and affects all parts of the body, eventually leading to acquired immunodeficiency syndrome (AIDS), its most deadly and advanced stage for which there is currently no cure. Yet there is hope for the many Americans living with HIV infection or AIDS. Improvements in medications and earlier diagnosis mean that those infected with HIV are living longer, healthier, and more productive lives.

HIV and AIDS Sourcebook, Eighth Edition offers basic consumer information about the HIV and AIDS, including information about the stages and types of the disease and about how it is transmitted. It includes guidelines for preventing disease transmission and details about how it is diagnosed and drug regimens used in its treatment. Information on co-occurring infections, complications, and tips for living with HIV infection are also included. The book concludes with a glossary of related terms and a list of resources for additional help and information.

HOW TO USE THIS BOOK

This book is divided into parts and chapters. Parts focus on broad areas of interest. Chapters are devoted to single topics within a part.

Part 1: Human Immunodeficiency Virus/Acquired Immunodeficiency Syndrome: An Overview defines HIV and AIDS, briefs up about what is known regarding the origin, facts and symptoms of the virus. It describes the life cycle, stages, and types of HIV infection, and explains how HIV causes AIDS. It also includes a brief discussion of the prevalence and incidence of HIV and AIDS in the United States and especially among specific populations.

Part 2: HIV/AIDS Transmission, Risk Factors, and Prevention presents the facts about the transmission of the human immunodeficiency virus. It explains the factors that put people at risk for HIV, provides tips for avoiding these risks, and answers questions related to transmission, risk, PrEP, and prevention.

Part 3: Receiving an HIV/AIDS Diagnosis describes the different types of HIV testing and explains consumer rights regarding confidentiality and counseling. It provides a detailed explanation of what the test results mean and how to determine if you have AIDS. It provides tips for choosing a provider and navigating the healthcare system and concludes with answers to frequently asked questions on testing and window period.

Part 4: Treatments and Therapies for HIV/AIDS gives an overview of treatment options, details the antiretroviral treatment process, describes the common side effects and complications of this treatment, and explains how the effectiveness of treatment is monitored and what to do in the event of treatment failure. It also discusses complementary and alternative HIV/AIDS treatments, other treatments currently being developed including the ones which are being researched, and how treatment varies in the special cases of children and pregnant women. It also offers information regarding paying for HIV care and provides answer to questions pertaining to treatment.

Part 5: Common Co-occurring Infections and Complications of HIV/AIDS describes the bacterial, fungal, parasitic, and viral infections that often accompany HIV and AIDS. It also offers tips on how to avoid these infections and explains how they are treated when they do occur. In addition, AIDS-related cancer, wasting syndrome, HIV-associated neurocognitive disorders, and other AIDS-related health concerns are discussed.

Part 6: Living with HIV Infection offers advice on coping with an HIV/AIDS diagnosis and explains how diet and exercise can help maintain health. It discusses legal responsibility for disclosure and provides tips for telling a spouse or sexual partners, family and friends, co-workers, and healthcare providers about HIV status. The part concludes with a discussion about laws that apply to people with HIV and a description of the public benefits, insurance, and housing options available, including information about providing home care for someone with AIDS.

Part 7: Additional Help and Information includes a glossary of terms related to AIDS and HIV and a directory of resources for additional help and support.

BIBLIOGRAPHIC NOTE

This volume contains documents and excerpts from publications issued by the following U.S. government agencies: ADA.gov; Centers for Disease Control and Prevention (CDC); Centers for Medicare & Medicaid Services (CMS); ClinicalInfo; Effective Health Care Program; Genetic and Rare Diseases Information Center (GARD); HIV.gov; HIVinfo; MedlinePlus; National Cancer Institute (NCI); National Center for Biotechnology Information (NCBI); National Institute of Allergy and Infectious Diseases (NIAID); National Institute of Dental and Craniofacial Research (NIDCR); National Institute of Mental Health (NIMH); National Institute of Neurological Disorders and Stroke (NINDS); National Institute on Drug Abuse (NIDA); National Institutes of Health (NIH); Office of Minority Health (OMH); U.S. Department of Labor (DOL); U.S. Department of Veterans Affairs (VA); U.S. Equal Employment Opportunity Commission (EEOC); U.S. Food and Drug Administration (FDA); and U.S. Social Security Administration (SSA).

It also contains original material produced by Infobase and reviewed by medical consultants.

ABOUT THE *HEALTH REFERENCE SERIES*

The *Health Reference Series* is designed to provide basic medical information for patients, families, caregivers, and the general public. Each volume provides comprehensive coverage on a particular topic. This is especially important for people who may be dealing with a newly diagnosed disease or a chronic disorder in themselves or in a family member. People looking for preventive guidance, information about disease warning signs, medical statistics, and risk factors for health problems will also find answers to their questions in the *Health Reference Series*. The *Series*, however, is not intended to serve as a tool for diagnosing illness, in prescribing treatments, or as a substitute for the physician–patient relationship. All people concerned about medical symptoms or the possibility of disease are encouraged to seek professional care from an appropriate healthcare provider.

A NOTE ABOUT SPELLING AND STYLE

Health Reference Series editors use *Stedman's Medical Dictionary* as an authority for questions related to the spelling of medical terms and *The Chicago Manual of Style* for questions related to grammatical structures, punctuation, and other editorial concerns. Consistent adherence is not always possible, however, because the individual volumes within the *Series* include many documents from a wide variety of different producers, and the editor's primary goal is to present material from each source as accurately as is possible. This sometimes means that information in different chapters or sections may follow other guidelines and alternate spelling authorities. For example, occasionally a copyright holder may require that eponymous terms be shown in possessive forms (Crohn's disease vs. Crohn disease) or that British spelling norms be retained (leukaemia vs. leukemia).

MEDICAL REVIEW

Infobase contracts with a team of qualified, senior medical professionals who serve as medical consultants for the *Health Reference Series*. As necessary, medical consultants review reprinted and originally written material for currency and accuracy. Citations including the phrase "Reviewed (month, year)" indicate material reviewed by this team. Medical consultation services are provided to the *Health Reference Series* editors by:

Dr. Vijayalakshmi, MBBS, DGO, MD
Dr. Senthil Selvan, MBBS, DCH, MD
Dr. K. Sivanandham, MBBS, DCH, MS (Research), PhD

HEALTH REFERENCE SERIES UPDATE POLICY

The inaugural book in the *Health Reference Series* was the first edition of *Cancer Sourcebook* published in 1989. Since then, the *Series* has been enthusiastically received by librarians and in the medical community. In order to maintain the standard of providing high-quality health information for the layperson the editorial staff at Infobase felt it was necessary to implement a policy of updating volumes when warranted.

Medical researchers have been making tremendous strides, and it is the purpose of the *Health Reference Series* to stay current with the most recent advances. Each decision to update a volume is made on an individual basis. Some of the considerations include how much new information

Part 1 | Human Immunodeficiency Virus/Acquired Immunodeficiency Syndrome: An Overview

Chapter 1 | Origin of HIV and AIDS

WHAT IS HUMAN IMMUNODEFICIENCY VIRUS?[1]

Human immunodeficiency virus (HIV) is a virus that attacks the body's immune system. If HIV is not treated, it can lead to AIDS (acquired immunodeficiency syndrome). Learning the basics about HIV can keep you healthy and prevent HIV transmission.

- There is currently no effective cure. Once people get HIV, they have it for life.
- But with proper medical care, HIV can be controlled. People with HIV who get effective HIV treatment can live long, healthy lives and protect their partners.

WHAT IS ACQUIRED IMMUNODEFICIENCY SYNDROME?[2]

- Acquired immunodeficiency syndrome is the most severe stage of HIV (Stage 3).
- People with AIDS have badly damaged immune systems. They get an increasing number of severe illnesses, called "opportunistic infections" (OIs).
- People receive an AIDS diagnosis when
  - They develop certain OIs, or
  - Their CD4 cell count drops below 200 cells per milliliter of blood.

This chapter includes text excerpted from documents published by two public domain sources. Text under the headings marked 1 are excerpted from "About HIV," Centers for Disease Control and Prevention (CDC), June 1, 2021; Text under the heading marked 2 is excerpted from "AIDS and Opportunistic Infections," Centers for Disease Control and Prevention (CDC), May 20, 2021.

WHERE DID HUMAN IMMUNODEFICIENCY VIRUS COME FROM?[1]

- HIV infection in humans came from a type of chimpanzee in Central Africa.
- The chimpanzee version of the virus (called "simian immunodeficiency virus," or "SIV") was probably passed to humans when humans hunted these chimpanzees for meat and came in contact with their infected blood.
- Studies show that HIV may have jumped from chimpanzees to humans as far back as the late 1800s.
- Over decades, HIV slowly spread across Africa and later into other parts of the world. We know that the virus has existed in the United States since at least the mid to late 1970s.

HOW DO YOU KNOW IF YOU HAVE HUMAN IMMUNODEFICIENCY VIRUS?[1]

The only way to know for sure whether you have HIV is to get tested. Knowing your HIV status helps you make healthy decisions to prevent getting or transmitting HIV.

ARE THERE SYMPTOMS?[1]

Some people have flu-like symptoms within 2–4 weeks after infection (called "acute HIV infection"). These symptoms may last for a few days or several weeks. Possible symptoms include:

- Fever
- Chills
- Rash
- Night sweats
- Muscle aches
- Sore throat
- Fatigue
- Swollen lymph nodes
- Mouth ulcers

But some people may not feel sick during acute HIV infection. These symptoms do not mean you have HIV. Other illnesses can cause these same symptoms.

Origin of HIV and AIDS

See a healthcare provider if you have these symptoms and think you may have been exposed to HIV. Getting tested for HIV is the only way to know for sure.

Chapter 2 | **HIV Stages and Types**

Chapter Contents

Section 2.1 | The HIV Life Cycle

This section includes text excerpted from "The HIV Life Cycle," HIVinfo, U.S. Department of Health and Human Services (HHS), August 4, 2021.

WHAT IS THE HIV LIFE CYCLE?

Human immunodeficiency virus (HIV) attacks and destroys the CD4 cells (CD4 T lymphocyte) of the immune system. CD4 cells are a type of white blood cell that play a major role in protecting the body from infection. HIV uses the machinery of the CD4 cells to multiply and spread throughout the body. This process, which is carried out in seven steps or stages, is called "the HIV life cycle."

WHAT IS THE CONNECTION BETWEEN THE HIV LIFE CYCLE AND HIV MEDICINES?

Antiretroviral therapy (ART) is the use of a combination of HIV medicines to treat HIV infection. People on ART take a combination of HIV medicines (called an "HIV treatment regimen") every day. HIV medicines protect the immune system by blocking HIV at different stages of the HIV life cycle. Figure 2.3 in Section 2.2 shows three stages of HIV infection. HIV medicines are grouped into different drug classes according to how they fight HIV. Each class of drugs is designed to target a specific step in the HIV life cycle.

Because an HIV treatment regimen includes HIV medicines from at least two different HIV drug classes, ART is very effective at preventing HIV from multiplying. Having less HIV in the body protects the immune system and prevents HIV from advancing to acquired immunodeficiency syndrome (AIDS).

ART cannot cure HIV, but HIV medicines help people with HIV live longer, healthier lives. HIV medicines also reduce the risk of HIV transmission (the spread of HIV to others).

WHAT ARE THE SEVEN STAGES OF THE HIV LIFE CYCLE?

The seven stages of the HIV life cycle are:
- Binding

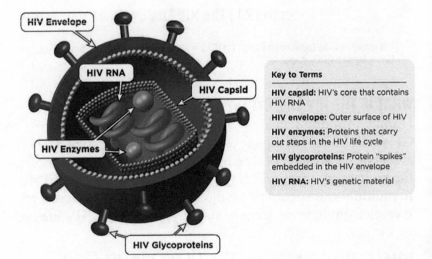

Figure 2.1. Human Immunodeficiency Virus

- Fusion
- Reverse transcription
- Integration
- Replication
- Assembly
- Budding

To understand each stage in the HIV life cycle, it helps to first imagine what HIV looks like. Figure 2.1 is an illustration of the virus.

Now, follow each stage in the HIV life cycle as HIV attacks a CD4 cell and uses the machinery of the cell to multiply as shown in Figure 2.2.

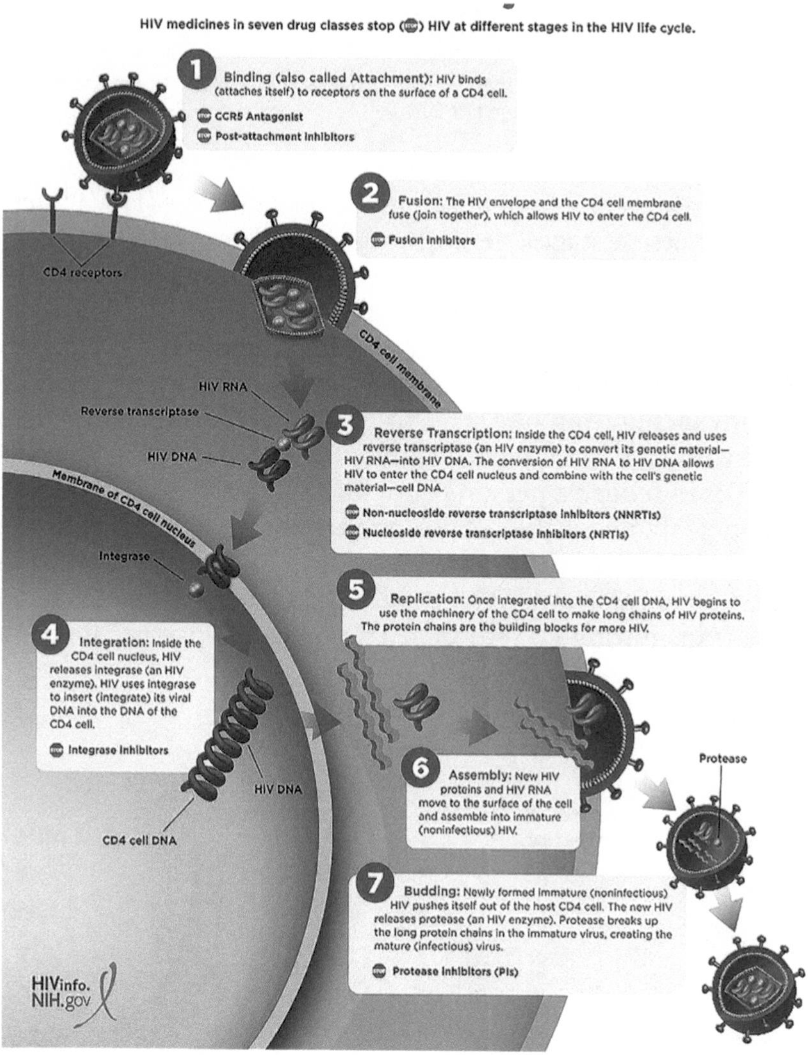

HIV medicines in seven drug classes stop (🚫) HIV at different stages in the HIV life cycle.

1 Binding (also called Attachment): HIV binds (attaches itself) to receptors on the surface of a CD4 cell.
- 🚫 CCR5 Antagonist
- 🚫 Post-attachment Inhibitors

2 Fusion: The HIV envelope and the CD4 cell membrane fuse (join together), which allows HIV to enter the CD4 cell.
- 🚫 Fusion Inhibitors

CD4 receptors

CD4 cell membrane

HIV RNA

Reverse transcriptase

HIV DNA

Membrane of CD4 cell nucleus

3 Reverse Transcription: Inside the CD4 cell, HIV releases and uses reverse transcriptase (an HIV enzyme) to convert its genetic material—HIV RNA—into HIV DNA. The conversion of HIV RNA to HIV DNA allows HIV to enter the CD4 cell nucleus and combine with the cell's genetic material—cell DNA.
- 🚫 Non-nucleoside reverse transcriptase inhibitors (NNRTIs)
- 🚫 Nucleoside reverse transcriptase inhibitors (NRTIs)

Integrase

5 Replication: Once integrated into the CD4 cell DNA, HIV begins to use the machinery of the CD4 cell to make long chains of HIV proteins. The protein chains are the building blocks for more HIV.

4 Integration: Inside the CD4 cell nucleus, HIV releases integrase (an HIV enzyme). HIV uses integrase to insert (integrate) its viral DNA into the DNA of the CD4 cell.
- 🚫 Integrase Inhibitors

HIV DNA

CD4 cell DNA

6 Assembly: New HIV proteins and HIV RNA move to the surface of the cell and assemble into immature (noninfectious) HIV.

Protease

7 Budding: Newly formed immature (noninfectious) HIV pushes itself out of the host CD4 cell. The new HIV releases protease (an HIV enzyme). Protease breaks up the long protein chains in the immature virus, creating the mature (infectious) virus.
- 🚫 Protease Inhibitors (PIs)

HIVinfo.
NIH.gov

Figure 2.2. HIV Life Cycle

Section 2.2 | **Stages of HIV Infection**

This section includes text excerpted from "The Stages of HIV Infection," HIVinfo, U.S. Department of Health and Human Services (HHS), August 20, 2021.

Without treatment, human immunodeficiency virus (HIV) infection advances in stages, getting worse over time. HIV gradually destroys the immune system and eventually causes acquired immunodeficiency syndrome (AIDS). Figure 2.3 shows HIV progression.

There is no cure for HIV, but treatment with HIV medicines (called "antiretroiral therapy" or "ART") can slow or prevent HIV from advancing from one stage to the next. HIV medicines help people with HIV live longer, healthier lives. One of the main goals of ART is to reduce a person's viral load to an undetectable level. An undetectable viral load means that the level of HIV in the blood is too low to be detected by a viral load test. People with HIV who maintain an undetectable viral load have effectively no risk of transmitting HIV to their HIV-negative partner through sex.

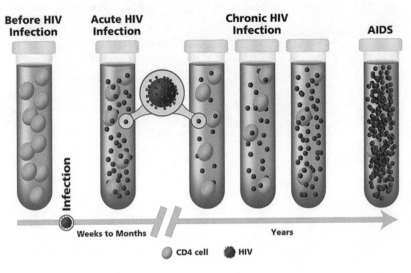

Figure 2.3. HIV Progression

THREE STAGES OF HIV INFECTION
Acute HIV Infection

Acute HIV infection is the earliest stage of HIV infection, and it generally develops within 2–4 weeks after infection with HIV. During this time, some people have flu-like symptoms, such as fever, headache, and rash. In the acute stage of infection, HIV multiplies rapidly and spreads throughout the body. The virus attacks and destroys the infection-fighting CD4 cells (CD4 T lymphocyte) of the immune system. During the acute HIV infection stage, the level of HIV in the blood is very high, which greatly increases the risk of HIV transmission. A person may experience significant health benefits if they start ART during this stage.

Chronic HIV Infection

The second stage of HIV infection is chronic HIV infection (also called "asymptomatic HIV infection" or "clinical latency"). During this stage, HIV continues to multiply in the body but at very low levels. People with chronic HIV infection may not have any HIV-related symptoms. Without ART, chronic HIV infection usually advances to AIDS in 10 years or longer, though in some people it may advance faster. People who are taking ART may be in this stage for several decades. While it is still possible to transmit HIV to others during this stage, people who take ART exactly as prescribed and maintain an undetectable viral load have effectively no risk of transmitting HIV to an HIV-negative partner through sex.

Acquired Immunodeficiency Syndrome

Acquired immunodeficiency syndrome is the final, most severe stage of HIV infection. Because HIV has severely damaged the immune system, the body cannot fight off opportunistic infections. (Opportunistic infections are infections and infection-related cancers that occur more frequently or are more severe in people with weakened immune systems than in people with healthy immune systems.) People with HIV are diagnosed with AIDS if they have a CD4 count of less than 200 cells/mm3 or if they have certain opportunistic infections. Once a person is diagnosed with AIDS, they can have a high viral load and are able to transmit HIV to others very easily. Without treatment, people with AIDS typically survive about 3 years.

Section 2.3 | Acute HIV Infection

This section includes text excerpted from "Early (Acute and Recent) HIV Infection," ClinicalInfo, U.S. Department of Health and Human Services (HHS), January 20, 2022.

Acute human immunodeficiency virus (HIV) infection occurs soon after transmission and is typically characterized by the lack of anti-HIV antibodies and the presence of viremia, which can be detected by HIV RNA or p24 antigen test. Recent HIV infection is considered the phase of ≤6 months after infection, during which anti-HIV antibodies become detectable. Throughout this section, the term "early HIV infection" is used to refer to either acute or recent HIV infection. Persons with acute HIV infection may experience fever, lymphadenopathy, pharyngitis, skin rash, myalgia, arthralgia, and other symptoms; however, illness is generally nonspecific and can be relatively mild or the person can be asymptomatic. Clinicians may fail to recognize acute HIV infection, because its manifestations are similar to those of many other viral infections, such as influenza and infectious mononucleosis.

DIAGNOSING ACUTE HIV INFECTION

Combination immunoassays that detect HIV-1 and HIV-2 antibodies and HIV p24 antigen (Ag/Ab assays) are part of the recommended initial laboratory HIV testing algorithm, primarily due to their enhanced ability to detect acute HIV infection. Specimens that are reactive on an initial Ag/Ab assay should be tested with an immunoassay that differentiates HIV-1 from HIV-2 antibodies. Specimens that are reactive on the initial assay and have either negative or indeterminate antibody differentiation test result should be tested for quantitative or qualitative HIV RNA; an undetectable

HIV RNA test result indicates that the original Ag/Ab test result was a false positive. Detection of HIV RNA in this setting indicates that acute HIV infection is highly likely. Patients presenting to care during the earliest days following HIV infection may have yet to develop a positive p24 Ag response, which typically occurs with viral load levels of >20,000 to 30,000 copies/mL. In clinical settings of high probability of infection, quantitative or qualitative HIV RNA testing should be considered even if the HIV Ag/Ab test result is negative. HIV infection should be confirmed by repeat quantitative HIV RNA testing or subsequent testing to document HIV antibody seroconversion. Persons receiving antiretroviral therapy (ART) during acute or very early HIV infection may demonstrate weaker reactivity to screening antibody assays or incomplete HIV antibody evolution; may remain nonreactive to confirmatory antibody assays; and in the setting of sustained virologic suppression, may have complete or partial seroreversion.

Some healthcare facilities may still be using HIV testing algorithms that test only for anti-HIV antibodies. In such settings, when acute HIV infection is suspected in a patient with a negative or indeterminate HIV antibody test result, a quantitative or qualitative HIV RNA test should be performed. A negative or indeterminate HIV antibody test result and a positive HIV RNA test result indicate that acute HIV infection is highly likely.

TREATING EARLY HIV INFECTION

The goals of ART during early HIV infection are to suppress plasma HIV RNA to undetectable levels (AI) and to prevent the transmission of HIV (AI). Importantly, as with chronic HIV infection, an individual's barriers to ART adherence and appointments should be assessed before the initiation of ART. ART should be initiated as soon as possible after a positive qualitative or quantitative HIV RNA test result. Same-day or rapid ART initiation in persons with acute HIV has been shown to be safe, acceptable, and effective. It is important to collect a new blood specimen for confirmatory HIV antibody test and quantitative plasma HIV RNA test to verify the HIV diagnosis. Given the sensitivity of current HIV RNA assays, a positive result by quantitative or qualitative plasma HIV RNA testing in the setting of a negative or indeterminate antibody test result indicates that acute HIV infection is highly likely. HIV treatment does not need to be delayed while awaiting confirmation of HIV diagnosis. Some individuals may not accept their diagnosis or may decline ART initially for other reasons. Individuals who do not begin ART immediately should be maintained in care, and every effort should be made to initiate therapy as soon as they are ready.

Considerations for Preventing HIV Transmission during Early HIV Infection

Persons with early HIV infection have a higher likelihood of sexual transmission of HIV to others. Prompt initiation of ART and sustained viral suppression to <200 copies/mL can prevent transmission of HIV to sexual partners. Individuals starting ART should use another form of prevention (e.g., condoms, PrEP for partners who are HIV negative, sexual abstinence) for at least the first 6 months of treatment and until they have a documented viral load of <200 copies/mL (AII). Many experts would recommend confirming sustained viral suppression before assuming no risk of sexual transmission of HIV (AIII).

Antiretroviral Regimens for Early HIV Infection

Antiretroviral therapy should be initiated with one of the combination regimens recommended for persons with chronic HIV infection (AIII). Providers should inform individuals starting ART of the importance of adherence to achieve and maintain viral suppression (AII). If available, the results of ARV drug-resistance testing or the resistance pattern of the source person's virus should be used to guide selection of the regimen. All persons of childbearing potential should have a pregnancy test before initiating ART (AIII).

If ART is to be initiated before the results of drug-resistance and HLA-B*5701 tests are available, one of the following regimens is an appropriate option (AIII):

- Dolutegravir with (emtricitabine (FTC) or lamivudine (3TC)) plus (tenofovir disoproxil fumarate (TDF) or tenofovir alafenamide (TAF))

- BIC/TAF/FTC
- Boosted darunavir (DRV) with (FTC or 3TC) plus (TAF or TDF)

Dolutegravir is a good treatment option because transmission of DTG-resistant HIV is rare, and DTG has a higher barrier to resistance than raltegravir and elvitegravir. Based on data from in vitro studies and clinical trials in ART-naive participants, it is anticipated that BIC also might have a high barrier to resistance. However, clinical data and experience defining the BIC barrier to resistance are relatively limited at this time.

A pharmacologically boosted protease inhibitor (PI)-based regimen (e.g., boosted DRV) is also an option because resistance to PIs emerges slowly, and clinically significant transmitted resistance to PIs is uncommon. Abacavir/3TC is not recommended for treatment of acute HIV infection, unless the patient is known to be HLA-B*5701 negative – information that is seldom available when individuals with acute infection are diagnosed. Therefore, TDF/FTC or TAF/FTC is generally recommended in this setting. Baseline laboratory testing recommended for individuals with chronic HIV infection should be performed. Individuals with hepatitis B virus/HIV coinfection should receive TDF/FTC or TAF/FTC as part of their ARV regimen.

Given the increasing use of TDF/FTC as PrEP, early HIV infection may be diagnosed in some persons while they are taking TDF/FTC. In this setting, drug-resistance test results are particularly important; however, the regimens listed above remain as reasonable treatment options pending drug-resistance test results.

Because the rate of transmitted drug resistance for NNRTIs is relatively high, agents in this drug class are not recommended as a component in the regimen of persons initiating ART before the results of drug-resistance tests are available.

TREATMENT REGIMENS OF EARLY HIV INFECTION DURING PREGNANCY

All persons of childbearing potential who receive a diagnosis of early HIV infection should have a pregnancy test (AIII). Because early HIV infection, especially in the setting of high-level viremia, is associated with a high risk of perinatal transmission, all pregnant persons with HIV should start combination ART as soon as possible to prevent perinatal transmission.

Section 2.4 | Drug Resistant HIV

This section includes text excerpted from "Drug Resistance," HIVinfo, U.S. Department of Health and Human Services (HHS), August 4, 2021.

WHAT IS HIV DRUG RESISTANCE?

Once a person gets human immunodeficiency virus (HIV), the virus begins to multiply in the body. As HIV multiplies, it sometimes changes form (mutates). Some HIV mutations that develop while a person is taking HIV medicines can lead to drug-resistant HIV.

Once drug resistance develops, HIV medicines that previously controlled the person's HIV are no longer effective. In other words, the HIV medicines cannot prevent the drug-resistant HIV from multiplying. Drug resistance can cause HIV treatment to fail.

Drug-resistant HIV can spread from person to person (called "transmitted resistance"). People with transmitted resistance have HIV that is resistant to one or more HIV medicines even before they start taking HIV medicines.

WHAT IS DRUG-RESISTANCE TESTING?

Drug-resistance testing identifies which, if any, HIV medicines that will not be effective against a person's HIV. Drug-resistance testing is done using a sample of blood.

People with HIV should start taking HIV medicines as soon as possible after their HIV is diagnosed. But before a person starts taking HIV medicines, drug-resistance testing is done.

Drug-resistance test results help determine which HIV medicines to include in a person's first HIV treatment regimen.

Once HIV treatment is started, a viral load test is used to monitor whether the HIV medicines are controlling a person's HIV. If viral load testing indicates that a person's HIV treatment regimen is not effective, drug-resistance testing is repeated. The test results can identify whether drug resistance is the problem and, if so, can be used to select a new HIV treatment regimen.

HOW CAN A PERSON TAKING HIV MEDICINES REDUCE THE RISK OF DRUG RESISTANCE?

Taking HIV medicines every day and exactly as prescribed (called "medication adherence") reduces the risk of drug resistance. Skipping HIV medicines allows HIV to multiply, which increases the risk that the virus will mutate and produce drug-resistant HIV.

Before starting HIV treatment, tell your healthcare provider about any issues that can make medication adherence difficult. For example, a busy schedule or lack of health insurance can make it hard to take HIV medicines consistently. Once you start treatment, use a 7-day pill box or other medication aid to stay on track.

Chapter 3 | **Symptoms of HIV**

There are several symptoms of human immunodeficiency virus (HIV). Not everyone will have the same symptoms. It depends on the person and what stage of the disease they are in.

Below are the three stages of HIV and some of the symptoms people may experience.

ACUTE HUMAN IMMUNODEFICIENCY VIRUS INFECTION

Within 2–4 weeks after infection with HIV, about two-thirds of people will have a flu-like illness. This is the body's natural response to HIV infection.

Flu-like symptoms can include:
- Fever
- Chills
- Rash
- Night sweats
- Muscle aches
- Sore throat
- Fatigue
- Swollen lymph nodes
- Mouth ulcers

These symptoms can last anywhere from a few days to several weeks. But some people do not have any symptoms at all during this early stage of HIV.

This chapter includes text excerpted from "Symptoms of HIV," HIV.gov, U.S. Department of Health and Human Services (HHS), July 1, 2020.

Do not assume you have HIV just because you have any of these symptoms – they can be similar to those caused by other illnesses. But if you think you may have been exposed to HIV, get an HIV test.

Here is what to do:

- **Find an HIV testing site near you**. You can get an HIV test at your primary care provider's office, your local health department, a health clinic, or many other places.
- **Request an HIV test for a recent infection**. Most HIV tests detect antibodies (proteins your body makes as a reaction to HIV), not HIV itself. But it can take a few weeks after you are infected for your body to produce them. There are other types of tests that can detect HIV infection sooner. Tell your doctor or clinic if you think you were recently exposed to HIV, and ask if their tests can detect early infection.
- **Know your status**. After you get tested, be sure to learn your test results. If you are HIV-positive, see a doctor as soon as possible so you can start treatment with HIV medicine. And be aware: when you are in the early stage of infection, you are at very high risk of transmitting HIV to others. It is important to take steps to reduce your risk of transmission. If you are HIV-negative, there are prevention tools such as pre-exposure prophylaxis (PrEP) that can help you stay negative.

CLINICAL LATENCY

In this stage, the virus still multiplies, but at very low levels. People in this stage may not feel sick or have any symptoms. This stage is also called "chronic HIV infection."

Without HIV treatment, people can stay in this stage for 10 or 15 years, but some move through this stage faster.

If you take HIV medicine every day, exactly as prescribed and get and keep an undetectable viral load, you can protect your health and have effectively no risk of transmitting HIV to your sexual partner(s).

But if your viral load is detectable, you *can* transmit HIV during this stage, even when you have no symptoms. It is important to see your healthcare provider regularly to get your viral load checked.

ACQUIRED IMMUNODEFICIENCY SYNDROME

If you have HIV and you are not on HIV treatment, eventually the virus will weaken your body's immune system and you will progress to acquired immunodeficiency syndrome (AIDS). This is the late stage of HIV infection.

Symptoms of AIDS can include:

- Rapid weight loss
- Recurring fever or profuse night sweats
- Extreme and unexplained tiredness
- Prolonged swelling of the lymph glands in the armpits, groin, or neck
- Diarrhea that lasts for more than a week
- Sores of the mouth, anus, or genitals
- Pneumonia
- Red, brown, pink, or purplish blotches on or under the skin or inside the mouth, nose, or eyelids
- Memory loss, depression, and other neurologic disorders

Each of these symptoms can also be related to other illnesses. The only way to know for sure if you have HIV is to get tested. If you are HIV-positive, a healthcare provider will diagnose if your HIV has progressed to AIDS based on certain medical criteria.

Many of the severe symptoms and illnesses of HIV disease come from the opportunistic infections that occur because your body's immune system has been damaged.

Chapter 4 | **How HIV Causes AIDS**

The human immunodeficiency virus (HIV) is a virus that functions by eliminating critical cells that fight disease and infection, eventually lowering a person's immune system. HIV is usually spread out over three stages. People with an acute infection are at stage 1. Asymptomatic HIV infection, often known as "clinical latency," is the second stage. The amount of HIV in the blood (known as "viral load") at this stage progresses, and the CD4 cell count decreases. As HIV level increases in the body, the person may develop symptoms and progress to stage 3. People with stage 3 HIV have severely weakened immune systems that can lead to acquired immunodeficiency syndrome (AIDS), which is a potentially life-threatening chronic condition. The condition reduces the efficacy of the human immune system since the virus impairs the body's ability to fight off infections and diseases. HIV is commonly termed as a "sexually transmitted infection (STI)" as it spreads through sexual interaction, via semen, vaginal and rectal fluids, and preseminal fluids. It can also be transmitted through blood and breast milk.

MECHANISM OF AN HIV INFECTION

- As soon as the virus enters the body after transmission, it attaches itself to several types of white blood cells (WBCs), the most important of which are specific helper T lymphocytes that are also known as "T cells." These cells are crucial because they assemble and coordinate the other cells of the human immune system, such as macrophages, neutrophils, and B-cells. T cells possess a receptor on their surfaces and are called "CD4 cells." The receptors make it easier for the HIV virion to attach to these cells, which is why they are also called "CD4+" cells.

- Being a retrovirus (a type of virus that inserts a duplicate of its ribonucleic acid (RNA) genome into the deoxyribonucleic acid (DNA) of the host cell that it invades, resulting in a change in its genome), HIV stores its genetic information in the form of RNA. After entering a CD4+ lymphocyte, the virus secretes an enzyme known as "reverse transcriptase" to help duplicate its RNA into copies that contain DNA.
- HIV mutates quickly and easily at this point since the enzyme is prone to making errors while replicating HIV RNA to DNA.
- HIV DNA is now infused into the DNA of the infected lymphocyte, which continues to reproduce the HIV. During this process, the cell produces thousands of HIV which then starts to deteriorate the cell itself. Similarly, other infected lymphocytes produce a large number of HIV and then deteriorate and die.
- Within a span of a few days or weeks, the blood and genital fluids of infected individuals begin to contain a large amount of HIV and show a possibility of a reduced CD4+ lymphocyte count.

An HIV infection occurs in three distinct stages namely:
- **Acute HIV infection**. This is the initial stage of the infection where people will experience flu-like symptoms and a rapid multiplication of HIV in the blood. In this stage, the HIV level in the blood is extremely high and it develops within 2–4 weeks after infection.
- **Chronic HIV infection**. It is the second stage of the infection and is also known as "asymptomatic HIV infection" or "clinical latency." At this stage, HIV continues to multiply in the blood at extremely low

levels and individuals in this stage will not have any HIV-related symptoms.

- **Acquired immunodeficiency syndrome (AIDS).** AIDS is the third and final stage, sometimes also referred to as the most advanced and severe stage of HIV. When the HIV infection starts to destroy CD4+ lymphocytes faster than they can be produced, the body's immune system begins to get severely compromised. Once AIDS occurs, the individual will become easily susceptible to infections or cancers.

An AIDS diagnosis is confirmed if the infected individual's CD4 count is less than 200 cells/mm3. Uninfected, healthy adults generally have a CD4 count of 500–1,600 cells/mm3. A person infected with AIDS can have a high viral load that makes it easy for them to transmit HIV to others.

HIV typically takes 8–10 years to progress to the AIDS stage if left untreated. Without any HIV treatment, infected individuals diagnosed with AIDS are expected to live for only about three years. The person living with AIDS is vulnerable to a wide range of illnesses, including pneumonia, tuberculosis, oral thrush, toxoplasmosis, cryptosporidiosis, and cancers such as Kaposi sarcoma and lymphoma.

Shortened life expectancy linked with untreated AIDS is not a direct result of the syndrome itself. Rather, it is a result of the diseases and complications that arise from having an immune system weakened by AIDS.

References

Cachay, Edward.R. "Human Immunodeficiency Virus (HIV) Infection," MSD Manual, April 2021.

"HIV and AIDS: The Basics," HIVinfo, U.S. Department of Health and Human Services (HHS), August 16, 2021.

"HIV/AIDS," Mayo Clinic, February 13, 2020.

"The Stages of HIV Infection," HIVinfo, U.S. Department of Health and Human Services (HHS), August 20, 2021.

Chapter 5 | **HIV/AIDS: A Statistical Overview**

A STATISTICAL OVERVIEW OF UNITED STATES

- Approximately 1.2 million people in the United States have human immunodeficiency virus (HIV). About 13 percent of them do not know it and need testing.
- HIV continues to have a disproportionate impact on certain populations, particularly racial and ethnic minorities and gay, bisexual, and other men who have sex with men (MSM).
- In 2019, an estimated 34,800 new HIV infections occurred in the United States.
- New HIV infections declined 8 percent from 37,800 in 2015 to 34,800 in 2019, after a period of general stability.
- In 2019, 36,801 people received an HIV diagnosis in the United States and 6 dependent areas – an overall 9 percent decrease compared with 2015.
- HIV diagnoses are not evenly distributed across states and regions. The highest rates of new diagnoses continue to occur in the South.

NEW HIV INFECTIONS

Human immunodeficiency virus incidence refers to the estimated number of new HIV infections during specified period of time (such as a year), which is different from the number of people diagnosed with HIV during a given year. (Some people may have

This chapter includes text excerpted from "U.S. Statistics," HIV.gov, U.S. Department of Health and Human Services (HHS), June 2, 2021.

HIV for some time but not know it, so the year they are diagnosed may not be the same as the year they acquired HIV.)

According to the estimates from the Centers for Disease Control and Prevention (CDC), approximately 34,800 new HIV infections occurred in the United States in 2019. Annual infections in the United States have been reduced by more than two-thirds since the height of the epidemic in the mid-1980s. Further, the CDC estimates of annual HIV infections in the United States show hopeful signs of progress in recent years. The CDC estimates show new HIV infections declined 8 percent from 37,800 in 2015 to 34,800 in 2019, after a period of general stability.

Much of this progress was due to larger declines among young gay and bisexual men in recent years. From 2015–2019, new infections among young gay and bisexual men (ages 13–24) dropped 33 percent overall, with declines in young men of all races, but African-Americans and Hispanics/Latinos continue to be severely and disproportionately affected.

Key Points: HIV Incidence

HIV incidence declined 8 percent from 2015–2019. In 2019, the estimated number of HIV infections in the United States was 34,800 and the rate was 12.6 (per 100,000 people).

By age group, the annual number of HIV infections in 2019, compared with 2015, decreased among persons aged 13–24 and persons aged 45–54 but remained stable among all other age groups. In 2019, the rate was highest for persons aged 25–34 (30.1), followed by the rate for persons aged 35–44 (16.5).

By race/ethnicity, the annual number of HIV infections in 2019, compared with 2015, decreased among persons of multiple races, but remained stable for persons of all other races/ethnicities. In 2019, the highest rate was for Blacks/African-American persons (42.1), followed by Hispanic/Latino persons (21.7) and persons of multiple races (18.4).

By sex at birth, the annual number of new HIV infections in 2019, as compared to 2015, decreased among males, but remained stable among females. In 2019, the rate for males (21.0) was 5 times the rate for females (4.5).

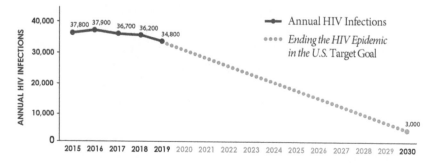

Figure 5.1. HIV Infection in the Unites States, 2015–2019. *(Source: Centers for Disease Control and Prevention (CDC), 2019 National HIV Surveillance System Reports, May 27, 2021.)*

By HIV transmission category, the annual number of HIV infections in 2019, compared with 2015, decreased among males with transmission attributed to male-to-male sexual contact, but remained stable among all other transmission categories. In 2019, the largest percentages of HIV infections were attributed to male-to-male sexual contact (66 percent overall and 81 percent among males.)

New HIV infections fell 8 percent from 2015–2019, after a period of general stability and is also expected to decrease moving forward as shown in Figure 5.1.

HIV DIAGNOSES

Human immunodeficiency virus diagnosis refers to the number of people who have received an HIV diagnosis during a year, regardless of when they acquired HIV. (Some people can live with HIV for years before they are diagnosed; others are diagnosed soon after acquiring HIV.)

According to the CDC data, in 2019, 36,801 people received an HIV diagnosis in the United States and dependent areas. From 2015 through 2019, HIV diagnoses decreased by 9 percent in the United States and 6 dependent areas. However, trends varied for different groups of people.

Key Points: HIV Diagnoses

Gay, bisexual and other men who have sex with men (MSM) are the population most affected by HIV in the United States:

- MSM accounted for 69 percent of new HIV diagnoses in the United States.
- From 2015 through 2019 in the United States and 6 dependent areas, Black/African-American MSM accounted for more than 36 percent and white MSM accounted for more than 30 percent of HIV diagnoses among MSM annually.
- In 2019, Black/African American MSM accounted for 26 percent (9,123) of new HIV diagnoses and 37.9 percent of diagnoses among all MSM.
- In 2019, Hispanic/Latino MSM made up 22 percent (7,820) of new HIV diagnoses and 32.5 percent of diagnosis among all MSM.

The number of HIV diagnoses decreased among MSM overall, but trends varied by race/ethnicity. From 2015 through 2019:

- Among MSM aged 13–24 years, HIV diagnoses decreased or were stable among all racial/ethnic groups.
- HIV diagnoses increased among American Indian/ Alaska Native and Native Hawaiian/other Pacific Islander MSM, ages 24 and older.

Transgender people accounted for approximately 2 percent of new HIV diagnoses in 2019.

- From 2015 through 2019 in the United States and 6 dependent areas, the number of diagnoses of HIV infection for transgender adults and adolescents increased.
- In 2019, among transgender adults and adolescents, the largest percentage (93 percent) of diagnoses of HIV infections was for transgender male-to-female (MTF) people.
- By age, in 2019, the largest percentage (24 percent) of diagnoses of HIV infection among transgender persons was for transgender MTF adults and adolescents aged 20–24 years, followed by transgender MTF adults and adolescents aged 25–29 years (23 percent).

Heterosexual people made up 23 percent of all HIV diagnoses in the United States and 6 dependent areas in 2019. Heterosexual men accounted for 7 percent of new HIV diagnoses and heterosexual women accounted for 16 percent.

People who inject drugs (PWID) accounted for 7 percent of new HIV infections in the United States and 6 dependent areas in 2019. Men who inject drugs accounted for 4 percent of new HIV diagnoses, and women who inject drugs accounted for 3 percent.

By race/ethnicity, Blacks/African Americans and Hispanics/Latinx continue to be severely and disproportionately affected by HIV:

- In 2019, Blacks/African Americans represented 13 percent of the U.S. population but accounted for 44 percent of new HIV diagnoses.
- In 2019, Hispanics/Latinx represented 18 percent of the U.S. population but accounted for 30 percent of new HIV diagnoses.
- From 2015–2019, the number of HIV diagnoses decreased among Black/African American, white, and Asian persons, and persons of multiple races. HIV diagnoses increased among American Indian/Alaska Natives, and remained stable among Hispanic/Latinos and Native Americans/other Pacific Islander persons.

By age group, in 2019, the number of new HIV diagnoses was highest among people aged 25–29. From 2015 through 2019, HIV diagnoses increased among persons aged 13–24 years, 35–44 years, and 45–54 years. Diagnoses remained stable among persons aged 25–35 years and persons aged 55 years and over.

By region, HIV diagnoses are not evenly distributed. From 2015 through 2019, the annual number and rate of diagnoses of HIV infection in the United States and 6 dependent areas decreased. In 2019, the rates were 15.2 in the South, 9.4 in the Northeast, 9.2 in the West, and 7.2 in the Midwest.

LIVING WITH HIV

At year-end 2019, an estimated 1.2 million people in the United States aged 13 and older had HIV in the United States.

According to the CDC data:

- About 13 percent of people with HIV in the United States do not know it and so need testing. Early HIV diagnosis is crucial. Everyone aged 13–64 should be tested at least once. People at higher risk of acquiring (or exposure to) HIV should be tested at least annually. Sexually active gay and bisexual men may benefit from more frequent testing (e.g., every 3–6 months).
- According to another CDC report, of the estimated 1.2 million people with HIV (diagnosed and undiagnosed) in 2019, about 65.9 percent received some HIV care, 50.1 percent were retained in care, and 56.8 percent were virally suppressed or undetectable. Having a suppressed or undetectable viral load protects the health of a person living with HIV, preventing disease progression. There is also a major prevention benefit. A person living with HIV who takes HIV medicine daily as prescribed and gets and stays virally suppressed can stay healthy and has effectively no risk of sexually transmitting HIV to HIV-negative partners.

DEATHS

In 2019, there were 15,815 deaths among adults and adolescents with diagnosed HIV in the United States and 6 dependent areas. These deaths may be due to any cause.

THE GLOBAL HUMAN IMMUNODEFICIENCY VIRUS/ACQUIRED IMMUNODEFICIENCY SYNDROME EPIDEMIC

Human immunodeficiency virus (HIV), the virus that causes acquired immunodeficiency syndrome (AIDS), is one of the world's most serious public health challenges. But, there is a global commitment to stopping new HIV infections and ensuring that everyone with HIV has access to HIV treatment.

According to the United Nations Programme on HIV/AIDS (UNAIDS):

- **Number of people with HIV.** There were approximately 37.7 million people across the globe with HIV in 2020. Of these, 36 million were adults and 1.7 million were children aged 0–14 years. More than half (53 percent) were women and girls.
- **New HIV infections.** An estimated 1.5 million individuals worldwide acquired HIV in 2020, marking a 31 percent decline in new HIV infections since 2010. (New HIV infections, or "HIV incidence," refers to the estimated number of people who newly acquired HIV during given period such as a year, which is different from the number of people *diagnosed with* HIV during a year. (Some people may have HIV but not know it.) Of these new HIV infections:
  - 1.3 million were individuals ages 15+
  - 160,000 were among children aged 0–14 years
- **HIV testing.** Approximately 84 percent of people with HIV globally knew their HIV status in 2020. The remaining 16 percent (about 6.0 million people) still need access to HIV testing services. HIV testing is an essential gateway to HIV prevention, treatment, care and support services.
- **HIV treatment access.** As of June 2020, 28.2 million people with HIV (75 percent) were accessing antiretroviral therapy (ART) globally. That means 9.5 million people are still waiting. HIV treatment access is key to the global effort to end AIDS as a public health threat. People with HIV who are aware of their status, take ART as prescribed, and get and keep an undetectable viral load can live long, healthy lives and have effectively no risk of sexually transmitting HIV to their HIV-negative partners.
- **HIV care continuum.** The term HIV care continuum refers to the sequence of steps a person with HIV takes from diagnosis through receiving treatment until her or his viral load is suppressed to undetectable levels. Each step in the continuum is marked by an assessment of the number of people who have reached that stage.

The stages are: being diagnosed with HIV; being linked to medical care; starting ART; adhering to the treatment regimen; and, finally, having HIV suppressed to undetectable levels in the blood. The UNAIDS reports that in 2020, of all people with HIV worldwide:

- 84 percent knew their HIV status
- 73 percent were accessing ART
- 66 percent were virally suppressed

- **Mother-to-child transmission**. In 2020, 85 percent of pregnant women with HIV received ART to prevent transmitting HIV to their babies during pregnancy and childbirth and to protect their own health.
- **Women and girls**. Every week, around 5,000 young women aged 15–24 years around the world acquire HIV. In sub-Saharan Africa, women and girls accounted for 63 percent of all new HIV infections in 2020.
- **AIDS-related deaths**. AIDS-related deaths have been reduced by 64 percent since the peak in 2004 and by 47 percent since 2010. In 2020, around 680,000 people died from AIDS-related illnesses worldwide, compared to 1.3 million in 2010.
- **Regional impact**. The vast majority of people with HIV are in low and middle-income countries. In 2020, there were 20.6 million people with HIV (55 percent) in eastern and southern Africa, 5.7 million (15 percent) in Asia and the Pacific, 4.7 million (13 percent) in western and central Africa, and 2.2 million (6 percent) in Western and Central Europe and North America.

CHALLENGES AND PROGRESS

Despite advances in our scientific understanding of HIV and its prevention and treatment as well as years of significant effort by the global health community and leading government and civil society organizations, too many people with HIV or at risk for HIV still do not have access to prevention, care, and treatment, and there is still no cure. Further, the HIV epidemic not only affects the health of individuals, it also impacts households, communities, and the development and economic growth of nations. Many of the countries hardest hit by HIV also suffer from other infectious diseases, food insecurity, and other serious problems.

Despite these challenges, there have been successes and promising signs. New global efforts have been mounted to address the epidemic, particularly in the last decade. The number of people with new HIV infections has declined over the years. In addition, the number of people with HIV receiving treatment in resource-poor countries has dramatically increased in the past decade and dramatic progress has been made in preventing mother-to-child transmission of HIV and keeping mothers alive.

However, despite the availability of a widening array of effective HIV prevention tools and methods and a massive scale-up of HIV treatment in recent years, the UNAIDS cautions there has been unequal progress in reducing new HIV infections, increasing access to treatment, and ending AIDS-related deaths, with too many vulnerable people and populations left behind. Stigma and discrimination, together with other social inequalities and exclusion, are proving to be key barriers.

THE UNITED STATES RESPONSE TO THE GLOBAL EPIDEMIC

The U.S. President's Emergency Plan for AIDS Relief (PEPFAR) is the U.S. government's response to the global HIV/AIDS epidemic and represents the largest commitment by any nation to address a single disease in history. Through PEPFAR, the U.S. has supported a world safer and more secure from infectious disease threats. It has demonstrably strengthened the global capacity to prevent, detect, and respond to new and existing risks – which ultimately enhances global health security and protects America's borders. Among other global results, PEPFAR provided HIV testing services for nearly 50 million people in the Fiscal Year 2020 and, as of September 30, 2020, supported lifesaving ART for nearly 18.2 million women, men, and children.

In addition, the National Institutes of Health (NIH) represents the largest public investment in HIV/AIDS research in the world. The NIH is engaged in research around the globe to understand, diagnose, treat, and prevent HIV infection and its many associated conditions, and to find a cure.

Chapter 6 | Impact of HIV on Racial and Ethnic Minorities in the United States

Chapter Contents

Section 6.1 | **HIV among African Americans**

This section contains text excerpted from the following sources: Text in this section begins with excerpts from "HIV/AIDS and African Americans," Office of Minority Health (OMH), U.S. Department of Health and Human Services (HHS), July 8, 2021; Text under the heading "Prevention Challenges" is excerpted from "HIV and African American People: Prevention Challenges," Centers for Disease Control and Prevention (CDC), February 4, 2022.

Although Black/African Americans represent almost 13 percent of the U.S. population, they account for 42.1 percent of human immunodeficiency virus (HIV) infection cases in 2019.

- In 2019, African Americans were 8.1 times more likely to be diagnosed with HIV infection, as compared to the white population.
- African-American males have 8.4 times the acquired immunodeficiency syndrome (AIDS) rate as compared to white males.
- African-American females have 15 times the AIDS rate as compared to white females.
- African-American men are 6.4 times as likely to die from HIV infection as non-Hispanic white men.
- African-American women are 14.5 times as likely to die from HIV infection as white women.

HIV INFECTION CASES AND RATES (ADULTS)

The below Table 6.1 compares estimated number of diagnosed cases and rates (per 100,000) of HIV infection between African American and white adult population.

Table 6.1. Estimated Number of Diagnosed Cases and Rates (per 100,000) of HIV Infection, 2019

	Cases	Rate	African American/White Ratio
African-American males	11,489	71.7	8.1
White males	7,498	8.9	
African-American females	3,810	21.3	12.5
White females	1,508	1.7	

Table 6.1. Continued

	Cases	Rate	African American/White Ratio
African American (total, all ages)	15,334	37.3	8.1
White (total, all ages)	9,013	4.6	

(Source: Centers for Disease Control and Prevention (CDC), 2021. HIV Surveillance Report: Diagnoses of HIV Infection in the United States and Dependent Areas, 2019.)

HIV INFECTION CASES AND RATES (CHILDREN LESS THAN 13 YEARS)

The below Table 6.2 compares estimated number of diagnosed cases and rates (per 100,000) of HIV infection between African American and white children less than 13 years.

Table 6.2. Estimated Number of Diagnosed Cases and Rates (per 100,000) of HIV Infection, 2019

	Cases	Rate
African American	35	0.5
White	7	0
Total Population	61	0.1

(Source: Centers for Disease Control and Prevention (CDC), 2021. HIV Surveillance Report: Diagnoses of HIV Infection in the United States and Dependent Areas, 2019.)

HIV INFECTION CASES (ADULTS AND CHILDREN)

The below Table 6.3 compares estimated number of cases of HIV infection by year of diagnosis between African American and white adults and children.

Table 6.3. Estimated Number of Cases of HIV Infection by Year of Diagnosis, 2019

	Cases	% of Total Cases
African American	15,334	42.1
White	9,013	24.7
Total Population	36,398	

(Source: Centers for Disease Control and Prevention (CDC), 2021. HIV Surveillance Report: Diagnoses of HIV Infection in the United States and Dependent Areas, 2019.)

The below Table 6.4 compares estimated number of persons living with HIV infection and rates (per 100,000) by year between African American and white adults and children.

Table 6.4. Estimated Number of Persons Living with HIV Infection and Rates (per 100,000) by Year, 2019

	Rate	Cases	% of Total Cases
African American	1,027.50	422,481	40.4
White	153.9	303,701	29
Total Population	318.4	1,044,977	

(Source: Centers for Disease Control and Prevention (CDC), 2021. HIV Surveillance Report: Diagnoses of HIV Infection in the United States and Dependent Areas, 2019.)

AIDS CASES AND RATES (ADULTS)

The below Table 6.5 compares estimated number of cases and rates (per 100,000) of AIDS between African American and white adult population.

Table 6.5. Estimated Number of Cases and Rates (per 100,000) of AIDS, 2019

	Cases	Rate	African American/White Ratio
African-American males	5,108	31.9	8.4
White males	3,190	3.8	
African-American females	2,157	12	15
White females	685	0.8	
African-American (both sexes)	7,265	21.4	9.3
White (both sexes)	3,875	2.3	

(Source: Centers for Disease Control and Prevention (CDC), 2021. National Center for HIV/AIDS, Viral Hepatitis, STD, and TB Prevention (NCHHSTP) Atlas Plus.)

The below Table 6.6 compares estimated number of cases of AIDS by year of diagnosis between African American and white adult population.

Table 6.6. Estimated Number of Cases of AIDS by Year of Diagnosis, 2019

	Cumulative Cases*	% of Total Cases
African American	520,919	39.8
White	444,613	34
Total Population	1,307,283	

Cumulative data are from the beginning of the epidemic through 2019.
(Source: Centers for Disease Control and Prevention (CDC), 2021. HIV Surveillance Report: Diagnoses of HIV Infection in the United States and Dependent Areas, 2019.)

DEATH RATE

The below Table 6.7 compares HIV infection death rates per 100,000 population between African American and white women and men.

Table 6.7. HIV Infection Death Rates per 100,000 Population, 2019

	African Americans	White	African American/White Ratio
All ages, Men	28.4	5	5.7
All ages, Women	11.6	0.8	14.5
Total Population	16.1	2.5	6.4

(Source: Centers for Disease Control and Prevention (CDC), 2021. HIV Surveillance Report: Diagnoses of HIV Infection in the United States and Dependent Areas, 2019.)

AIDS DEATHS

The below Table 6.8 provides estimated number of deaths, and death rates, of persons with AIDS by year of death.

Table 6.8. Estimated Number of Deaths, and Death Rates, of Persons with AIDS by Year of Death, 2019

	Deaths 2019	Rate 2019	Cumulative Deaths*	% of Total Cases
African Americans	5,099	15	306,003	39.9
White	3,637	2.1	293,444	38.3

Table 6.8. Continued

	Deaths 2019	Rate 2019	Cumulative Deaths*	% of Total Cases
Total Population	11,899	4.3	766,380	

*Cumulative data are from the beginning of the epidemic through 2019.
(Source: Centers for Disease Control and Prevention (CDC), 2021. National Center for HIV/AIDS, Viral Hepatitis, STD, and TB Prevention (NCHHSTP) Atlas Plus; Centers for Disease Control and Prevention (CDC), 2021. HIV Surveillance Report: Diagnoses of HIV Infection in the United States and Dependent Areas, 2019.)

HIV TESTING

The below Table 6.9 compares the age-adjusted percent of HIV testing status among persons 18 years of age and over between Non-Hispanic Black and Non-Hispanic white population.

Table 6.9. Age-Adjusted Percent of HIV Testing Status among Persons 18 Years of Age and Over, 2018

	Non-Hispanic Black	Non-Hispanic White	Non-Hispanic Black/ Non-Hispanic White Ratio
Ever tested	62.8	39.9	1.6
Never tested	37.2	60.1	0.6

(Source: Centers for Disease Control and Prevention (CDC), 2021. Summary Health Statistics for the U.S. Adults: 2018.)

PREVENTION CHALLENGES

Racism, discrimination, HIV stigma, and homophobia have a negative impact on the overall health and well-being of African-American people. Additionally, poverty and the associated socioeconomic factors – including limited access to high-quality healthcare, housing, and HIV prevention education – directly and indirectly increase the risk for HIV. Addressing these social and structural barriers and encouraging safe and supportive communities can help improve health outcomes for African-American people.

Other factors that can increase African-American people's chances of getting or transmitting HIV include:

- **Low percentages of viral suppression**. African-American people have lower percentages of viral suppression compared to all people with HIV. Getting and keeping an undetectable viral load (or staying virally suppressed) can prevent transmission to others.
- **Mistrust in the healthcare system**. African-American people experience high levels of mistrust of the healthcare system. Lower levels of trust can reduce the likelihood of engaging in HIV treatment and care.
- **Other sexually transmitted diseases (STDs)**. African-American people are disproportionately affected by chlamydia, gonorrhea, and syphilis. Having another STD can increase a person's chance of getting or transmitting HIV.

Section 6.2 | HIV among American Indians and Alaska Natives

This section contains text excerpted from the following sources: Text in this section begins with excerpts from "HIV/AIDS and American Indians/Alaska Natives," Office of Minority Health (OMH), U.S. Department of Health and Human Services (HHS), July 8, 2021; Text under the heading "Prevention Challenges" is excerpted from "HIV and American Indian/Alaska Native People: Prevention Challenges," Centers for Disease Control and Prevention (CDC), January 12, 2022.

- Asian Americans have lower HIV infection rates as compared to their white counterparts, and they are less likely to die of HIV Infection.
- National surveillance data for HIV infection in Asian subgroups is limited.

HIV INFECTION CASES AND RATES (ADULTS)

The below Table 6.10 compares estimated number of diagnosed cases and rates (per 100,000) of HIV infection between American Indian/Alaska Native adult population.

Table 6.10. Estimated Number of Diagnosed Cases and Rates (per 100,000) of HIV Infection, 2019

	Cases	Rate	American Indian/Alaska Native/White Ratio
American Indian/Alaska Native males	165	16.9	1.9
White males	7,498	8.9	
American Indian/Alaska Native females	44	4.3	2.5
White females	1,508	1.7	
American Indian/Alaska Native (total, all ages)	210	8.6	1.9
White (total, all ages)	9,013	4.6	

(Source: Centers for Disease Control and Prevention (CDC), 2021. HIV Surveillance Report: Diagnoses of HIV Infection in the United States and Dependent Areas, 2019.)

HIV INFECTION CASES AND RATES (CHILDREN LESS THAN 13 YEARS)

The below Table 6.11 compares estimated number of diagnosed cases and rates (per 100,000) of HIV infection between American Indian/Alaska Native and white children less than 13 years.

Table 6.11. Estimated Number of Diagnosed Cases and Rates (per 100,000) of HIV Infection, 2019

	Cases	Rate
American Indians/Alaska Natives	1	0.2
White	7	0
Total Population	61	0.1

(Source: Centers for Disease Control and Prevention (CDC), 2021. HIV Surveillance Report: Diagnoses of HIV Infection in the United States and Dependent Areas, 2019.)

HIV INFECTION CASES (ADULTS AND CHILDREN)

The below Table 6.12 compares estimated number of cases of HIV infection by year of diagnosis between American Indian/Alaska Native and white adults and children.

Table 6.12. Estimated Number of Cases of HIV Infection By Year of Diagnosis, 2019

	Cases	% of Total Cases
American Indians/Alaska Natives	210	0.6
White	9,013	24.8
Total Population	36,398	

(Source: Centers for Disease Control and Prevention (CDC), 2021. HIV Surveillance Report: Diagnoses of HIV Infection in the United States and Dependent Areas, 2019.)

The below Table 6.13 compares estimated number of persons living with HIV infection and rates (per 100,000) by year, between American Indian/Alaska Native and white adults and children.

Table 6.13. Estimated Number of Persons Living with HIV Infection and Rates (per 100,000) by Year, 2019

	Rate	Cases	% of Total Cases
American Indians/Alaska Natives	132	3,215	0.3
White	153.9	303,701	29
Total Population	318.4	1,044,977	

(Source: Centers for Disease Control and Prevention (CDC), 2021. HIV Surveillance Report: Diagnoses of HIV Infection in the United States and Dependent Areas, 2019.)

AIDS CASES AND RATES (ADULTS)

The below Table 6.14 compares estimated number of cases and rates (per 100,000) of AIDS between American Indian/Alaska Native and white adults.

Table 6.14. Estimated Number of Cases and Rates (per 100,000) of AIDS, 2019

	Cases	Rate	American Indians/Alaska Natives/White Ratio
American Indians/Alaska Natives males	48	4.9	1.3
White males	3,190	3.8	

Table 6.14. Continued

	Cases	Rate	American Indians/Alaska Natives/White Ratio
American Indians/Alaska Natives females	17	1.7	2.1
White females	685	0.8	
American Indians/Alaska Natives (both sexes)	65	3.3	1.4
White (both sexes)	3,975	2.3	

Source: Centers for Disease Control and Prevention (CDC), 2021. National Center for HIV/AIDS, Viral Hepatitis, STD, and TB Prevention (NCHHSTP) Atlas Plus.)

The below Table 6.15 compares estimated number of cases of AIDS by year of diagnosis between American Indian/Alaska Native and white adults.

Table 6.15. Estimated Number of Cases of AIDS by Year of Diagnosis, 2019

	Cumulative Cases*	% of Total Cases
American Indian/Alaska Native	3,562	0.3
White	444,613	34
Total Population	1,307,283	

*Cumulative data are from the beginning of the epidemic through 2019.
(Source: Centers for Disease Control and Prevention (CDC), 2021. HIV Surveillance Report: Diagnoses of HIV Infection in the United States and Dependent Areas, 2019.)

DEATH RATE

The below Table 6.16 compares HIV infection death rates between American Indian/Alaska Native and white population.

Table 6.16. HIV Infection Death Rates per 100,000 Population, 2019

	American Indian/ Alaska Native	White	American Indian/Alaska Native/White Ratio
All ages, Men	3.4	5	0.7
All ages, Women	1.8	0.6	2.3
Total Population	2.1	2.5	0.8

(Source: Centers for Disease Control and Prevention (CDC), 2021. HIV Surveillance Report: Diagnoses of HIV Infection in the United States and Dependent Areas, 2019.)

AIDS DEATHS

The below Table 6.17 compares estimated number of deaths, and death rates, of persons with AIDS by year of death between American Indian/Alaska Native and white population.

Table 6.17. Estimated Number of Deaths, and Death Rates, of Persons with AIDS by Year of Death, 2019

	Deaths 2019	Rate 2019	Cumulative Deaths*	% of Total Cases
American Indian/Alaska Native	41	2.1	2,087	0.3
White	3,637	2.1	293,444	38.3
Total Population	11,899	4.3	766,380	

*Cumulative data are from the beginning of the epidemic through 2019.
(Source: Centers for Disease Control and Prevention (CDC), 2021. National Center for HIV, Viral Hepatitis, STD, and TB Prevention (NCHHSTP) Atlas Plus; Centers for Disease Control and Prevention (CDC), 2021. HIV Surveillance Report: Diagnoses of HIV Infection in the United States and Dependent Areas, 2019.)

HIV TESTING

The below Table 6.18 compares the age-adjusted percent of HIV testing status among persons 18 years of age and over between American Indian/Alaska Native and white population.

Table 6.18. Age-Adjusted Percent of HIV Testing Status among Persons 18 Years of Age and Over, 2018

	American Indian/ Alaska Native	Non-Hispanic White	American Indian/Alaska Native/ Non-Hispanic White Ratio
Ever tested	46.6	39.9	1.2
Never tested	53.4	60.1	0.9

(Source: Centers for Disease Control and Prevention (CDC) 2021. Summary Health Statistics for U.S. Adults: 2018.)

PREVENTION CHALLENGES

There are more than 574 federally recognized American Indians/ Alaska Natives (AI/AN) tribes and many different languages.

Because each tribe has its own culture, beliefs, and practices, creating culturally appropriate prevention programs for each group can be challenging. Additionally, racial misidentification of AI/AN people may lead to the undercounting of this population in HIV surveillance systems and may contribute to the underfunding of targeted services for AI/AN people.

Some AI/AN people experience social, cultural, and economic barriers such as stigma, confidentiality concerns, and poverty. These issues could limit opportunities for HIV testing, treatment, and other prevention services, especially among AI/AN people who live in rural communities or on reservations. Addressing these barriers and encouraging supportive communities can help improve health outcomes for AI/AN people.

Other factors that can increase the chances of getting or transmitting HIV include:

- **Sexually transmitted diseases (STDs).** In 2018, AI/AN people had the second highest rates of chlamydia and gonorrhea among all racial/ethnic groups. Having another STD increases a person's risk for getting or transmitting HIV.
- **Knowledge of HIV status.** It is important for everyone to know their HIV status. People who do not know they have HIV cannot take advantage of HIV care and treatment and may unknowingly pass HIV to others.
- **Alcohol and illicit drug use.** Alcohol and substance use can impair judgment and lead to behaviors that increase the risk of HIV. Injection drug use can directly increase the risk of HIV if a person shares needles, syringes, and other drug injection equipment – for example, cookers – with someone who has the virus. Compared with other racial/ethnic groups, AI/AN people tend to use alcohol and drugs at a younger age and use them more often and in higher quantities.

Section 6.3 | **HIV among Asians**

This section includes text excerpted from "HIV and Asians," Centers for Disease Control and Prevention (CDC), January 12, 2022.

Between 2014 and 2018 the Asian population in the United States grew around 10 percent, which is more than three times as fast as the total U.S. population. During the same period, in the United States and dependent areas, the number of Asians receiving an HIV diagnosis remained stable, driven primarily by HIV diagnoses among Asian gay, bisexual, and other men who have sex with men remaining stable. Asians, who make up 6 percent of the population, accounted for about 2 percent of HIV diagnoses in 2018 in the United States and dependent areas.

THE NUMBERS

Two percent of the 37,968 HIV diagnoses in the United States and dependent areas in 2018, 2 percent were among Asians.

New HIV diagnoses among adult and adolescent Asians in the United States and dependent areas by transmission category and sex,* (Figure 6.2) 2018.

Most new HIV diagnoses were among Asian gay and bisexual men (Figure 6.1), than Asian gay and bisexual women (Figure 6.2).

From 2014 to 2018, annual HIV diagnoses in the United States and dependent areas remained stable among Asians overall, with trends varying by age and age and sex as shown in Figure 6.3 and Figure 6.4.

HIV diagnoses among adult and adolescent Asians in the United States and dependent areas, 2014–2018* (Figure 6.4).

LIVING WITH HIV

Adult and adolescent Asians with HIV in the 50 states and the District of Columbia

At the end of 2018, an estimated 1.2 million people had HIV. Of those 17,600 were Asian.

Four in 5 Asians knew they had the virus.

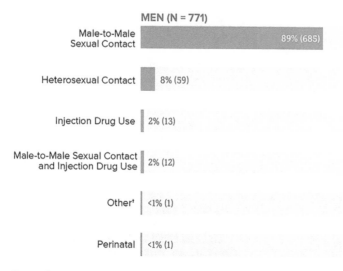

Figure 6.1. HIV Diagnoses Were among Gay and Bisexual Men *(Source: Centers for Disease Control and Prevention (CDC). Diagnoses of HIV infection in the United States and dependent areas, 2018. HIV Surveillance Report 2020.)*

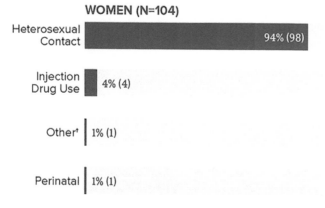

Figure 6.2. HIV Diagnoses Were among Gay and Bisexual Women *(Source: Centers for Disease Control and Prevention (CDC). Diagnoses of HIV infection in the United States and dependent areas, 2018. HIV Surveillance Report 2020.)*

*Based on sex at birth and includes transgender people.
†Includes hemophilia, blood transfusion, perinatal exposure, and risk factors not reported or not identified.

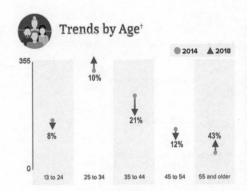

Figure 6.3. HIV Diagnoses – Trends by Age *(Source: Centers for Disease Control and Prevention (CDC). Diagnoses of HIV infection in the United States and dependent areas, 2018. HIV Surveillance Report 2020.)*

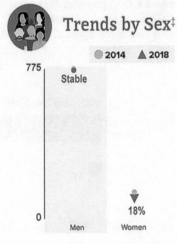

Figure 6.4. HIV Diagnoses – Trends by Sex *(Source: Centers for Disease Control and Prevention (CDC). Diagnoses of HIV infection in the United States and dependent areas, 2018. HIV Surveillance Report 2020.)*

*Changes in populations with fewer HIV diagnoses can lead to a large percentage increase or decrease.
†Does not include perinatal and other categories.
‡Based on sex at birth and includes trans-gender people.

It is important for Asians to know their HIV status so they can take medicine to treat HIV if they have the virus. Taking HIV medicine every day can make the viral load undetectable. People who get and keep an undetectable viral load (or stay virally suppressed) have effectively no risk of transmitting HIV to HIV-negative sex partners.

When compared to other people with HIV, Asians were less likely to have received some HIV care. More work is needed to increase these. In 2016 for every 100 Asians with HIV:

- 59 received some HIV care
- 49 were retained in care*
- 54 were virally suppressed[†]

For comparison for every 100 people overall with HIV, 64 received some HIV care, 49 were retained in care, and 53 were virally suppressed.

*Had 2 viral load or CD4 tests at least 3 months apart in a year.
[†]Based on most recent viral load test.

DEATHS

During 2018, there were 79 deaths among Asians with diagnosed HIV in the United States and dependent areas. These deaths may be due to any cause.

PREVENTION CHALLENGES

There are some behaviors that put everyone at risk for HIV. These include having anal or vaginal sex without protection (such as a condom or medicine to prevent or treat HIV) or sharing injection drug equipment with someone who has HIV. Other factors that affect Asians particularly include:

- **Undiagnosed HIV**. People with undiagnosed HIV cannot obtain the care they need to stay healthy and may unknowingly transmit HIV to others. A lower percentage of Asians with HIV have received a diagnosis, compared to other races/ethnicities.
- **Cultural factors**. Some Asians may avoid seeking testing, counseling, or treatment because of language

barriers or fear of discrimination, the stigma of homosexuality, immigration issues, or fear of bringing shame to their families.

- **Limited research**. Limited research about Asian health and HIV infection means there are few targeted prevention programs and behavioral interventions for this population.
- **Data limitations**. The reported number of HIV cases among Asians may not reflect the true HIV diagnoses in this population because of race/ethnicity misidentification. This could lead to the underestimation of HIV infection in this population.

Section 6.4 | **HIV among Hispanics/Latinos**

This section includes text excerpted from "HIV and Hispanic/Latino People," Centers for Disease Control and Prevention (CDC), October 12, 2021.

Hispanic/Latinx people are disproportionately affected by human immunodeficiency virus (HIV). Social and structural issues – such as racism, HIV stigma, homophobia, poverty, and limited access to high-quality healthcare – influence health outcomes and continue to drive inequities.

HIV RISK BEHAVIORS

The risk of getting or transmitting HIV varies widely depending on the type of exposure or behavior. Most commonly, people get or transmit HIV through anal or vaginal sex, or sharing needles, syringes, or other drug-injection equipment – for example, cookers.

Sexual behaviors among Hispanic/Latinx people with diagnosed HIV in the United States, 2019[*][†]

Getting and keeping an undectable viral load is the best way for people with HIV to stay healthy and protect others.

- 7 percent of all people with HIV and

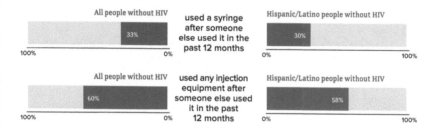

Figure 6.5. Injection Behaviors among Hispanic/Latinx People Who Inject Drugs in 23 U.S. Cities, 2018*† *(Source: Centers for Disease Control and Prevention (CDC). HIV infection risk, prevention, and testing behaviors among persons who inject drugs – National HIV Behavioral Surveillance: injection drug use, 23 U.S. Cities, 2018. HIV Surveillance Special Report 2020.)*

Hispanic/Latinx people can be of any race.
†Among people aged 18 and older

- 7 percent of Hispanic/Latinx people with HIV had sex without using any HIV prevention strategy in the past 12 months‡

Hispanic/Latinx people can be of any race.
†Among people aged 18 and older.
‡Had sex while not virally suppressed with a partner whose HIV status was negative or unknown, a condom was not used, and the partner was not taking PrEP.

Injection behaviors among Hispanic/Latinx people who inject drugs in 23 U.S. cities, 2018*†

Sharing needles, syringes and other drug injection equipment puts people at high risks for HIV and other infections.

The percentage of Hispanic/Latino people who used syringes, and other equipment after someone else used it in the past 12 months is shown in Figure 6.5.

PrEP COVERAGE

Pre-exposure prophylaxis (PrEP) coverage is one of the six *Ending the HIV Epidemic in the United States* indicators. PrEP coverage is the estimated percentage of people with indications for PrEP classified as having been prescribed PrEP.

PrEP is highly effective for preventing HIV from sex or injection drug use.

- 14 percent of Hispanic/Latinx people who could benefit from PrEP were prescribed PrEP in 2019. 23 percent of people overall who could benefit from PrEP were prescribed PrEP in 2019.

HIV INCIDENCE

HIV incidence is one of the six *Ending the HIV Epidemic in the United States* indicators. HIV incidence is the estimated number of new HIV infections in a given year.

Ending the HIV pandemic. Overall goal: Decrease the estimated number of new HIV infections to 9,300 by 2025 and 3,000 by 2030.

- 29 percent of the 34,800 estimated new HIV infections in the United States in 2019, 29 percent (10,200) were among Hispanic/Latinx people.

The number of estimated HIV infections has decreased in 2019 compared to 2015, as shown in Figure 6.6.

HIV DIAGNOSES

HIV diagnosis is one of the six *Ending the HIV Epidemic in the United States* indicators. HIV diagnosis refers to the number of people who received an HIV diagnosis during a given year. In 2019, Hispanic/Latinx people made up 29 percent (10,494) of the 36,801 new HIV diagnoses in the United States and Dependent Areas.

Ending the HIV epidemic. Overall goal: Decrease the number of new HIV diagnoses to 9,588 by 2025 and 3000 by 2030.

- 29 percent of the 36,801 new HIV diagnoses in the United States and dependent areas in 2019, 29 percent (10,494) were among Hispanic/Latinx people.

Hispanic/Latinx gay and bisexual men accounted for most new HIV diagnoses in 2019 as shown in Figure 6.7, while heterosexual women accounted for most new HIV diagnoses as shown in Figure 6.8.

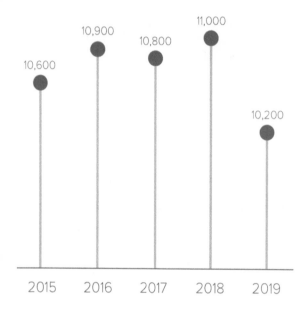

Figure 6.6. Estimated HIV Infections among Hispanic/Latinx People in the United States, 2015–2019*

Hispanic/Latinx people can be of any race.

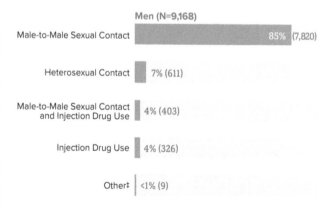

Figure 6.7. HIV Diagnoses among Hispanic/Latino in Men, 2019*†
(Source: Centers for Disease Control and Prevention (CDC). Diagnoses of HIV infection in the United States and dependent areas, 2019. HIV Surveillance Report 2021.)

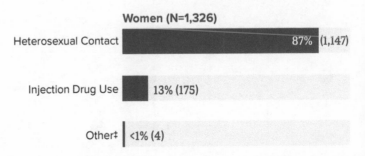

Figure 6.8. HIV Diagnoses among Hispanic/Latino in Women, 2019*† *(Source: Centers for Disease Control and Prevention (CDC). Diagnoses of HIV infection in the United States and dependent areas, 2019. HIV Surveillance Report 2021.)*

*Hispanic/Latinx people can be of any race.
†Based on sex assigned at birth and includes transgender people.
‡Includes perinatal exposure, blood transfusion, hemophilia, and risk factors not reported or not identified.

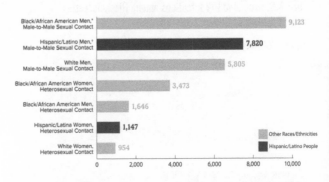

Figure 6.9. New HIV Diagnoses in the United States and Dependent Areas for the Most-Affected Subpopulations, 2019 *(Source: Centers for Disease Control and Prevention (CDC). Diagnoses of HIV infection in the United States and dependent areas, 2019. HIV Surveillance Report 2021.)*

*Black *refers to people having origins in any of the Black racial groups of* Africa. African American *is a term often used for people of African descent with ancestry in North America.*
†Hispanic/Latinx people can be of any race.

Subpopulations representing 2 percent or less of all people who received an HIV diagnosis in 2019 are not represented in Figure 6.9.

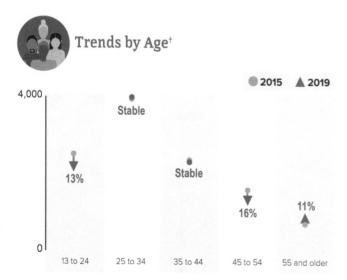

Figure 6.10. HIV Diagnoses among Hispanic/Latino – Trend by Age *(Source: Centers for Disease Control and Prevention (CDC). Diagnoses of HIV infection in the United States and dependent areas, 2019. HIV Surveillance Report 2021)*

HIV disproportionately affects Hispanic/Latinx communities.
From 2015–2019, HIV diagnoses remained stable among Hispanic/Latinx people overall. Although trends varied for different groups of Hispanic/Latinx people, HIV diagnoses declined for some groups, including Hispanic/Latinx youth aged 13–24 as shown in Figure 6.10 and Hispanic/Latinx women as shown in Figure 6.11.

KNOWLEDGE OF STATUS

Knowledge of status is one of the six *Ending the HIV epidemic in the United States* indicators. Knowledge of status refers to the estimated percentage of people with HIV who have received an HIV diagnosis.

Ending the HIV epidemic. Overall goal: Increase the estimated percentage of people with HIV who have received an HIV diagnosis to 95 percent by 2025 and remain stable at 95 percent by 2020.

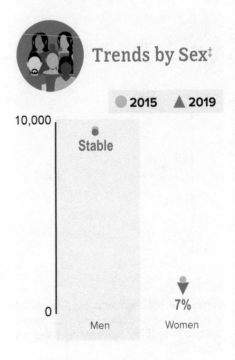

Figure 6.11. HIV Diagnoses among Hispanic/Latino – Trend by Sex[t] *(Source: Centers for Disease Control and Prevention (CDC). Diagnoses of HIV infection in the United States and dependent areas, 2019. HIV Surveillance Report 2021)*

**Hispanic/Latinx people can be of any race.
[t]Does not include perinatal and other transmission categories.
[‡]Based on sex assigned at birth and includes transgender people.*

Hispanic/Latinx people with HIV in the United States, 2019*

In 2019 an estimated 1.2 million people had HIV. Of those 294,200 were Hispanic/Latinx people.

- For every 100 people with HIV 87 knew their HIV status. For every 100 Hispanic/Latinx people with HIV 84 their HIV status.

*Hispanic/Latinx people can be of any race.

VIRAL SUPPRESSION

Viral suppression is one of the six *Ending the HIV Epidemic in the United States* indicators. Viral suppression refers to the percentage of people with diagnosed HIV who have less than 200 copies of HIV per milliliter of blood.

Ending the HIV epidemic. Overall goal: Increase the percentage of people with diagnosed HIV who are virally suppressed to 95 percent by 2025 and remain stable at 95 percent by 2030.

It is important for Hispanic/Latinx people to know their HIV status so they can take medicine to treat HIV if they have the virus. Taking HIV medicine every day can make the viral load undetectable. People who get and keep an undetectable viral load (or remain virally suppressed) can stay healthy for many years and have effectively no risk of transmitting HIV to their sex partners.

Hispanic/Latinx people with diagnosed HIV in 44 states and the District of Columbia, 2019*

Compared to all people with diagnosed HIV Hispanic/Latinx people have about the same viral suppression rates.

For every 100 Hispanic/Latinx people with diagnosed HIV in 2019:

- 74 received some HIV care
- 59 were retained in care[†]
- 65 were virally suppressed[‡]

For comparison for every 100 people overall with dignosed HIV 76 received some HIV care, 58 were retained in care and 66 were virally suppressed.

Hispanic/Latinx people can be of any race.
[†]*Had two viral load or CD4 tests at least three months apart in a year.*
[‡]*Based on most recent viral load test.*

Many people with HIV experience challenges with achieving and maintaining viral suppression over time. Some of these challenges include missing HIV medical appointments, needing but not receiving other important healthcare services, or missing doses of HIV treatment.

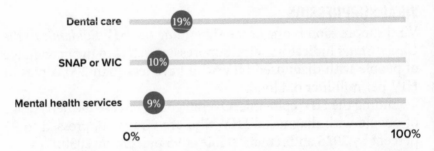

Figure 6.12. Needed HIV Ancillary Care Services among Hispanic/Latino People with Diagnosed HIV in the United States, 2019*†‡ *(Source: Centers for Disease Control and Prevention (CDC).) Medical Monitoring Project.*

*Hispanic/Latinx people can be of any race.
†Among people aged 18 and older.
‡HIV ancillary care services, such as case management and mental health services, are services that support retention in HIV care.

Missed HIV medical care appointments among Hispanic/Latinx people with diagnosed HIV in the United States, 2019*†

Staying in HIV care is important to achieving and maintaining viral suppression.

- 24 percent of all people with HIV and 27 percent of Hispanic/Latinx people with HIV missed at least one medical appointment in the past 12 months.

*Hispanic/Latinx people can be of any race.
†Among people aged 18 and older.

HIV ancillary care services are essential for supporting people in staying in HIV care and maintaining viral suppression.

About 38 percent of all people with HIV needed at least 1 HIV ancillary care service such as dental care, SNAP or WIC, and mental health, in the 12 months as shown in Figure 6.12.

HIV treatment among Hispanic/Latinx people with diagnosed HIV in the United States, 2019*†

Taking HIV medicine consistently and as prescribed is the best way to achieve and maintain viral suppression.

- 61 percent of all people with HIV and 57 percent of Hispanic/Latinx People with HIV took all their doses of HIV medicine over the last 30 days.

*Hispanic/Latinx people can be of any race.
†Among people aged 18 and older.

Depression and anxiety among Hispanic/Latinx people with diagnosed HIV in the United States, 2019*†

People who experience symptoms of depression or anxiety may face challenges maintaining viral suppression.

- 22 percent of all people with HIV and 22 percent of Hispanic/Latinx people with HIV experienced symptoms of depression and anxiety is the past 12 months.

*Hispanic/Latinx people can be of any race.
†Among people aged 18 and older.

Homelessness among Hispanic/Latinx people with diagnosed HIV in the United States, 2019*†

People who experience homelessness may find it difficult to get HIV care and treatment.

- 9 percent of all people with HIV and 7 percent of Hispanic/Latinx people with HIV reported homelessness in the past 12 months.

*Hispanic/Latinx people can be of any race.
†Among people aged 18 and older.

Below Figure 6.13 shows median HIV stigma score for Hispanic/Latinx people with HIV.

DEATHS

In 2019, there were 3,047 deaths among Hispanic/Latinx people with diagnosed HIV in the United States and Dependent Areas. These deaths could be from any cause.

PREVENTION CHALLENGES

Racism, discrimination, HIV stigma, and homophobia have a negative impact on the overall health and well-being of Hispanic/Latinx people. Additionally, poverty, migration patterns, lower educational level, and language barriers may make it harder for some

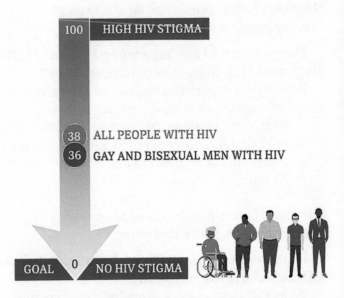

Figure 6.13. Median HIV Stigma Score among Hispanic/Latinx People with Diagnosed HIV in the United States, 2019*† *(Source: Centers for Disease Control and Prevention (CDC).) Medical Monitoring Project.*

***Note:** Ten-item ranging from 0 (no stigma) to 100 (high stigma) that measures personalized stigma, disclosure concerns, negative self-image, and perceived public attitudes about people with HIV.*
*Hispanic/Latinx people can be of any race.
†Among people aged 18 and older.

Hispanic/Latinx people to seek and receive high-quality healthcare, including HIV testing, treatment, and other prevention services. Addressing these social and structural barriers and encouraging safe and supportive communities can help improve health outcomes for Hispanic/Latinx people.

Other factors that can increase the chances of getting or transmitting HIV include:

- **Knowledge of HIV status.** It is important for everyone to know their HIV status. People who do not know they have HIV cannot take advantage of HIV care and treatment and may pass HIV to others without knowing it.

- **Other sexually transmitted diseases (STDs).** Having another STD can increase a person's chance of getting or transmitting HIV.
- **Immigration status.** Some Hispanic/Latinx people may not use HIV prevention services, get an HIV test, or get treatment if they have HIV due to fear of disclosing their immigration status.
- **Mistrust of the healthcare system.** Hispanic/Latinx people experience high levels of mistrust of the healthcare system. Lower levels of trust can reduce the likelihood of clinic visits and result in lower use of and adherence to antiretroviral medications.

Section 6.5 | HIV among Native Hawaiians and Other Pacific Islanders

This section includes text excerpted from "HIV and Native Hawaiians and Other Pacific Islanders," Centers for Disease Control and Prevention (CDC), January 12, 2022.

Although Native Hawaiians and Other Pacific Islanders (NHOPI) account for a very small percentage of new HIV diagnoses in the United States and dependent areas, HIV affects NHOPI in ways that are not always apparent because of their small population size. In 2018, NHOPI made up 0.2 percent of the U.S. population.

HIV DIAGNOSES

One percent of the 37,968 new HIV diagnoses in the United States and dependent areas in 2018, < one percent (68) were among Native Hawaiians and Other Pacific Islanders (NHOPI).

Most new HIV diagnoses among NHOPI men were due to male-to-male sexual contacts as shown in Figure 6.14.

All new HIV diagnoses among NHOPI were attributed to heterosexual contact in women as shown in Figure 6.15.

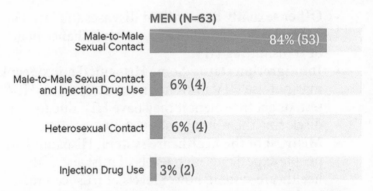

Figure 6.14. New HIV Diagnoses among NHOPI Men *(Source: Centers for Disease Control and Prevention (CDC).) Diagnoses of HIV infection in the United States and dependent areas, 2018. HIV Surveillance Report 2020)*

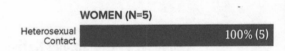

Figure 6.15. New HIV Diagnoses among NHOPI Women *(Source: Centers for Disease Control and Prevention (CDC).) Diagnoses of HIV infection in the United States and dependent areas, 2018. HIV Surveillance Report 2020)*

*Based on sex at birth and includes transgender people. Total for men may not equal 100 percent due to rounding.

HIV diagnoses increased among NHOPI men, while decreased for women during 2014–2018 as shown in Figure 6.16.

LIVING WITH HIV
Adult and adolescent NHOPI with HIV in the 50 states and District of Columbia

At the end of 2018, an estimated 1.2 million people had HIV. Of those, 1,100 were NHOPI.

It is important for NHOPI to know their HIV status so they can take medicine to treat HIV if they have the virus. Taking HIV medicine every day can make the viral load undetectable. People who

Trends by Sex

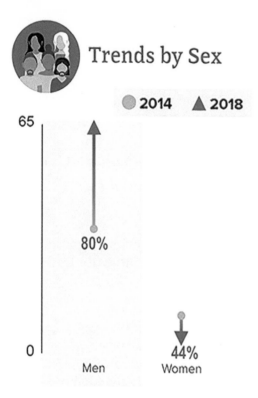

● **2014**   ▲ **2018**

65

80%

0

44%

Men   Women

Figure 6.16. HIV Diagnoses among NHOPI in the
United States and Dependent Areas, 2014–2018*†
*(Source: Centers for Disease Control and Prevention
(CDC).) Diagnoses of HIV infection in the United States
and dependent areas, 2018. HIV Surveillance Report
2020*

*Changes in subpopulations with fewer HIV diagnoses
can lead to a large percentage increase or decrease.
†Based on sex at birth and includes transgender people.*

get and keep an undetectable viral load (or stay virally suppressed)
have effectively no risk of transmitting HIV to HIV-negative sex
partners.

Compared to all people with HIV, NHOPI have about the same
viral suppression rates. But, more work is needed to increase these
rates. For every 100 NHOPI with HIV in 2016.

- 60 received some HIV care.
- 43 were retained in care*
- 54 were virally suppressed†

For comparison, for every 100 people overall with HIV, 64 received some HIV care, 49 were retained in care and 53 were virally suppressed.

*Had two viral load or CD4 tests at least three months apart in a year.
†Based on the most recent viral load test.

DEATHS

In 2018, there were 15 deaths among NHOPI with diagnosed HIV in the United States and Dependent Areas. These deaths may be due to any cause.

PREVENTION CHALLENGES

- **Socioeconomic issues**. Poverty, inadequate or no healthcare coverage, language barriers, and lower educational attainment may make it harder for some NHOPI to get HIV testing and care.
- **Cultural factors**. NHOPI cultural customs, such as not talking about sex across generations, may stigmatize sexuality in general and homosexuality specifically. This could result in lower use of HIV prevention methods such as condoms.
- **Limited research**. With limited research about NHOPI health and HIV, creating targeted HIV prevention programs and behavioral interventions for this population can be challenging.
- **Data limitations**. The reported number of HIV cases among NHOPI may not reflect the true HIV diagnoses in this population because of race/ethnicity misidentification. This could lead to an underestimation of HIV infection in this population.

Chapter 7 | **HIV/AIDS among Specific Populations**

Chapter Contents

Section 7.1 | **HIV among Children and Adolescents**

This section includes text excerpted from "HIV and Children and Adolescents," HIVinfo, U.S. Department of Health and Human Services (HHS), August 19, 2021.

DOES HIV AFFECT CHILDREN AND ADOLESCENTS?

Yes, children and adolescents are among the people living with HIV in the United States.

- According to the Centers for Disease Control and Prevention (CDC), 87 cases of human immunodeficiency virus (HIV) in children younger than 13 years of age were diagnosed in the United States in 2018.
- The CDC reports that youth 13–24 years of age accounted for 21 percent of all new HIV diagnoses in the United States and dependent areas in 2018.

HOW DO MOST CHILDREN GET HIV?

Human immunodeficiency virus can pass from a mother with HIV to her child during pregnancy, childbirth, or breastfeeding, called "perinatal transmission" of HIV. In the United States, this is the most common way children under 13 years of age get HIV. Perinatal transmission of HIV is also called "mother-to-child transmission" of HIV.

The use of HIV medicines and other strategies have helped to lower the rate of perinatal transmission of HIV to one percent or less in the United States and Europe.

HOW DO ADOLESCENTS GET HIV?

Some adolescents, 13–19 years of age, with HIV in the United States acquired the virus as infants through perinatal transmission. But, most youth who acquire HIV during adolescence get it through sexual transmission. Many adolescents with HIV do not know they are HIV positive.

WHAT FACTORS INCREASE THE RISK OF HIV IN ADOLESCENTS?

Several factors make it challenging to prevent adolescents from getting HIV. Many adolescents lack basic information about HIV and how to protect themselves from HIV.

The following are some factors that put adolescents at risk of HIV:

- **Low rates of condom use.** Always using a condom correctly during sex reduces the risk of HIV and some other sexually transmitted diseases (STDs).
- **High rates of STDs among youth.** An STD increases the risk of getting or spreading HIV.
- **Alcohol or drug use.** Adolescents under the influence of alcohol or drugs may engage in risky behaviors, such as having sex without a condom.

WHAT FACTORS AFFECT HIV TREATMENT IN CHILDREN AND ADOLESCENTS?

Treatment with HIV medicines (called "antiretroviral therapy" or "ART") is recommended for everyone with HIV, including children and adolescents. HIV medicines help people with HIV live longer, healthier lives and reduce the risk of HIV transmission.

Several factors affect HIV treatment in children and adolescents, including a child's growth and development. For example, because children grow at different rates, dosing of an HIV medicine may depend on a child's weight rather than their age. Children who are too young to swallow a pill may use HIV medicines that come in liquid form.

Issues that make it difficult to take HIV medicines every day and exactly as prescribed (called "medication adherence") can affect HIV treatment in children and adolescents. Effective HIV treatment depends on good medication adherence.

WHY CAN MEDICATION ADHERENCE BE DIFFICULT FOR CHILDREN AND ADOLESCENTS?

Several factors can make medication adherence difficult for children and adolescents with HIV. For example, a child may refuse to take an HIV medicine because it tastes unpleasant.

Negative beliefs and attitudes about HIV (called "stigma") can make adherence especially difficult for adolescents living with HIV. They may skip medicine doses to hide their HIV-positive status from others.

The following factors can also affect medication adherence in children and adolescents:

- A busy schedule that makes it hard to take HIV medicines on time every day
- Side effects from HIV medicines
- Issues within a family, such as physical or mental illness, an unstable housing situation, or alcohol or drug abuse
- Lack of health insurance to cover the cost of HIV medicines
- A child's age and developmental stage.

Section 7.2 | HIV among Women

This section includes text excerpted from "HIV and Women," HIVinfo, U.S. Department of Health and Human Services (HHS), August 13, 2021.

DOES HIV AFFECT WOMEN?

Yes. According to the Centers for Disease Control and Prevention (CDC), in 2018, 19 percent of the new human immunodeficiency virus (HIV) diagnoses in the United States and dependent areas were among women. In addition, 57 percent of women with HIV were Black/African American.

The most common way that women get HIV is through sex with a male partner who has HIV without using a condom. Most women who have HIV know that they are HIV-positive, but some women are not getting the HIV care and treatment they need.

WHAT FACTORS PUT WOMEN AT RISK FOR HIV?

Human immunodeficiency virus is spread through blood, preseminal fluids, semen, vaginal fluids, rectal fluids, and breast milk.

In the United States, the main risk factors for HIV transmission are the following:

- Having anal or vaginal sex with a person who has HIV without using a condom or taking medicines to prevent or treat HIV. Anal sex is the riskiest type of sex for getting HIV, because the rectum's lining is thin and may allow HIV to enter the body during anal sex.
- Sharing injection drug equipment (works), such as needles, with a person who has HIV.

In women, several factors can increase the risk of HIV transmission. For example, during vaginal or anal sex, a woman has a greater risk for getting HIV because, in general, receptive sex is riskier than insertive sex. Age-related thinning and dryness of the vagina may also increase the risk of HIV in older women, because these can cause a tear in the vagina during sex and lead to HIV transmission. A woman's risk of HIV can also increase if her partner engages in high-risk behaviors, such as injection drug use or having sex with other partners without using condoms.

ARE THERE ANY ISSUES THAT AFFECT HIV TREATMENT IN WOMEN?

Treatment with HIV medicines (called "antiretroviral therapy" or "ART") is recommended for everyone with HIV. Treatment with HIV medicines helps people with HIV live longer, healthier lives. ART also reduces the risk of HIV transmission.

People should start taking HIV medicines as soon as possible after HIV is diagnosed. However, birth control and pregnancy are two issues that can affect HIV treatment in women.

Birth Control

Some HIV medicines may reduce the effectiveness of hormonal contraceptives, such as birth control pills, patches, rings, or implants. Women taking certain HIV medicines may have to use an additional or different form of birth control.

Pregnancy

Women with HIV take HIV medicines during pregnancy and childbirth to reduce the risk of perinatal transmission of HIV and to protect their own health.

The choice of an HIV treatment regimen to use during pregnancy depends on several factors, including a woman's current or past use of HIV medicines, other medical conditions she may have, and the results of drug-resistance testing. In general, pregnant women with HIV can use the same HIV treatment regimens recommended for nonpregnant adults – unless the risk of any known side effects to a pregnant woman or her baby outweighs the benefits of a regimen.

Sometimes a woman's HIV treatment regimen may change during pregnancy. Women and their healthcare providers should discuss whether any changes need to be made to an HIV treatment regimen during pregnancy.

Section 7.3 | HIV among Older Adults

This section includes text excerpted from documents published by two public domain sources. Text under the headings marked 1 are excerpted from "HIV and Older Americans," Centers for Disease Control and Prevention (CDC), January 12, 2022; Text under the headings marked 2 are excerpted from "HIV and Older People," HIVinfo, U.S. Department of Health and Human Services (HHS), August 23, 2021.

HIV DIAGNOSES[1]

In 2018, over half (51 percent) of people in the United States and dependent areas with diagnosed HIV were aged 50 and older. Though new HIV diagnoses are declining among people aged 50 and older, around 1 in 6 HIV diagnoses in 2018 were in this group. People aged 50 and older with diagnosed HIV are living longer, healthier lives because of effective HIV treatment.

17 Percent of the 37,968 new HIV diagnoses in the United States and dependent areas in 2018, 17 percent were among people aged 50 and older.

Among people aged 50 and older most new HIV diagnoses were among men as shown in Figure 7.1 and Figure 7.2.

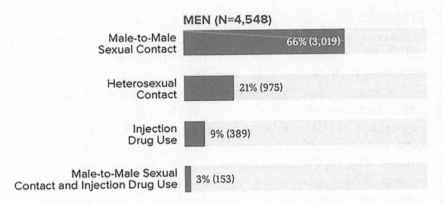

Figure 7.1. New HIV Diagnoses among Men Aged 50 and Older in the United States and Dependent Areas by Transmission Category and Sex, 2018* *(Source: Centers for Disease Control and Prevention (CDC). Diagnoses of HIV infection in the United States and dependent areas, 2018. HIV Surveillance Report 2020.)*

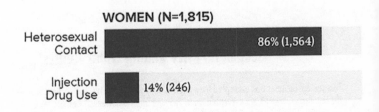

Figure 7.2. New HIV Diagnoses among Women Aged 50 and Older in the United States and Dependent Areas by Transmission Category and Sex, 2018*(Source: Centers for Disease Control and Prevention (CDC). Diagnoses of HIV infection in the United States and dependent areas, 2018. HIV Surveillance Report 2020.)*

Total for men may not equal 100 percent due to rounding.
*Based on sex at birth and includes transgender people.

1 in 6 new HIV diagnoses was among people aged 50 and older. Figure 7.3 shows HIV diagnoses across various age groups.

From 2014–2018, HIV diagnoses decreased 6 percent overall among people aged 50 and older, with trends varying by sex and transmission category as shown in Figure 7.4 and Figure 7.5.

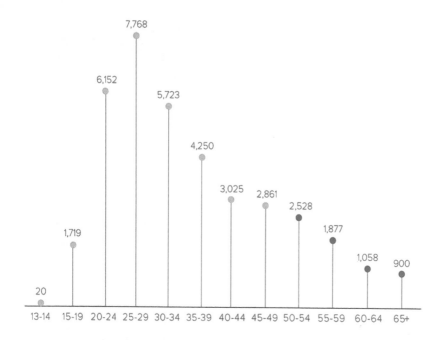

Figure 7.3. New HIV Diagnoses among Adults and Adolescents in the United States and Dependent Areas by Age, 2018 *(Source: Centers for Disease Control and Prevention (CDC). Diagnoses of HIV infection in the United States and dependent areas, 2018. HIV Surveillance Report 2020.)*

LIVING WITH HIV[1]

People aged 55 and older with HIV in the 50 states and the District of Columbia

At the end of 2018, an estimated 1.2 million Americans had HIV. Of those 3,79,000 were aged 55 and older. 9 in 10 people aged 55 and older knew they had the virus.

It is important for people aged 50 and older to know their HIV status so they can take medicine to treat HIV if they have the virus. Taking HIV medicine every day can make the viral load undetectable. People who get and keep an undetectable viral load (or stay virally suppressed) can live a long and healthy life. They also have effectively no risk of transmitting HIV to HIV-negative sex partners.

Compared to all people with HIV, people aged 55 and older have higher viral suppression rates. In 2018, for every 100 people aged 55 and older with HIV:

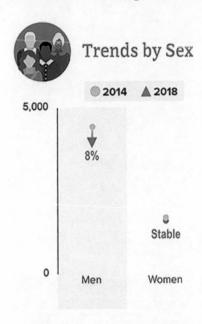

Figure 7.4. HIV Diagnoses among People Aged 50 and Older in the United States and Dependent Areas, 2014–2018*: Trends by Sex *(Source: Centers for Disease Control and Prevention (CDC). Diagnoses of HIV infection in the United States and dependent areas, 2018. HIV Surveillance Report 2020.)*

Based on sex at birth and includes transgender people.

- 71 received some HIV care
- 57 were retained in care*
- 64 were viral suppressed†

For comparison, for every 100 people overall with HIV, 65 received some HIV care, 50 were retained in care, 56 were virally suppressed.

*Had 2 viral load or CD4 tests at least 3 months apart in a year.
†Based on the most recent viral load test.*

Over half of people with diagnosed HIV were aged 50 and older as shown in Figure 7.6.

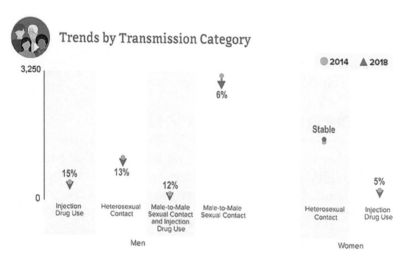

Figure 7.5. HIV Diagnoses among People Aged 50 and Older in the United States and Dependent Areas, 2014–2018*: Trends by Commission Category *(Source: Centers for Disease Control and Prevention (CDC). Diagnoses of HIV infection in the United States and dependent areas, 2018. HIV Surveillance Report 2020.)*

*Based on sex at birth and includes transgender people.

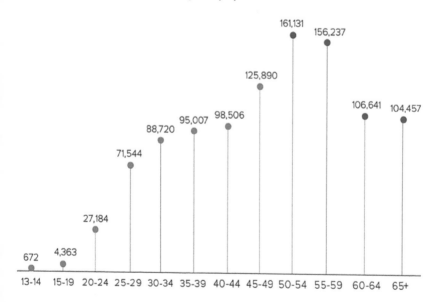

Figure 7.6. Adults and Adolescents with Diagnosed HIV in the United States and Dependent Areas by Age, 2018 *(Source: Centers for Disease Control and Prevention (CDC). Diagnoses of HIV infection in the United States and dependent areas, 2018. HIV Surveillance Report 2020)*

DEATHS[1]

In 2018, there were 11,425 deaths among people aged 50 and older with diagnosed HIV in the United States and dependent areas. These deaths could be from any cause.

SHOULD OLDER PEOPLE GET TESTED FOR HIV?[2]

The CDC recommends that everyone 13–64 years old get tested for HIV, at least once, as part of routine healthcare, and that people at higher risk of HIV get tested more often. Your healthcare provider may recommend HIV testing if you are over 64 and at risk for HIV.

For several reasons, older people are less likely to get tested for HIV:

- In general, older people are often considered at low risk of getting HIV. For this reason, healthcare providers may not always think to test older people for HIV.
- Some older people may be embarrassed or afraid to be tested for HIV.
- In older people, signs of HIV may be mistaken for symptoms of aging or of age-related conditions. Consequently, testing to diagnose the condition may not include HIV testing.

For these reasons, HIV is more likely to be diagnosed at an advanced stage in many older people. Diagnosing HIV at a late stage also means a late start to treatment with HIV medicines and possibly more damage to the immune system.

ARE THERE ANY ISSUES THAT AFFECT HIV TREATMENT IN OLDER PEOPLE?[2]

Treatment with HIV medicines is recommended for everyone with HIV. As for anyone with HIV, the choice of an HIV treatment regimen for an older person is based on the person's individual needs.

However, the following factors can complicate HIV treatment in older people.

- Conditions, such as heart disease or cancer, that are more common in older people and require additional medical care.

- Side effects from HIV medicines and other medicines may occur more frequently in older people with HIV than in younger people with HIV.
- The increased risk of drug interactions in an older person taking HIV medicines and medicines for another condition.
- Age-related changes that can affect an older person's ability to think or remember, which can make it harder to stick to an HIV treatment regimen.

PREVENTION CHALLENGES[1]

There are some behaviors that put everyone at risk for HIV. These include having anal or vaginal sex without protection (like a condom or medicine to prevent or treat HIV) or sharing injection drug equipment with someone who has HIV. Other factors that affect older people particularly include:

- Although they visit their doctors more frequently, older people and their providers are less likely to discuss sexual or drug use behaviors. Healthcare providers may not ask patients aged 50 and older about these issues or test them for HIV. Also, older people may not consider themselves to be at risk for HIV, may be embarrassed to discuss sex, or may mistake HIV symptoms for those of normal aging.
- Older people may have many of the same HIV risk factors as younger people, including a lack of knowledge about HIV prevention and sexual risk, such as having multiple sex partners, and may be less likely to use a condom or other prevention options.
- Older people in the United States are more likely than younger people to have late-stage HIV infection at the time of diagnosis. People aged 50 and older may start treatment late, which may put this population at risk of more immune system damage. Among people aged 55 and older who received an HIV diagnosis in 2015, 50 percent had HIV for 4.5 years before they were diagnosed – the longest diagnosis delay for any age group.

- Stigma is common among adults with HIV and negatively affects people's quality of life, self-image, and behaviors. People aged 50 and older may avoid getting the care they need or disclosing their HIV status because they may already face isolation due to illness or loss of family, friends, or community support.
- Aging with HIV presents special challenges for preventing other diseases. Both age and HIV increase the risk for cardiovascular disease, lung disease (specifically chronic obstructive pulmonary disease), bone loss, and certain cancers. People aged 50 and older also need to be careful about interactions between medications used to treat HIV and those used to treat common age-related conditions such as hypertension, diabetes, elevated cholesterol, and obesity.

Section 7.4 | HIV among Gay and Bisexual Men

This section includes text excerpted from "HIV and Gay and Bisexual Men," Centers for Disease Control and Prevention (CDC), September 16, 2021.

Gay, bisexual, and other men who reported male-to-male sexual contact are disproportionately affected by human immunodeficiency virus (HIV). Social and structural issues – such as HIV stigma, homophobia, discrimination, poverty, and limited access to high-quality healthcare – influence health outcomes and continue to drive inequities.

HIV RISK BEHAVIORS

The risk of getting or transmitting HIV varies widely depending on the type of exposure or behavior. Most commonly, people get or transmit HIV through anal or vaginal sex, or sharing needles, syringes, or other drug injection equipment – for example, cookers.

Sexual Behaviors among Gay and Bisexual Men with Diagnosed HIV in the United States, 2019*

Getting and keeping an undetectable viral load is the best way for people with HIV to stay healthy and protect others.

- 7 percent of people with HIV had sex without using any HIV prevention strategy in the past 12 months[†]
- 8 percent of gay and bisexual men with HIV had sex without using any HIV prevention strategy in the past 12 months[†]

Among people aged 18 and older.
[†]*Had sex while not virally suppressed with a partner whose HIV status was negative or unknown, a condom was not used, and the partner was not taking pre-exposure prophylaxis (PrEP).*

HIV PREVENTION

There are many HIV prevention strategies available, including condoms; pre-exposure prophylaxis (PrEP); post-exposure prophylaxis (PEP); as well as interventions focused on risk reduction; adherence to HIV medicine; linkage to, retention in, and re-engagement in care; structural approaches; and engagement in PrEP care. Additionally, for people with HIV, treatment provides substantial benefits for personal health and reduces HIV transmission to others. This is sometimes called "HIV treatment" as prevention.

PrEP Awareness and Use among Gay and Bisexual Men in 23 United States Cities, 2017

PrEP is highly effective for preventing HIV from sex or injection drug use.

- 85 percent of gay and bisexual men without HIV were aware of PrEP.
- 25 percent of gay and bisexual men without HIV used PrEP.

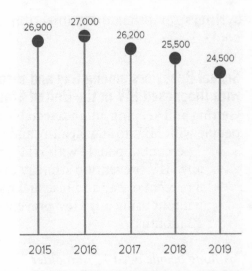

Figure 7.7. Estimated HIV Infections Among Gay and Bisexual Men in the United States, 2015–2019 (Source: Centers for Disease Control and Prevention (CDC). Estimated HIV incidence and prevalence in the United States 2015–2019. HIV Surveillance Supplemental Report 2021)

HIV INCIDENCE

HIV incidence is one of the six ending the HIV epidemic in the United States indicators. HIV incidence is the estimated number of new HIV infections in a given year.

Ending the HIV epidemic. Overall goal: Decrease the estimated number of new HIV infections to 9,300 by 2025 and 3000 by 2030.

70 percent of the 34800 estimated new HIV infections in the United States in 2019, 70 percent (24,500) were among gay and bisexual men.

The number of estimated HIV infections has decreased in 2019 compared to 2015 as shown in Figure 7.7.

HIV DIAGNOSES

HIV diagnoses is one of the six ending the HIV epidemic in the United States indicators. HIV diagnoses refers to the number of people who received an HIV diagnosis during a given year. In 2019,

HIV/AIDS among Specific Populations

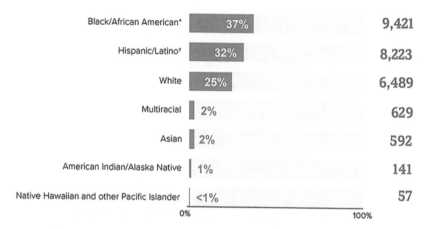

Figure 7.8. New HIV Diagnoses among Gay and Bisexual Men in the United States and Dependent Areas by Race/Ethnicity, 2019 *(Source: Centers for Disease Control and Prevention (CDC). Diagnoses of HIV infection in the United States and dependent areas, 2019. HIV Surveillance Report 2021)*

*Black refers to people having origins in any of the Black racial groups of Africa. African-American is a term often used for people of African descent with ancestry in North America. ʸHispanic/Latinx people can be of any race.

gay and bisexual men made up 69 percent (25,552) of the 36,801 new HIV diagnoses in the United States and dependent areas.

Ending the HIV epidemic. Overall goal: Decrease the estimated number of new HIV diagnose to 9588 by 2025 and 3000 by 2030.

69 percent of the 36801 estimated new HIV diagnose in the United States and dependent areas in 2019, 69 percent (25,552) were among gay and bisexual men.

Among gay and bisexual men who received an HIV diagnosis in 2019, racial and ethnic disparities continue to exist as shown in Figure 7.8.

Gay and bisexual men aged 13 to 34 made up most new HIV diagnoses among all gay and bisexual men as shown in Figure 7.9.

From 2015 to 2019, HIV diagnoses decreased 9 percent among gay and bisexual men overall, trends by age groups shown in Figure 7.10 But, trends varied for different groups of gay and bisexual men as shown in Figure 7.11.

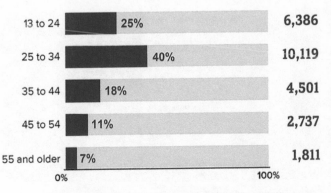

Figure 7.9. New HIV Diagnoses among Gay and Bisexual Men in the United States and Dependent Areas by Age, 2019 *(Source: Centers for Disease Control and Prevention (CDC). Diagnoses of HIV infection in the United States and dependent areas, 2019. HIV Surveillance Report 2021)*

Note: *Total may not equal 100 percent due to rounding.*

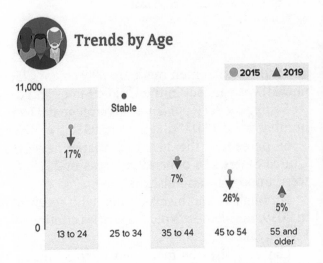

Figure 7.10. HIV Diagnoses among Gay and Bisexual Men in the United States and Dependent Areas, 2019: Trends by Age *(Source: Centers for Disease Control and Prevention (CDC). Diagnoses of HIV infection in the United States and dependent areas, 2019. HIV Surveillance Report 2021).*

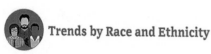

Trends by Race and Ethnicity

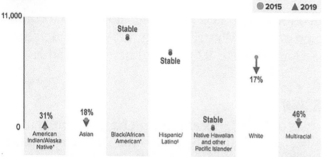

Figure 7.11. HIV Diagnoses among Gay and Bisexual Men in the United States and Dependent Areas, 2019: Trends by Race and Ethnicity *(Source: Centers for Disease Control and Prevention (CDC). Diagnoses of HIV infection in the United States and dependent areas, 2019. HIV Surveillance Report 2021)*

*Changes in subpopulations with fewer HIV diagnoses can lead to a large percentage increase or decrease.
†Black refers to people having origins in any of the Black racial groups of Africa. African-American is a term often used for people of African descent with ancestry in North America.
‡Hispanic/Latinx people can be of any race.

KNOWLEDGE OF STATUS

Knowledge of status is one of the six ending the HIV epidemic in the United States indicators. Knowledge of status refers to the estimated percentage of people with HIV who have received an HIV diagnosis.

Ending the HIV epidemic. Overall goal: Increase the estimated percentage of people with HIV who have received an HIV diagnosis to 95 percent by 2025 and remain stable at 95 percent by 2030.

Gay and Bisexual Men with HIV in the United States, 2019

- In 2019 an estimated 1.2 million people had HIV. Of those 754,700 were gay and bisexual men.
- For every people with HIV 87 percent knew their HIV status.

- For every 100 gay and bisexual men with HIV 85 percent knew their HIV status

including infections attributed to male-to-male sexual contact only. Among men with HIV attributed to male-to-male sexual contact and injection drug use, 92 percent knew they had HIV.

VIRAL SUPPRESSION

Viral suppression is one of the six ending the HIV epidemic in the United States indicators. Viral suppression refers to the percentage of people with diagnosed HIV who have less than 200 copies of HIV per milliliter of blood.

Ending the HIV epidemic. Overall goal: Increase the percentage of people with diagnosed HIV who are virally suppressed to at least 95 percent by 2025 and remain stable at 95 percent by 2030.

It is important for women to know their HIV status so they can take medicine to treat HIV if they have the virus. Taking HIV medicine every day can make the viral load undetectable. People who get and keep an undetectable viral load (or remain virally suppressed) can stay healthy for many years and have effectively no risk of transmitting HIV to their sex partners.

Gay and Bisexual Men with Diagnosed HIV in 44 states and the District of Columbia, 2019

Compared to all people with diagnosed HIV, gay and bisexual men have higher viral suppression rates. For every 100 gay and bisexual men with diagnosed HIV in 2019:

- 78 received some HIV care
- 59 were retained in care*
- 68 were virally suppressed[†]

Had 2 viral load or CD4 tests at least 3 months apart in a year.
[†]*Based on most recent viral load test.*

Many people with HIV may experience challenges with achieving and maintaining viral suppression over time. Some of these challenges include missing HIV medical appointments, needing,

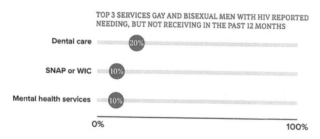

Figure 7.12. Needed HIV Ancillary Care Services among Gay and Bisexual Men with Diagnosed HIV in the United States, 2019*† *(Source: Centers for Disease Control and Prevention (CDC). Medical Monitoring Project.)*

*Among people aged 18 and older.
†HIV ancillary care services, such as case management and mental-health services, are services that support retention in HIV care.

but not receiving other important healthcare services, or missing doses of HIV treatment.

Missed HIV Medical Care Appointments among Gay and Bisexual Men with Diagnosed HIV in the United States, 2019

Staying in HIV care is important to achieving and maintaining viral suppression.

- 24 percent of all people with HIV missed at least one medical appointment in the past 12 months.
- 22 percent of gay and bisexual men with HIV at least one medical appointment in the past 12 months.

HIV ancillary care services are essential for supporting people in staying in HIV care and maintaining viral suppression.

Nearly half (45 percent) of all people with HIV needed at least 1 HIV ancillary care service including dental care, SNAP or WIC, or mental health, in the past 12 months (See Figure 7.12).

HIV Treatment among Gay and Bisexual Men with Diagnosed HIV in the United States, 2019*

Taking HIV medicines consistently and as prescribed in the best way to achieve and maintain viral suppression.

- 58 percent cisgender women and 59 percent of people overall reported talking all of their doses of HIV medicines

Among people aged 18 and older.

Depression and Anxiety among Gay and Bisexual Men with Diagnosed HIV in the United States, 2019*

People who have experience symptoms of depression or anxiety may face challenges maintaining viral suppression.

- 22 percent of all people with HIV and 22 percent of gay and bisexual men with HIV experienced symptoms of depression and anxiety in the past 12 months.

Among people aged 18 and older.

Homelessness among Gay and Bisexual Men with Diagnosed HIV in the United States, 2019*

People who may experience homelessness may find it difficult to get HIV care and treatment.

- 9 percent of people with HIV and 8 percent of gay and bisexual men with HIV reported homeless in the past 12 months.

Among people aged 18 and older.

Below Figure 7.13 shows median HIV stigma score for gay and bisexual men with HIV.

Deaths

In 2019, there were 8,253 deaths among gay and bisexual men with diagnosed HIV in the United States and dependent areas. These deaths could be from any cause.

PREVENTION CHALLENGES

Racism, discrimination, HIV stigma, and homophobia affect the overall health and well-being of some gay and bisexual men.

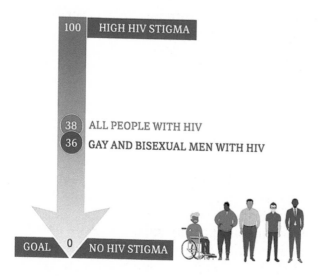

Figure 7.13. Median HIV Stigma Scores among Gay and Bisexual Men with Diagnosed HIV in the United States, 2019* *(Source: Centers for Disease Control and Prevention (CDC). Medical Monitoring Project.)*

Note: *Ten-item scale ranging from 0 (no stigma) to 100 (high stigma) that measures personalized stigma, disclosure concerns, negative self-image, and perceived public attitudes about people with HIV. *Among people aged 18 and older.*

Additionally, lower income and educational levels, and higher rates of unemployment and incarceration may place some gay and bisexual men at higher risk for HIV and make it harder to seek and receive high-quality healthcare, including HIV testing, treatment, and other prevention services. Addressing these social and structural barriers and encouraging safe and supportive communities can help improve health outcomes for gay and bisexual men.

Other factors that can increase the chances of getting or transmitting HIV include:

- **HIV prevalence.** A higher proportion of gay and bisexual men have HIV compared to any other group in the United States. Therefore, gay and bisexual men have an increased chance of having a partner who has HIV.

- **Knowledge of HIV status**. It is important for everyone to know their HIV status. People who do not know they have HIV cannot take advantage of HIV care and treatment and may pass HIV to others without knowing it.
- **Sexual behaviors**. Some factors put gay and bisexual men at higher risk for HIV, including having anal sex with someone who has HIV without using protection (such as condoms or medicines to prevent or treat HIV). Anal sex is the riskiest type of sex for getting or transmitting HIV. Receptive anal sex is 13 times as risky for getting HIV as insertive anal sex.
- **Low PrEP (pre-exposure prophylaxis) use**. PrEP use among gay and bisexual men, especially Black/African-American and Hispanic/Latinx gay and bisexual men, remains low. If taken as prescribed, PrEP is highly effective for preventing HIV.
- **Other sexually transmitted diseases (STDs)**. Gay and bisexual men are at increased risk for other STDs, such as syphilis, gonorrhea, and chlamydia. Having another STD can increase a person's chance of getting or transmitting HIV. Condoms can protect from some STDs, including HIV.

Section 7.5 | **HIV among Transgender People**

This section includes text excerpted from "HIV and Transgender People," Centers for Disease Control and Prevention (CDC), September 20, 2021.

Nearly 1 million people identify as transgender in the United States; and, adult and adolescent transgender people made up 2 percent (601) of new HIV diagnoses in the United States and dependent areas in 2018. Get the data on HIV among transgender people and find out how CDC is making a difference.

TERMINOLOGY

- **Transgender**. A person whose gender identity or expression is different from their sex assigned at birth.
- **Transgender man**. A person assigned female at birth and identifies as a male.
- **Transgender woman**. A person assigned male at birth and identifies as a female.
- **Cisgender**. A person whose sex assigned at birth is the same as their gender identity or expression.
- **Gender expression**. A person's outward presentation of their gender (e.g., how they act or dress).
- **Gender identity**. A person's internal understanding of their own gender.

HIV TESTING

HIV testing is the gateway to care for people who have HIV and to prevention services for people who do not have HIV. The CDC recommends that everyone between the ages of 13 and 64 get tested for HIV at least once as part of routine healthcare. People with certain risk factors should get tested at least once a year. A recent study found that transgender women have high rates of recent and lifetime HIV testing.

HIV Testing among Transgender Women in 7 United States Cities, 2019–2020

Getting tested for HIV is the only way for people to learn their status.

- 96 percent of transgender women have ever tested for HIV
- 82 percent of transgender women were tested for HIV in the past 12 months

HIV PREVENTION

There are many HIV prevention strategies available, including condoms; pre-exposure prophylaxis (PrEP); post-exposure prophylaxis (PEP); as well as interventions focused on risk reduction; adherence to HIV medicine; linkage to, retention in, and re-engagement in care; structural approaches; and engagement in PrEP care. Additionally, for people with HIV, treatment provides substantial benefits for personal health and reduces HIV transmission to others. This is sometimes called "HIV treatment" as prevention.

HIV Prevention Interventions among Transgender Women in 7 United States Cities, 2019–2020

HIV prevention interventions can reduce risk behaviors.
- 61 percent of transgender women who do not have HIV participated in an individual or group level HIV prevention intervention

PrEP Awareness and Use among Transgender Women in 7 United States Cities, 2019–2020

PrEP is highly effective for preventing HIV from sex or injection drug use.
- 92 percent of transgender women without HIV were aware of PrEP
- 32 percent of transgender women without HIV used PrEP

HIV DIAGNOSES

HIV diagnoses refer to the number of people who received an HIV diagnosis during a given year. Adult and adolescent transgender people accounted for 2 percent (601) of the 37,968 new HIV diagnoses in the United States and dependent areas in 2018.

Ending the HIV epidemic. Overall Goal: Decreases the number of new HIV diagnoses to 9588 by 2025 and 3000 by 2030.
- 2 percent of the 37968 new HIV diagnoses in the united states and dependent areas in 2018, 2 percent (601) were among transgender people.

Most new HIV diagnoses among transgender people were among Black/African-American women and men as shown in Figure 7.14 and Figure 7.15.

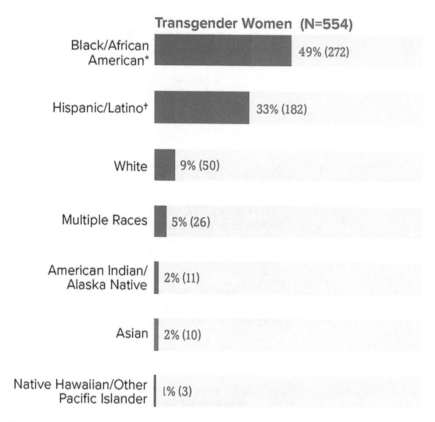

Figure 7.14. New HIV Diagnoses among Transgender Women by Race/Ethnicity in the United States and Dependent Areas, 2018 *(Source: Centers for Disease Control and Prevention (CDC). Diagnoses of HIV infection in the United States and dependent areas, 2018 (updated). HIV Surveillance Report 2020;31.)*

Among transgender people, most new HIV diagnoses were among people aged 25 to 34 as shown in Figure 7.16.

The highest number of new HIV diagnoses among transgender people were in the south as shown in Figure 7.17.

Though HIV diagnoses increased 9 percent among transgender people overall from 2014 to 2018, trends varied by age for the same period as shown in Figure 7.18.

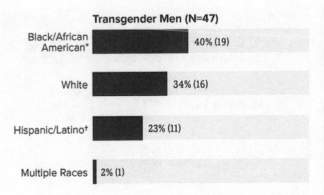

Figure 7.15. New HIV Diagnoses among Transgender Men by Race-Ethnicity in the United States and Dependent Areas, 2018 *(Source: Centers for Disease Control and Prevention (CDC). Diagnoses of HIV infection in the United States and dependent areas, 2018. HIV Surveillance Report 2020)*

Note: *Total may not equal 100 percent due to rounding.*
*Black refers to people having origins in any of the Black racial groups of Africa. African-American is a term often used for people of African descent with ancestry in North America.
†Hispanic/Latinx people can be of any race.

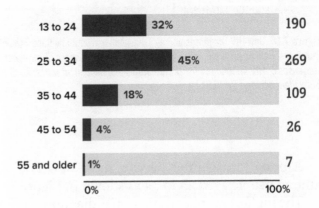

Figure 7.16. New HIV Diagnoses among Transgender People by Age in the United States and Dependent Areas, 2018 *(Source: Centers for Disease Control and Prevention (CDC). Diagnoses of HIV infection in the United States and dependent areas, 2018. HIV Surveillance Report 2020)*

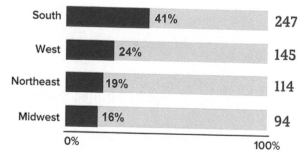

Figure 7.17. New HIV Diagnoses among Transgender People by Region in the United States and Dependent Areas, 2018* *(Source: Centers for Disease Control and Prevention (CDC). Diagnoses of HIV infection in the United States and dependent areas, 2018. HIV Surveillance Report 2020)*

*Regions used in CDC's National HIV Surveillance System:
Northeast: CT, ME, MA, NH, NJ, NY, PA, RI, VT
Midwest: IL, IN, IA, KS, MI, MN, MO, NE, ND, OH, SD, WI
South: AL, AR, DE, DC, FL, GA, KY, LA, MD, MS, NC, OK, SC, TN, TX, VA, WV
West: AK, AZ, CA, CO, HI, ID, MT, NV, NM, OR, UT, WA, WY*

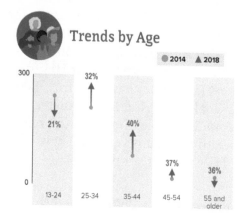

Figure 7.18. HIV Diagnoses among Transgender People in the United States and Dependent Areas, 2014-2018* *(Source: Centers for Disease Control and Prevention (CDC). Diagnoses of HIV infection in the United States and dependent areas, 2018. HIV Surveillance Report 2020)*

Changes in sub populations with fewer HIV diagnoses can lead to a large percentage increase or decrease.

HiV PREVALENCE

HIV prevalence is the number of people with HIV at a given time regardless of the time of infection.

HIV Prevalence among Transgender Women in 7 United States Cities, 2019–2020

Racial and ethnic disparities exists among transgender women with HIV.

Among transgender women interviewed, 42 percent had HIV.

- 62 percent of Black/American transgender women had HIV.
- 35 percent of Hispanic/Latina transgender women had HIV.
- 17 percent of white transgender women had HIV.

VIRAL SUPPRESSION

Viral suppression is the percentage of people with diagnosed HIV who have less than 200 copies of HIV per milliliter of blood.

Ending the HIV epidemic. Overall goal: Increase the percentage of people with diagnosed HIV who are virally suppressed to 95 percent by 2025 and remain stable at 95 percent by 2030.

It is important for transgender people to know their HIV status so they can take medicine to treat HIV if they have the virus. Taking HIV medicine every day can make the viral load undetectable. People who get and keep an undetectable viral load (or remain virally suppressed) can stay healthy for many years and have effectively no risk of transmitting HIV to their sex partners.

Transgender People with Diagnosed HIV in 41 States and the District of Columbia, 2018

Compared to all people with diagnosed HIV in 2018, transgender women have about the same viral suppression rates and transgender men have high viral suppression rates. More work is needed to increase these rates.

For every 100 transgender women with diagnosed HIV in 2018:

- 84 received some HIV care
- 66 were retained in care*
- 65 were virally suppressed†

For every 100 transgender men with diagnosed HIV in 2018:
- 87 received some HIV care
- 61 were retained in care*
- 72 were virally suppressed†

For comparison, for every 100 people overall with diagnosed HIV, 76 received some HIV care, 58 were retained in care, 66 were virally suppressed.

*Had 2 viral load or CD4 tests at least 3 months apart in a year.
†Had less than 200 copies of HIV per milliliter of blood on most recent viral load test.

Although many people taking HIV medicine are virally suppressed, some people with HIV who are taking HIV medicine are currently not virally suppressed or do not maintain viral suppression over time. Some challenges with achieving and maintaining viral suppression include missing multiple doses of HIV treatment, missing medical appointments, or needing other important health-care services.

Missed HIV Medical Care Appointments among Transgender People with Diagnosed HIV in the United States, 2018

Staying in HIV care is important to achieving and maintaining viral suppression.
- 39 percent of transgender people and 24 percent of people overall missed at least one medical appointment in the past 12 months.

HIV Treatment among Transgender People with Diagnosed HIV in the United States, 2018

Taking HIV medicines consistently and as prescribed in the best way to achieve and maintain viral suppression.

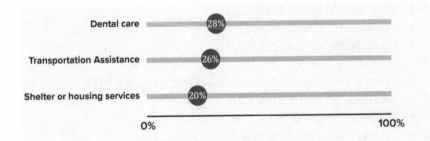

Figure 7.19. Top 3 Services Transgender People Reported Needing, but Not Receiving in the Past 12 Months *(Source: Centers for Disease Control and Prevention (CDC). Medical Monitoring Project.)*

- 43 percent of transgender people and 59 percent of people overall reported talking all of their doses of HIV medicine over the last 30 days.

Needed Care Services among Transgender People with Diagnosed HIV in the United States, 2018*

People who have experienced symptoms of depression or anxiety may face challenges maintaining viral suppression.

Top 3 services transgender person reported needing, but not receiving in the past 12 months.

Among people aged 18 and older.

Homelessness among Gay and Bisexual Men with Diagnosed HIV in the United States, 2019*

People who may experience homelessness may find it difficult to get HIV care and treatment.

- 9 percent of people with HIV and 8 percent of gay and bisexual men with HIV reported being homeless in the past 12 months.

Among people aged 18 and older.

Having access to needed healthcare services could reduce barriers to achieving and maintaining viral suppression.

Dental care, transportation assistance, and shelter or housing services are three top services transgender people reported needing, but not receiving percentage as shown in Figure 7.19.

Social and economic issues – such as homelessness, depression, and stigma – have prevented some transgender people from getting the HIV care and treatment they need. These factors make it difficult for some transgender people with HIV to achieve and maintain viral suppression.

Homelessness among Transgender People with Diagnosed HIV in the United States, 2018

People who may experience homelessness may find it difficult to get HIV care and treatment.

- 15 percent of transgender people and 10 percent of people overall reported homelessness in the past 12 months.

Depression and Anxiety among Transgender People with Diagnosed HIV in the United States, 2018

Some transgender people with diagnosed HIV may have difficulty getting treatment for depression and anxiety.

- 38 percent of transgender people and 24 percent of people reported being treated for depression and anxiety.

Below Figure 7.20 shows median HIV stigma score for transgender people with diagnosed HIV.

Ten-item scale ranging from 0 (no stigma) to 100 (high stigma) that measures personalized stigma, disclosure concerns, negative self-image, and perceived public attitudes about people with HIV.

Deaths

In 2018, there were 113 deaths among transgender people with diagnosed HIV in the United States and dependent areas. These deaths could be from any cause.

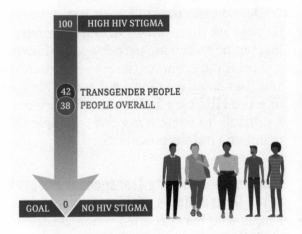

Figure 7.20. HIV Stigma among Transgender People with Diagnosed HIV in the United States, 2018 *(Source: Centers for Disease Control and Prevention (CDC). Medical Monitoring Project.)*

PREVENTION CHALLENGES

There are many prevention challenges that may impact the HIV health outcomes for some transgender people.

- Racism and discrimination may increase HIV risk-related behaviors and lead to health disparities in HIV. According to a study, young minority transgender women experienced racial discrimination more often than young white transgender women. Issues associated with racism and discrimination – including limited access to healthcare, employment, and housing – can increase the risk for HIV and affect the health and well-being of transgender people.
- HIV stigma may prevent transgender people from learning their HIV status. One study found that anticipated HIV stigma was associated with delaying regular HIV testing among some young transgender women.
- Transphobic discrimination (transphobia) occurs when transgender people face stigma and oppression directed toward them. Findings from the CDC's National HIV Behavioral Surveillance (NHBS) shows that most

transgender women have experienced some form of abuse or harassment because of their gender identity or presentation. This may negatively impact accessing testing, care, or getting treatment for HIV.

- Transgender and other gender minority youth may be less likely to engage in HIV prevention and treatment services. One study found that transgender youth were more likely to miss HIV care appointments if they did not feel supported through medical gender affirmation or were treated negatively because of their gender identity. Understanding these factors may help improve engagement in HIV prevention and treatment services for transgender youth.

- Multilevel interventions for transgender people may be needed to address disparities. According to a 2017 review, evidence-based multilevel interventions that address the structural, biomedical, and behavioral risks for HIV among transgender women and men are needed to address HIV disparities. Evidence-based behavioral interventions for transgender women have been found to be effective and are included in the CDC's Compendium of Evidence-Based Interventions and Best Practices for HIV Prevention.

- Unmet need for gender affirmation, including not being on hormones, may impact or delay HIV treatment. A study found that unmet surgical needs and not being on hormones were significantly associated with HIV treatment interruptions. Similarly, another study found that hormone use lowered the odds of not being on HIV treatment.

Section 7.6 | **HIV among Sex Workers**

This section includes text excerpted from "HIV Risk among Persons Who Exchange Sex for Money or Nonmonetary Items," Centers for Disease Control and Prevention (CDC), January 12, 2022.

The term "people who exchange sex for money or nonmonetary items" (hereinafter referred to as "people who exchange sex") includes a broad range of persons who trade sex for income or other items including food, drugs, medicine, and shelter. Persons who exchange sex are at increased risk of getting or transmitting human immunodeficiency virus (HIV) and other sexually transmitted diseases (STDs) because they are more likely to engage in risky sexual behaviors (e.g., sex without a condom, sex with multiple partners) and substance use. Those who exchange sex more regularly as a source of ongoing income are at higher risk for HIV than those who do so infrequently. Persons who engage in such activities include escorts; people who work in massage parlors, brothels, and the adult film industry; exotic dancers; state-regulated prostitutes (in Nevada); and men, women, and transgender persons who participate in survival sex, that is, trading sex to meet basic needs of daily life. For any of the above, sex can be consensual or nonconsensual.

It is important for people who exchange sex to get tested for HIV regularly and know their status. Knowing one's status helps determine the best prevention or care options:

- Condoms are highly effective in preventing a person from getting or transmitting HIV infection if used the right way every time during sex.
- For persons who are HIV-negative, prevention options like pre-exposure prophylaxis (PrEP), taking HIV medicines as prescribed to prevent getting HIV, may be beneficial.
- For people who are living with HIV, taking medicines to treat HIV (called "antiretroviral therapy" or "ART") the right way every day can help keep them healthy and greatly reduce their chance of transmitting HIV to others.

PREVENTION CHALLENGES
Lack of Data
There is a lack of population-based studies on persons who exchange sex, although some studies have been done in singular settings such as prisons and exotic dance clubs. However, the illegal – and often criminalized – nature of exchange sex makes it difficult to gather population-level data on HIV risk among this population. This lack of data creates significant barriers to developing targeted HIV prevention efforts.

Socioeconomic Factors
Many persons who exchange sex face stigma, poverty, and lack of access to healthcare and other social services – all of which pose challenges to HIV prevention efforts. Existing research shows that,

- Many persons who exchange sex may have a history of homelessness, unemployment, incarceration, mental-health issues, violence, emotional/physical/sexual abuse, and drug use.
- Some transgender persons may turn to exchange sex because of discrimination and lack of economic opportunities. They may exchange sex to generate income for rent, drugs, medicines, hormones, and gender-related surgeries.

Sexual Risk Factors
Persons who exchange sex may not use condoms consistently. Several factors may contribute to this behavior, including:

- **Economics**. Persons who exchange sex may receive more money for sex without a condom.
- **Partner type**. Persons who exchange sex may use condoms less often with regular clients than with one-time clients and even less frequently with intimate partners.
- **Power dynamics**. Unequal power in a relationship with clients may make it difficult for persons who exchange sex to negotiate condom use.

Other risk factors for this population include:
- Multiple high-risk sex partners, for example, partners who do not know they are living with HIV or other STDs.
- More money for sex with partners known to be HIV-positive.

Drug and Alcohol Use

There is a strong link between exchange sex and drug and alcohol use. Persons who exchange sex, if under the influence of drugs or alcohol, may have impaired judgment, engage in riskier forms of sex such as anal sex, and have difficulty negotiating safer sex (e.g., condom use) with their customers. People who trade sex for drugs tend to have more clients, use condoms less often, and are more likely to share needles and other drug works.

Knowledge of HIV Status

Many persons who exchange sex may not know their HIV status because they,
- Do not know where to access available services.
- Are uncomfortable sharing information about sexual and substance use histories as part of HIV testing protocol.

Some persons who know their HIV status may be reluctant to seek or stay in care because of:
- Mistrust of the healthcare system.
- Concern that they may lose income if identified as being HIV-positive.
- Financial circumstances and other barriers (e.g., health insurance) that affect healthcare access.

Part 2 | HIV/AIDS Transmission, Risk Factors, and Prevention

Chapter 8 | **HIV Transmission: Questions and Answers**

HOW IS HIV PASSED FROM ONE PERSON TO ANOTHER?

Most people who get human immunodeficiency virus (HIV) get it through anal or vaginal sex, or sharing needles, syringes, or other drug-injection equipment (e.g., cookers). But there are powerful tools that can help prevent HIV transmission.

CAN YOU GET HIV FROM ANAL SEX?

You can get HIV if you have anal sex with someone who has HIV without using protection (such as condoms or medicine to treat or prevent HIV).

- Anal sex is the riskiest type of sex for getting or transmitting HIV.
- Being the receptive partner (bottom) is riskier for getting HIV than being the insertive partner (top).
- The bottom's risk of getting HIV is very high because the rectum's lining is thin and may allow HIV to enter the body during anal sex.
- The top is also at risk because HIV can enter the body through the opening at the tip of the penis (or urethra),

This chapter contains text excerpted from the following sources: Text beginning with the heading "How Is HIV Passed from One Person to Another?" is excerpted from "Ways HIV Can Be Transmitted," Centers for Disease Control and Prevention (CDC), April 21, 2021; Text beginning with the heading "Does HIV Viral Load Affect Getting or Transmitting HIV?" is excerpted from "How Is HIV Transmitted?" HIV.gov, U.S. Department of Health and Human Services (HHS), June 24, 2019.

the foreskin if the penis is not circumcised, or small cuts, scratches, or open sores anywhere on the penis.

CAN YOU GET HIV FROM VAGINAL SEX?

You can get HIV if you have vaginal sex with someone who has HIV without using protection (such as condoms or medicine to treat or prevent HIV).

- Vaginal sex is less risky for getting HIV than receptive anal sex.
- Either partner can get HIV during vaginal sex.
- Most women who get HIV get it from vaginal sex. HIV can enter a woman's body during vaginal sex through the mucous membranes that line the vagina and cervix.
- Men can also get HIV during vaginal sex. This is because vaginal fluid and blood can carry HIV. Men get HIV through the opening at the tip of the penis (or urethra), the foreskin if the penis is not circumcised, or small cuts, scratches, or open sores anywhere on the penis.

CAN HIV BE TRANSMITTED FROM A MOTHER TO HER BABY?

HIV can be transmitted from a mother to her baby during pregnancy, birth, or breastfeeding. However, it is less common because of advances in HIV prevention and treatment.

- This is called "perinatal transmission" or "mother-to-child transmission."
- Mother-to-child transmission is the most common way that children get HIV.
- Recommendations to test all pregnant women for HIV and start HIV treatment immediately have lowered the number of babies who are born with HIV.
- If a mother with HIV takes HIV medicine daily as prescribed throughout pregnancy and childbirth, and gives HIV medicine to her baby for four to six weeks after giving birth, the risk of transmitting HIV to the baby can be less than one percent.

CAN YOU GET HIV FROM SHARING NEEDLES, SYRINGES, OR OTHER DRUG INJECTION EQUIPMENT?

You are at high risk for getting HIV if you share needles, syringes, or other drug-injection equipment (e.g., cookers) with someone who has HIV. Never share needles or other equipment to inject drugs, hormones, steroids, or silicone.

- Used needles, syringes, and other injection equipment may have someone else's blood on them, and blood can carry HIV.
- People who inject drugs are also at risk for getting HIV (and other sexually transmitted diseases) because they may engage in risky sexual behaviors such as having sex without protection (such as condoms or medicine to prevent or treat HIV).
- You are also at risk for getting hepatitis B and C, and other infections if you share needles, syringes, or other injection equipment.

WHAT ARE SOME RARE WAYS THAT HIV HAS BEEN TRANSMITTED?

There is little to no risk of getting HIV from the activities below. For transmission to occur, something very unusual would have to happen.

Oral Sex

- Oral sex involves putting the mouth on the penis (fellatio), vagina (cunnilingus), or anus (rimming).
- Factors that may affect this risk include ejaculation in the mouth with oral ulcers, bleeding gums, or genital sores, and the presence of other sexually transmitted diseases (STDs).
- You can get other STDs from oral sex. And if you get feces in your mouth during anilingus, you can get hepatitis A and B, parasites such as *Giardia*, and bacteria such as *Shigella*, *Salmonella*, *Campylobacter*, and *E. coli*.

Workplace

- The most likely cause is being stuck with a contaminated needle or another sharp object.
- Careful practice of standard precautions protects patients and healthcare personnel from possible occupational HIV transmission.

Medical Care

- The U.S. blood supply and donated organs and tissues are thoroughly tested, so it is very unlikely that you would get HIV from blood transfusions, blood products, or organ and tissue transplants.
- You cannot get HIV from donating blood. Blood collection procedures are highly regulated and safe.

Pre-chewed Food

- The only known cases are among infants. Contamination occurs when blood from a caregiver's mouth mixes with food that is pre-chewed before feeding to an infant.
- You cannot get HIV from consuming food handled by someone with HIV.

Biting

- Each of the very small number of documented cases has involved severe trauma with extensive tissue damage and the presence of blood. Transmission can occur when there is contact between broken skin, wounds, or mucous membranes and blood or body fluids mixed with the blood of a person who has HIV.
- There is no risk of transmission if the skin is not broken.

Deep, Open-Mouth Kissing

- Although very rare, transmission can occur if both partners have sores or bleeding gums, and blood from the partner with HIV gets into the bloodstream of the HIV-negative partner.

- HIV is not transmitted through closed-mouth or "social" kissing with someone who has HIV.
- HIV is not transmitted through saliva.

Female-to-Female

- Case reports of female-to-female transmission of HIV are rare.
- Vaginal fluids and menstrual blood may carry the virus and exposure to these fluids through mucous membranes (in the vagina or mouth) could potentially lead to HIV infection.

Tattoos and Body Piercings

- There are no known cases in the United States of anyone getting HIV this way.
- However, it is possible to get HIV from tattooing or body piercing if the equipment used for these procedures has someone else's blood in it or if the ink is shared. This is more likely to happen when the person doing the procedure is unlicensed because of the potential for unsanitary practices such as sharing needles or ink.
- If you get a tattoo or a body piercing, be sure that the person doing the procedure is properly licensed and that they use only new or sterilized needles, ink, and other supplies.

DOES HIV VIRAL LOAD AFFECT GETTING OR TRANSMITTING HIV?

Yes. Viral load is the amount of HIV in the blood of someone who has HIV. Taking HIV medicine (called "antiretroviral therapy" or "ART") daily as prescribed can make the viral load very low – so low that a test cannot detect it (this is called an "undetectable viral load").

People with HIV who take HIV medicine daily as prescribed and get and keep an undetectable viral load have effectively no risk of transmitting HIV to an HIV-negative partner through sex.

HIV medicine is a powerful tool for preventing sexual transmission of HIV. But it works only as long as the HIV-positive partner gets and keeps an undetectable viral load. Not everyone taking HIV medicine has an undetectable viral load. To stay undetectable, people with HIV must take HIV medicine every day as prescribed and visit their healthcare provider regularly to get a viral load test.

WHAT ARE THE WAYS HIV CANNOT BE SPREAD?

HIV is not spread by:

- Air or water
- Mosquitoes, ticks, or other insects
- Saliva, tears, or sweat that is not mixed with the blood of a person with HIV
- Shaking hands, hugging, sharing toilets, sharing dishes, silverware, or drinking glasses; or engaging in closed-mouth or "social" kissing with a person with HIV
- Drinking fountains
- Other sexual activities that do not involve the exchange of body fluids (e.g., touching).

HIV cannot be passed through healthy, unbroken skin.

Chapter 9 | Risky Behaviors and HIV

Chapter Contents

Section 9.1 | Alcohol, Drugs, and HIV Risk

This section includes text excerpted from "Alcohol and HIV Risk," HIV.gov, U.S. Department of Health and Human Services (HHS), August 27, 2018. Reviewed February 2022.

HOW CAN ALCOHOL PUT YOU AT RISK FOR GETTING OR TRANSMITTING HIV?

Drinking alcohol, particularly binge drinking, affects your brain, making it hard to think clearly. When you are drunk, you may be more likely to make poor decisions that put you at risk for getting or transmitting HIV, such as having sex without a condom.

You also may be more likely to have a harder time using a condom the right way every time you have sex, have more sexual partners or use other drugs. Those behaviors can increase your risk of exposure to HIV and other sexually transmitted diseases. Or, if you have HIV, they can also increase your risk of transmitting HIV to others.

WHAT CAN YOU DO?

- If you drink alcohol:
  - Drink in moderation. Moderate drinking is up to 1 drink per day for women and up to 2 drinks per day for men. One drink is a 12-ounce bottle of beer, a 5-ounce glass of wine, or a shot of liquor.
  - Visit Rethinking Drinking (www.rethinkingdrinking. niaaa.nih.gov), a website from the National Institutes of Health's (NIH) National Institute on Alcohol Abuse and Alcoholism (NIAAA). This website can help you evaluate your drinking habits and consider how alcohol may be affecting your health.
- Do not have sex if you are drunk or high from other drugs.
- Use a condom every time you have sex. You can also consider sexual activities that are lower risk for HIV than anal or vaginal sex (such as oral sex).

- If you are HIV-negative, talk to your healthcare provider about pre-exposure prophylaxis (PrEP). PrEP is when people at very high risk for HIV take HIV medicine (called "antiretroviral therapy" or "ART") daily to lower their chances of getting HIV. PrEP must be taken every day as prescribed and alcohol use can make it hard to stick to a daily HIV regimen. Be open and honest about your alcohol use so you and your doctor can develop a plan for you to stick to your HIV medicine.
- If you are living with HIV, taking ART every day, exactly as prescribed is also important to stay healthy and prevent transmission. People living with HIV who take HIV medication daily as prescribed and get and keep an undetectable viral load have effectively no risk of sexually transmitting HIV to their HIV-negative partners. Like PrEP, ART must be taken every day, exactly as prescribed.

NEED HELP?

- Therapy and other methods are available to help you stop or cut down on your alcohol use if you have a problem. Talk with a counselor, doctor, or other healthcare provider about options that might be right for you.
- To find a treatment center near you, use the Substance Abuse and Mental Health Services Administration (SAMHSA) Behavioral Health Treatment Locator (findtreatment.samhsa.gov) or call 800-662-HELP (800-662-4357). Open 24/7.

STAYING HEALTHY

If you are living with HIV, alcohol use can be harmful to your brain and body and affect your ability to stick to your HIV treatment. Learn about the health effects of alcohol and other drug use (www.hiv.gov/hiv-basics/staying-in-hiv-care/other-related-health-issues/alcohol-and-drug-use) and how to access alcohol treatment programs if you need them.

HOW CAN USING DRUGS PUT YOU AT RISK FOR GETTING OR TRANSMITTING HIV?

Using drugs affects your brain, alters your judgment, and lowers your inhibitions. When you are high, you may be more likely to make poor decisions that put you at risk for getting or transmitting HIV, such as having sex without a condom, have a hard time using a condom the right way every time you have sex, have more sexual partners, or use other drugs. These behaviors can increase your risk of exposure to HIV and other sexually transmitted diseases. Or, if you have HIV, they can increase your risk of spreading HIV to others.

And if you inject drugs, you are at risk for getting or transmitting HIV and hepatitis B and C if you share needles or equipment (or "works") used to prepare drugs, such as cotton, cookers, and water. This is because the needles or works may have blood in them, and blood can carry HIV. You should not share needles or works for injecting silicone, hormones, or steroids for the same reason.

Here are some commonly used substances and their link to HIV risk:

- **Alcohol**. Excessive alcohol consumption, notably binge drinking, can be an important risk factor for HIV because it is linked to risky sexual behaviors and, among people living with HIV, can hurt treatment outcomes.
- **Opioids**. Opioids, a class of drugs that reduce pain, include both prescription drugs and heroin. They are associated with HIV risk behaviors such as needle sharing when infected and risky sexual behaviors, and have been linked to outbreaks of HIV and viral hepatitis. People who are addicted to opioids are also at risk of turning to other ways to get the drug, including trading sex for drugs or money, which increases HIV risk.
- **Methamphetamine**. "Meth" is linked to risky sexual behaviors, such as having more sexual partners or sex without a condom, that place people at greater risk for HIV and other sexually transmitted diseases. Meth can

be injected, which also increases HIV risk if people share needles and other injection equipment.

- **Crack cocaine**. Crack cocaine is a stimulant that can create a cycle in which people quickly exhaust their resources and may engage in behaviors to obtain the drug that increase their HIV risk.
- **Inhalants**. Use of amyl nitrite ("poppers") has long been linked to risky sexual behaviors, illegal drug use, and sexually transmitted diseases among gay and bisexual men.

Therapy, medicines, and other methods are available to help you stop or cut down on drinking or using drugs. Talk with a counselor, doctor, or other healthcare provider about options that might be right for you. To find a substance abuse treatment center near you, visit SAMHSA's treatment locator or call 800-662-HELP (800-662-4357).

HOW CAN YOU PREVENT GETTING OR TRANSMITTING HIV FROM INJECTION DRUG USE?

Your risk is high for getting or transmitting HIV and hepatitis B and C if you share needles or equipment (or "works") used to prepare drugs, such as cotton, cookers, and water. This is because the needles or works may have blood in them, and blood can carry HIV.

If you inject drugs, you are also at risk of getting HIV (and other sexually transmitted diseases) because you may be more likely to take risks with sex when you are high.

The best way to lower your chances of getting HIV is to stop injecting drugs. You may need help to stop or cut down using drugs, but there are many resources available to help you. To find a substance abuse treatment center near you, visit SAMHSA's treatment locator or call 800-662-HELP (800-662-4357).

If you keep injecting drugs, here are some ways to lower your risk for getting HIV and other infections:

- Use only new, sterile needles and works each time you inject. Many communities have needle exchange programs where you can get new needles and works, and some pharmacies may sell needles without a prescription.

- Never share needles or works.
- Clean used needles with bleach only when you cannot get new ones. Bleaching a needle may reduce the risk of HIV, but does not eliminate it.
- Use sterile water to fix drugs.
- Clean your skin with a new alcohol swab before you inject.
- Be careful not to get someone else's blood on your hands or your needle or works.
- Dispose of needles safely after one use. Use a sharps container, or keep used needles away from other people.
- Get tested for HIV at least once a year.
- Ask your doctor about taking daily medicine to prevent HIV called "PrEP."
- If you think you have been exposed to HIV within the last 3 days, ask a healthcare provider about post-exposure prophylaxis (PEP) right away. PEP can prevent HIV, but it must be started within 72 hours.
- Do not have sex if you are high. If you do have sex, make sure to protect yourself and your partner by using a condom the right way every time or by using other effective methods.

WHAT ARE SYRINGE SERVICES PROGRAMS?

Many communities have syringe services programs (SSPs), also called "syringe exchange programs" or "needle exchange programs." SSPs are places where injection drug users can get new needles and works, along with other services such as help with stopping substance abuse; testing and, if needed, linkage to treatment for HIV, hepatitis B, and hepatitis C; and education on what to do for an overdose. SSPs have been demonstrated to be an effective component of a comprehensive approach to prevent HIV and viral hepatitis among people who inject drugs, while not increasing illegal drug use.

STAYING HEALTHY

If you are living with HIV, substance use can be harmful to your brain and body and affect your ability to stick to your HIV treatment regimen. Learn about the health effects of alcohol and other substance use (www.hiv.gov/hiv-basics/staying-in-hiv-care/other-related-health-issues/alcohol-and-drug-use) and how to access substance abuse treatment programs if you need them.

Section 9.2 | Sexually Transmitted Diseases and HIV Risk

This section contains text excerpted from the following sources: Text under the heading "What Are Sexually Transmitted Diseases?" is excerpted from "Diseases and Related Conditions," Centers for Disease Control and Prevention (CDC), December 8, 2021; Text beginning with the heading "STDs and HIV" is excerpted from "Detailed STD Facts – STDs and HIV," Centers for Disease Control and Prevention (CDC), April 5, 2021.

WHAT ARE SEXUALLY TRANSMITTED DISEASES?

Sexually transmitted diseases (STDs), also known as "sexually transmitted infections" (STIs), are very common. Millions of new infections occur every year in the United States.

STDs pass from one person to another through vaginal, oral, and anal sex. They also can spread through intimate physical contact such as heavy petting, though this is not very common.

STDs do not always cause symptoms or may only cause mild symptoms. Therefore, it is possible to have an infection and not know it. That is why getting an STD test is important if you are having sex. If you receive a positive STD diagnosis, know that all are treatable with medicine and some are curable entirely.

STDs are preventable. If you have sex, know how to protect yourself and your sex partner(s) from STDs.

STDs AND HIV

People who have an STD may be at an increased risk of getting HIV. One reason is the behaviors that put someone at risk for one infection (not using condoms, multiple partners, anonymous partners) often put them at risk for other infections. Also, because STDs and HIV tend to be linked, when someone gets an STD it suggests they got it from someone who may be at risk for other STDs and HIV. Finally, a sore or inflammation from an STD may allow infection with HIV that would have been stopped by intact skin.

STDs CAN INCREASE THE RISK OF SPREADING HIV

People with HIV are more likely to shed HIV when they have urethritis or a genital ulcer. When a person with HIV gets another STD, such as gonorrhea or syphilis, it suggests that they were having sex without using condoms. If so, they may have spread HIV to their partners. Antiretroviral treatment for HIV can prevent the transmission of HIV even from persons who have other STDs.

SOME STDs ARE MORE CLOSELY LINKED TO HIV THAN OTHERS

In the United States, both syphilis and HIV are highly concentrated epidemics among gay, bisexual, and other men who have sex with men (MSM). In MSM only men who have sex with both women and men (MSMW) accounted for 47 percent of all primary and secondary syphilis cases among males in which sex of sex partner was known. In Florida, among all persons diagnosed with infectious syphilis, 42 percent were also HIV infected. Men who get syphilis are at very high risk of being diagnosed with HIV in the future; among HIV-uninfected men who got syphilis in Florida in 2003, 22 percent were newly diagnosed with HIV by 2011. HIV is more closely linked to gonorrhea than chlamydia (which is particularly common among young women). Herpes is also commonly associated with HIV; a meta-analysis found persons infected with HSV-2 are at 3-fold increased risk for acquiring HIV infection.

SOME ACTIVITIES CAN PUT PEOPLE AT INCREASED RISK FOR BOTH STDs AND HIV

- Having anal, vaginal, or oral sex without a condom
- Having multiple sex partners

- Having anonymous sex partners
- Having sex while under the influence of drugs or alcohol can lower inhibitions and result in greater sexual risk-taking.

DOES TREATING STDs PREVENT HIV?

Not by itself. Given the close link between STDs and HIV in many studies, it seems obvious that treating STDs should reduce the risk of HIV. However, most studies that have treated STDs to prevent HIV has not lowered the risk of HIV.

Screening for STDs can help assess a person's risk for getting HIV. Treatment of STDs is important to prevent the complications of those infections, and to prevent transmission to partners, but it should not be expected to prevent spread of HIV.

WHAT CAN PEOPLE DO TO REDUCE THEIR RISK OF GETTING STDs AND HIV?

The only 100 percent effective way to avoid STDs is to not have vaginal, anal, or oral sex. If people are sexually active, they can do the following things to lower their chances of getting STDs and HIV:

- Choose less risky sexual behaviors
- Use a new condom, consistently and correctly, for every act of vaginal, anal, and oral sex throughout the entire sex act (from start to finish)
- Reduce the number of people with whom they have sex
- Limit or eliminate drug and alcohol use before and during sex
- Have an honest and open talk with their healthcare provider and ask whether they should be tested for STDs and HIV
- Talk with their healthcare provider and find out if either pre-exposure prophylaxis, or PrEP, or post-exposure prophylaxis, or PEP, is a good option for them to prevent HIV infection.

IF SOMEONE ALREADY HAS HIV AND SUBSEQUENTLY GETS AN STD, DOES THAT PUT THEIR SEX PARTNER(S) AT AN INCREASED RISK FOR GETTING HIV?

If the person living with HIV gets and maintains an undetectable viral load by taking antiretroviral treatment, then an STD does not increase the risk of transmitting HIV. However, HIV-infected persons who are not taking antiretroviral treatment may be more likely to transmit HIV when they have another STD.

HIV-negative sex partners of people with HIV can prevent HIV if:

- HIV-positive people use antiretroviral therapy (ART) as prescribed. ART reduces the amount of virus (viral load) in blood and body fluids. People with HIV who take ART, as prescribed, to achieve and maintain an undetectable viral load can stay healthy for many years, and have effectively no risk of transmitting HIV to sexual partners.
- Sex partners take PrEP medications, as prescribed, after discussing this option with their healthcare provider and determining whether it is appropriate.
- Partners choose less risky sex activities.
- Partners use a new condom for every act of vaginal, anal, and oral sex throughout the entire sex act (from start to finish).

WILL TREATING SOMEONE FOR STDs PREVENT THEM FROM GETTING HIV?

No. It is not enough. Screening for STDs can help assess a person's risk for getting HIV. Treatment of STDs is important to prevent the complications of those infections, and to prevent transmission to partners, but it should not be expected to prevent spread of HIV.

If someone is HIV-positive and is diagnosed with an STD, they should receive counseling about risk reduction and how to protect their sex partner(s) from getting re-infected with the same STD or getting HIV.

Chapter 10 | **HIV Risk in the Healthcare Setting**

Chapter Contents

Section 10.1 | **Occupational Exposure**

This section contains text excerpted from the following sources: Text in this section begins with excerpts from "Occupational HIV Transmission and Prevention among Health Care Workers," Centers for Disease Control and Prevention (CDC), June 2015. Reviewed February 2022; Text beginning with the heading "The Risk of Occupational HIV Transmission" is excerpted from "HIV and Occupational Exposure," Centers for Disease Control and Prevention (CDC), September 5, 2019.

The proper use of gloves and goggles, along with safety devices to prevent injuries from sharp medical devices, can help minimize the risk of exposure to HIV in the course of caring for patients with HIV. When workers are exposed, the Centers for Disease Control and Prevention (CDC) recommends immediate treatment with a short course of antiretroviral drugs to prevent infection.

Healthcare workers who are exposed to a needlestick involving HIV-infected blood at work have a 0.23 percent risk of becoming infected. In other words, 2.3 of every 1,000 such injuries, if untreated, will result in infection. Risk of exposure due to splashes with body fluids is thought to be near zero even if the fluids are overtly bloody. Fluid splashes to intact skin or mucous membranes are considered to be extremely low risk of HIV transmission, whether or not blood is involved.

THE RISK OF OCCUPATIONAL HIV TRANSMISSION

The risk of occupational HIV transmission varies by the type of exposure.

- The risk of exposure due to splashes with body fluids is thought to be near zero even if the fluids have blood in them.
- Fluid splashes to intact skin or mucous membranes are considered to be extremely low risk of HIV transmission, whether or not blood is involved.
- Percutaneous (needlestick) injury has less than 1 percent risk of transmission.

HOW CAN YOU PREVENT OCCUPATIONAL HIV TRANSMISSION?

Follow Standard Precautions at all times. Assume that blood and other body fluids are potentially infectious.

- Use gloves, goggles, and other barriers when anticipating contact with blood or body fluids.
- Wash hands and other skin surfaces immediately after contact with blood or body fluids.
- Be careful when handling and disposing of sharp instruments during and after use.
- Use safety devices to prevent needlestick injuries.
- Dispose of used syringes or other sharp instruments in a sharps container.

WHAT IF AN HIV EXPOSURE HAPPENS AT WORK

- If you are exposed to HIV at work, report your exposure to the appropriate person, and see a doctor or visit an emergency room right away.
- Post-exposure prophylaxis (PEP) can reduce your chance of getting HIV infection. It must be started within 72 hours (three days) after you may have been exposed to HIV. But, the sooner you start PEP, the better. Every hour counts!
- Clinicians caring for personnel who have had a possible exposure can call the PEPline (888-448-4911) for advice on managing the exposure. Clinicians who administer PEP should tell patients about possible side effects and follow patients closely to make sure they take their medicine correctly.

HOW CAN ORGANIZATIONS MAKE A DIFFERENCE?

Occupational exposure is considered an urgent medical concern and should be managed immediately after possible exposure – the sooner the better; every hour counts.

- Review the CDC's guidelines for the management of occupational HIV exposures. When personnel is exposed, the CDC recommends immediate treatment with PEP or a short course of antiretroviral drugs to prevent infection.

- Train personnel in infection control procedures.
- Remind personnel to occupational exposures immediately after they occur.
- Develop and distribute written policies for the management of occupational exposures.
- Promote the use of safety devices to prevent sharps injuries.
- Report all cases of occupational HIV exposure to state health department HIV surveillance staff and the CDC coordinator at 404-639-2050.

Section 10.2 | Blood Transfusion

"Blood Transfusion," © 2022 Infobase. Reviewed February 2022.

A blood transfusion is a standard medical procedure that replaces the blood lost as a result of injury or surgery or due to a medical condition that affects blood and its components. The blood used in transfusion is typically from donors, and the blood or blood components are administered to the patient with the help of an intravenous (IV) line.

TYPES OF BLOOD AND BLOOD TRANSFUSIONS

There are four types of blood (A, B, AB, and O), and each blood type can be either positive or negative:

Administering the incorrect blood type to the patient can lead to the body rejecting the blood and causing severe consequences. The blood components include:

- **Red blood cells (RBCs).** These carry oxygen and remove waste products from the blood.
- **White blood cells (WBCs).** They help fight infections.

- **Plasma**. It is the liquid part of the blood that contains the necessary proteins required for good health.
- **Platelets**. Allows blood to clot properly.

The American Red Cross (ARC) highlights four types of transfusions:
- **RBC transfusion**. This procedure helps restore blood in case of blood loss, anemia, or to treat a blood disorder.
- **Platelet transfusion**. This procedure benefits patients with low platelet count as a result of chemotherapy or a platelet disorder.
- **Plasma transfusion**. This procedure benefits patients who have suffered liver damage, severe burns, or infections.
- **Whole blood transfusion**. This procedure benefits those who have suffered severe blood loss and requires RBCs, WBCs, and platelets.

WHY ARE BLOOD TRANSFUSIONS NEEDED?

The blood transfusion may take 1–3 hours, depending on how much blood or components are needed. Conditions and disorders requiring blood transfusions include:
- Cancer
- Anemia (kidney disease, iron deficiency, etc.)
- Hemophilia
- Sickle cell disease (SCD)
- Liver disease
- Blood disorder
- Leukemia
- Bleeding in the digestive tract

RISKS AND COMPLICATIONS

The healthcare industry takes strict measures to ensure the safety and proper storage of donated blood. As a result, blood transfusions are considered safe. However, mild complications or, in rare cases, severe complications might occur. In some people, a reaction to new blood may occur soon after the transfusion, and in some, it may occur after several days. Some complications are:

- **Fever.** It is not considered serious if a person gets a fever within six hours of a transfusion. However, if accompanied by chest pain and nausea, it is advised to see a doctor as soon as possible.
- **Allergies.** Even with the right blood type, it is possible to develop an allergic reaction such as itching or hives. They can occur during or shortly after the transfusion.
- **Hemolytic reaction.** The immune system attacks the new RBCs if the donor blood is not a good match. It can occur during the transfusion or right after and can cause symptoms such as nausea, chills, chest or lower back pains, dark urine, or fever.
- **Anaphylactic reaction.** This can be life-threatening and takes place minutes into the transfusion process. It results in swelling in the throat or face, low blood pressure, and shortness of breath.
- **Transfusion-related acute lung injury (TRALI).** This type of reaction is rare but potentially fatal and is caused by antibodies or other substances in the new blood. It occurs within hours of the transfusion process, and symptoms include low blood pressure and fever.
- **Bloodborne infections.** Even with all the precautions taken by blood banks, a rare chance of infection by viruses, bacteria, and parasites still exists. The chances of someone catching a bloodborne infection are:
  - **Human immunodeficiency virus (HIV).** 1 in 2 million.
  - **Hepatitis B.** 1 in 300,000.
  - **Hepatitis C.** 1 in 1.5 million.
  - **Zika virus.** Though most people do not show symptoms anymore, the U.S. Food and Drug Administration (FDA) recommends blood centers to scan for the virus.

- **West Nile virus.** 1 in 350,000.
- **Hemochromatosis.** Multiple blood transfusions can lead to iron overload in the blood and cause damage to the heart and liver.
- **Graft-versus-host disease**. This is a rare condition where the WBCs from the transfused blood begin to attack the bone marrow. It is potentially fatal and likely to affect people with a weak immune system.

Blood donors are asked a set of questions, and their blood is assessed for HIV risk status. Regulations in the United States require all donor blood to be tested for HIV antibodies and HIV ribonucleic acid (RNA). If blood is tested positive for HIV, it is safely disposed of and not used for transfusions. If a donor is tested positive for HIV, they are informed of their status and are not allowed to donate blood in the future. An HIV infection can take three months to show up after a person has been infected. For this reason, those in high-risk groups are not allowed to donate blood for a certain period (or in some cases for a lifetime) despite their test results being HIV negative. People considered a part of the high-risk group includes:

- Sex workers
- Men who engage in sex with men
- People who do injectable drugs

An individual who falls in these categories should inform the healthcare provider, who can then advise them if it is safe for them to donate or not. Factors such as having tattoos, body piercings, certain illnesses that may put a person at considerable risk for HIV also may be banned from donating blood. Contracting HIV by donating blood is unlikely as blood donations are highly regulated in most countries.

References
"Blood Transfusion," Cleveland Clinic, October 29, 2020.
"Blood Transfusion," Mayo Clinic, April 15, 2020.

"Blood Transfusion: What to Know If You Get One,"
WebMD, November 1, 2021.
Robertson, Sally. "HIV and Blood Transfusions," News-
Medical.net, February 26, 2019.

Section 10.3 | Organ Transplantation

"Organ Transplantation," © 2022 Infobase. Reviewed February 2022.

The Public Health Service guidelines of 2013 mandate all people who donate organs, whether living or deceased, be tested for risk factors such as human immunodeficiency virus (HIV), hepatitis B, and hepatitis C virus infections. Although HIV testing is extremely accurate, there have been cases when the testing failed to detect the HIV virus in people who had been exposed to the virus recently. Earlier, medical institutions used to decline organs available for transplant due to concerns regarding the transmission of HIV and other infections, especially when donors had risk factors such as intravenous drug use.

THE HOPE ACT (2013)

The concept of transplanting organs from HIV-positive individuals to other HIV-positive individuals was only made possible by the passing of the HIV Organ Policy Equity (HOPE) ACT in 2013. The guidelines for the transplantation of organs from individuals affected by HIV into other HIV-positive patients with end-stage organ failure were adopted in 2015. Johns Hopkins Medicine became the first hospital in the United States to perform a living donor HIV-to-HIV kidney transplantation on March 25, 2019.

SOME KEY FACTS

- Around 120,000 people are waiting for a lifesaving organ transplant in the United States.

- The addition of HIV positive donors will significantly decrease the wait time for both HIV positive recipients and patients not infected with HIV.
- The HOPE Act has made it possible for more organs to be made available for transplantation.
- The estimated 600 HIV positive donors annually in the United States could make possible the transplantation of 1,000 more organs and the saving of lives in the country.

ORGAN PROCUREMENT

Several federal agencies oversee activities relating to organ donation, procurement, selection of candidates, and transplantation. The Centers for Disease Control and Prevention (CDC), in partnership with the United States Public Health Service (USPHS), makes recommendations for the testing of organ donors and the monitoring of organ recipients. The Organ Procurement and Transplantation Network (OPTN), contracted by the Health Resources and Services Administration (HRSA), formulates policies regarding the following:

- Organ donation safety
- Selection and evaluation of recipients
- Organ allocation, procurement, and transportation
- Getting informed consent of the recipient
- Follow-up monitoring for outcomes and safety

The beneficial consequences of the HOPE Act are far-reaching and will be felt for a long time to come. The availability of organs harvested from HIV+ individuals will significantly decrease the waiting time for all individuals who need an organ transplant, regardless of whether they have HIV or not.

TRANSPLANTATION DURING THE PANDEMIC

The COVID-19 pandemic has severely impacted medical operations and resources at numerous hospitals, organ procurement organizations, and organ transplant centers across the United

States. The organ procurement community (OPO) has been carefully evaluating the risk of Coronavirus among potential organ donors and candidates waiting for an organ transplant. Although there was a decline in the number of organ transplants being conducted in the United States due to the COVID-19, the numbers are expected to rise eventually.

References

"Can I Donate if I'm HIV+?" Life-Source.org, January 30, 2021.

Carter, Michael. "Kidney Transplant between People with HIV Is Safe," NAM, August 26, 2020.

"HHS Announces New Organ Transplant Guidance," HIV.gov, June 29, 2020.

Robertson, Sally. "HIV and Organ Transplants," News-Medical.net, February 26, 2019.

Chapter 11 | **HIV/AIDS Prevention Strategies**

There are now more options than ever before to reduce the risk of acquiring or transmitting human immunodeficiency virus (HIV). Using medicines to treat HIV, using medicines to prevent HIV, using condoms, having only low-risk sex, only having partners with the same HIV status, and not having sex can all effectively reduce risk. Some options are more effective than others. Combining prevention strategies maybe even more effective. But in order for any option to work, it must be used correctly and consistently.

The following topics provide the best estimates of effectiveness for various strategies to prevent HIV acquisition or transmission. Each estimate was identified from the published scientific literature and represents the effectiveness of each strategy when used optimally. Available measures of optimal use vary by strategy.

ANTIRETROVIRAL THERAPY FOR HIV-POSITIVE PERSONS TO PREVENT SEXUAL TRANSMISSION
Heterosexual Women and Men
For HIV-positive heterosexual women and men, taking ART regularly greatly reduces the risk of HIV transmission to an HIV-negative partner. For persons who achieve and maintain viral suppression, there is effectively no risk of transmitting HIV to their HIV-negative sexual partner. This translates to an effectiveness estimate of 100 percent for taking ART regularly as prescribed and

This chapter contains text excerpted from the following sources: Text in this chapter begins with excerpts from "Effectiveness of Prevention Strategies to Reduce the Risk of Acquiring or Transmitting HIV," Centers for Disease Control and Prevention (CDC), December 8, 2021; Text beginning with the heading "Protect Yourself during Sex" is excerpted from "HIV Prevention," Centers for Disease Control and Prevention (CDC), June 1, 2021.

achieving and maintaining viral suppression. Effectiveness is lower, and there is a risk of transmitting HIV when persons do not take ART as prescribed or stop taking ART, if viral suppression is not achieved, or if viral suppression is not maintained.

Men Who Have Sex with Men

For HIV-positive men who have sex with men (MSM), taking ART regularly greatly reduces the risk of HIV transmission to an HIV-negative partner. For persons who achieve and maintain viral suppression, there is effectively no risk of transmitting HIV to their HIV-negative sexual partner. This translates to an effectiveness estimate of 100 percent for taking ART regularly as prescribed and achieving and maintaining viral suppression. Effectiveness is lower, and there is a risk of transmitting HIV when persons do not take ART as prescribed or stop taking ART, if viral suppression is not achieved, or if viral suppression is not maintained.

ORAL DAILY PRE-EXPOSURE PROPHYLAXIS FOR HIV-NEGATIVE PERSONS
Men Who Have Sex with Men

When taking PrEP daily or consistently (at least four times per week), the risk of acquiring HIV is reduced by about 99 percent among MSM. While daily use is recommended in the United States, taking PrEP consistently (at least four times per week) appears to provide similar levels of protection among MSM. The effectiveness of oral PrEP is highly dependent on PrEP adherence. When taking oral PrEP daily or consistently, HIV acquisition is extremely rare and has not been observed in any of the studies described below. In clinical practice, a few cases of new HIV infections have been confirmed while HIV-negative individuals were on PrEP with verified adherence.

Heterosexual Women and Men

There is evidence for the effectiveness of PrEP when used recently (based on detecting Tenofovir in plasma), which is estimated to be 88–90 percent as described below. There is no effectiveness estimate of PrEP when taken daily or consistently among heterosexuals; however, it is likely to be greater than the estimates corresponding to recent use and similar to what has been observed for MSM. The effectiveness of oral daily PrEP is highly dependent on PrEP adherence, with maximum effectiveness when taking PrEP daily and lower effectiveness when not taken consistently.

Persons Who Inject Drugs

Persons who inject drugs (PWIDs) face HIV risks from both injecting and sex behaviors. Studies on the effectiveness of PrEP, when taken daily among PWID, are limited. However, when taking PrEP consistently, the risk of acquiring HIV is reduced by an estimated 74–84 percent among PWID. These estimates are based on tenofovir alone and among a subset of PWID taking PrEP consistently, as verified by directly observed therapy or daily diary plus monthly pill count. The effectiveness of two-drug oral therapy has not been assessed among PWID but may be higher. The effectiveness of oral daily PrEP is highly dependent on PrEP adherence, with maximum effectiveness when taking PrEP daily and lower effectiveness when missing doses.

MALE CONDOM USE
MSM or Heterosexual Women and Men

Condoms provide an impermeable barrier to HIV. The U.S. Food and Drug Administration (FDA) quality control standards and laboratory studies indicate leaks due to product failure are extremely rare. In practice, it is difficult, if not impossible, to measure optimal use of condoms during sex. No studies have been able to provide accurate estimates for the effectiveness of condoms in preventing HIV, when used consistently and correctly, in practice. However, such an estimate is likely to be greater than the estimates provided in studies where participants self-reported consistent condom use during sex.

Heterosexual Women and Men

Always using condoms, based on self-report, during sex with an HIV-positive partner reduces the risk of HIV acquisition by an estimated 80 percent among heterosexual women and men. Self-report may not be entirely accurate, resulting in an underestimate of the true effectiveness of consistent condom use. Condom effectiveness is also likely to be higher when condoms are used correctly every time during sex.

MSM, Receptive Anal Sex

Always using condoms, based on self-report, during receptive anal sex with HIV-positive partners reduces the risk of HIV acquisition by an estimated 72 percent and an estimated 91 percent among HIV-negative MSM. Self-report may not be entirely accurate, resulting in an underestimate of the true effectiveness of consistent condom use. Condom effectiveness is also likely to be higher when condoms are used correctly every time during sex.

MSM, Insertive Anal Sex

Always using condoms, based on self-report, during insertive anal sex with HIV-positive partners reduces the risk of HIV acquisition by an estimated 63 percent among HIV-negative MSM. Self-report may not be entirely accurate, resulting in an underestimate of the true effectiveness of consistent condom use. Condom effectiveness is also likely to be higher when condoms are used correctly every time during sex.

CIRCUMCISION OF ADULT MALES
MSM, Insertive Anal Sex

Based on observational studies of circumcision among adult males, there is insufficient evidence at this time to conclude that male circumcision reduces the risk of the insertive partner acquiring HIV during anal sex among MSM.

MSM, Receptive Anal Sex

Based on observational studies of circumcision among adult males, there is insufficient evidence at this time to conclude that male circumcision (of the insertive partner) reduces the risk of the receptive partner acquiring HIV during anal sex among MSM.

Heterosexual Men

Based on trials of circumcision among adult males, male circumcision reduces the risk of heterosexual men acquiring HIV during sex by 50 percent.

Heterosexual Women

Based on several trials and observational studies of circumcision among adult males, there is insufficient evidence at this time to conclude that male circumcision reduces the risk of heterosexual women acquiring HIV during sex.

PROTECT YOURSELF DURING SEX
Choose Sexual Activities with Little to No Risk

- Choose sex that is less risky than anal or vaginal sex. There is little to no risk of getting HIV through oral sex.
- You cannot get HIV from sexual activities that do not involve contact with body fluids (semen, vaginal fluid, or blood).

Use Condoms the Right Way Every Time You Have Sex

- Condoms are highly effective in preventing HIV and other sexually transmitted diseases (STDs), such as gonorrhea and chlamydia.
- Use water-based or silicone-based lubricants to help prevent condoms from breaking or slipping during sex.

Take PrEP

- PrEP is medicine people at risk for HIV take to prevent HIV.
- If taken as prescribed, PrEP is highly effective for preventing HIV from sex.
- PrEP is much less effective when it is not taken as prescribed.

Decide Not to Have Sex

- Not having sex (also known as "being abstinent") is a 100 percent effective way to make sure you will not get HIV through sex.

- You can be abstinent at different times in your life for different reasons that may change over time.
- Not having sex also prevents other STDs and pregnancy.

Get Tested and Treated for Other STDs

- If you have another STD, you are more likely to get HIV. Getting tested and treated for other STDs can lower your chances of getting HIV.
- Many people with an STD may not know they have one because they do not have symptoms.

If Your Partner Has HIV, Encourage Your Partner to Get and Stay in Treatment

- This is the most important thing your partner can do to stay healthy.
- If your partner takes HIV medicine and gets and keeps an undetectable viral load, there is effectively no risk of you getting HIV from sex with your partner.

PROTECT YOURSELF IF YOU INJECT DRUGS
Never Share Needles, Syringes, or Other Drug Injection Equipment

- Use new, clean syringes and injection equipment every time you inject.
- Many communities have syringe services programs (SSPs) where you can get new needles and syringes and safely dispose of used ones.
- Some pharmacies sell needles without a prescription.

Take PrEP

- PrEP is medicine people at risk for HIV take to prevent HIV.
- If taken as prescribed, PrEP is highly effective for preventing HIV from injection drug use.

- PrEP is much less effective when it is not taken as prescribed.

Do Not Have Sex When You Are High on Drugs
- You are more likely to engage in risky sexual behaviors.
- If you do have sex, use condoms the right way every time.

Use Bleach to Clean Needles, Syringes, or Other Drug Injection Equipments
- A disinfected syringe is not as good as a new, sterile syringe, but it can greatly reduce your risk for HIV and viral hepatitis.

Decide Not to Inject Drugs
- This is the best way to prevent getting HIV through injection drug use.
- Talk with a counselor, doctor, or other healthcare providers about treatment for substance use disorder, including medication-assisted treatment.

Chapter 12 | HIV/AIDS Prevention

Chapter Contents

Section 12.1 | Safer Sex

This section includes text excerpted from "Safer Sexual Behavior," Centers for Disease Control and Prevention (CDC), November 4, 2020.

A growing number of people are living longer with human immunodeficiency virus (HIV), with fewer acquired immunodeficiency syndrome (AIDS)-related complications and deaths. Preventing transmission of HIV to others remains a critical element of care to protect both the health of those living with HIV and that of their partners.

The Centers for Disease Control and Prevention (CDC) recommends that clinicians who treat patients living with HIV infection integrate routine discussions about safer sexual practices into every office visit.

Research suggests that healthcare provider-initiated brief conversations about sexual behavior at every visit, with every patient, can help HIV-infected patients adopt positive behavior changes, including:

- Decline in sex without a condom
- Fewer sexual partners
- Decline in sexually transmitted disease (STD) acquisition, including syphilis, chlamydia, and gonorrhea

Data from the CDC's STD Surveillance Network (SSuN) indicate that the burden of STDs is greater among HIV-infected men who have sex with men (MSM) than among uninfected MSM. In fact, MSM comprised 72 percent of all primary and secondary syphilis cases in the United States. Regular screening for STDs provides a benchmark for sexual behavioral assessment for both men and women living with HIV. However, a published Morbidity and Mortality Weekly Report (MMWR) report from the CDC showed that fewer than 20 percent of all HIV-infected patients were tested annually for STDs and less than half of them received counseling about available HIV and STD prevention strategies.

WHAT PREVENTS SOME PATIENTS FROM PRACTICING SAFER SEXUAL BEHAVIORS?

Some patients living with HIV do not realize that their behaviors are not "safe." Others may not understand the virus or how it is transmitted. They may be uncomfortable or unable to disclose their HIV status to sexual or drug-injecting partners. Or they may use alcohol or drugs or have undiagnosed depression, any of which can cause disinhibition and lapses in judgment.

WHY ARE SOME HEALTHCARE PROFESSIONALS UNCOMFORTABLE TALKING ABOUT SEX?

Sometimes healthcare providers ascribe the difficulty of talking about sex to the patient, but it may be the clinician who is uncomfortable with this subject. Healthcare professionals cite several barriers to discussing sex, including:

- Overall discomfort discussing sex and sexuality
- Belief that discussing sex will take a lot of time
- Belief that patients are uncomfortable discussing sex
- Concerns about cultural differences or saying the "wrong thing"
- Belief that older (age 60+) patients are "probably not having sex"

HOW DO BRIEF CONVERSATIONS ABOUT SAFER SEXUAL BEHAVIORS BENEFIT HEALTHCARE PROVIDERS?

When healthcare providers are open to talking to patients about their sexual behaviors, patients may be more willing to confide with their healthcare providers, fostering trust and empathy and building a therapeutic relationship.

Brief conversations offer clinicians unique opportunities to educate patients and normalize discussions about safer sexual behaviors by:

- Using teachable moments to impart factual information about all of the risk-reduction strategies available today
- Helping patients understand how to reduce their risk of HIV transmission

- Helping patients better understand the benefits of safer sex to their own health
- Helping patients feel more comfortable discussing sexual behavior

WHICH SAFER SEXUAL BEHAVIORS AND RISK-REDUCTION STRATEGIES SHOULD HEALTHCARE PROVIDERS DISCUSS WITH PATIENTS?

Patients' health status, relationship status, and personal needs change over time. Therefore, conversations about sexual behaviors should continue and evolve for as long as the patient remains in care.

Topics include:
- Adhering to antiretroviral therapy (ART) and ongoing medical care, even if viral load is undetectable
- Communicating HIV status with others
- Correctly and consistently using condoms (to prevent STDs) and appropriate nonoil-based lubricants, even when negotiation of use occurs in the heat of the moment
- Assessing relative risk of HIV transmission associated with various sexual activities (e.g., oral sex is less risky than receptive anal sex)
- Discussing how alcohol and/or drug use can impair judgment
- Using pre-exposure prophylaxis (PrEP) for some HIV-negative partners, including women planning to become pregnant
- Using PEP for emergencies for HIV-negative or unknown status partners (e.g., if a condom breaks or is not used and the patient is not virally suppressed)

WHAT ARE SOME SUGGESTED CONVERSATION STARTERS ABOUT SAFER SEXUAL BEHAVIORS?

Following are a few conversation starters to assist healthcare providers with initiating brief conversations with patients.

Disclosing HIV Status to Others

- "Some of my patients have told me how hard it is to decide who to tell about their HIV status, and what the best way is to tell someone. Are you comfortable disclosing your HIV status to your sexual partners?"

Relative Risk of HIV Transmission Associated with Type of Sexual Activity

- "You have said that you do not always use condoms during anal sex. Did you know anal sex is the highest-risk sexual activity for HIV transmission? Overall, oral sex is much less risky. What do you think about that?"

Advice to Serodiscordant Couples

- "You said your spouse (or partner) is HIV-negative. Has (she/he) talked with (her/his) doctor about additional ways to protect herself/himself, including PrEP as an extra protective step?"
- "I know you always use condoms, and that is terrific. But, what do you do if your condom breaks while you are having sex with an HIV-negative partner?"

Once clinicians have started a brief conversation, they can use the teachable moment to help the patient understand how to protect their overall health and prevent transmission to partners.

Section 12.2 | **Circumcision**

This section contains text excerpted from the following sources: Text beginning with the heading "What Is Circumcision?" is excerpted from "Circumcision," MedlinePlus, National Institutes of Health (NIH), March 22, 2016. Reviewed February 2022; Text beginning with the heading "Heterosexually Active Adolescent and Adult Males" is excerpted from "CDC Provides Information to Male Patients and Parents," Centers for Disease Control and Prevention (CDC), September 2018. Reviewed February 2022.

WHAT IS CIRCUMCISION?

Circumcision is a surgical procedure to remove the foreskin, the skin that covers the tip of the penis. In the United States, it is often done before a new baby leaves the hospital. According to the American Academy of Pediatrics (AAP), there are medical benefits and risks to circumcision.

WHAT ARE THE MEDICAL BENEFITS OF CIRCUMCISION?

The possible medical benefits of circumcision include:
- A lower risk of HIV
- A slightly lower risk of other sexually transmitted diseases
- A slightly lower risk of urinary tract infections and penile cancer. However, these are both rare in all males.

WHAT ARE THE RISKS OF CIRCUMCISION?

The risks of circumcision include:
- A low risk of bleeding or infection
- Pain. The AAP suggests that providers use pain medicines to reduce pain from circumcision.

CIRCUMCISION AND THE PREVENTION OF HIV INFECTION, STIs, AND OTHER HEALTH OUTCOMES

The Centers for Disease Control and Prevention (CDC) has released new information to share with male patients and parents of patients about voluntary medically performed male circumcision for the prevention of HIV, STIs, and other health outcomes in the United States.

Personal decisions about circumcision are influenced by information on the preventive health benefits, safety and risk of the procedures as well as ethical, religious, cultural, familial, and economic considerations.

HETEROSEXUALLY ACTIVE ADOLESCENT AND ADULT MALES

Healthcare providers should inform all uncircumcised adolescent and adult males that male circumcision reduces, but does not eliminate, the risk of acquiring HIV and other STIs during heterosexual sex. Additionally, they should be informed of the potential risks associated with the procedure. Healthcare providers should assess the sexual risk behaviors of their male patients and those at increased risk of HIV infection should be counseled about voluntary male circumcision as another potential strategy for HIV risk reduction. Those who choose to be circumcised should be offered medically performed circumcision services and HIV risk-reduction information. Heterosexual men at increased risk for HIV include:

- Men who are in sexual relationships with HIV-infected female partners
- Men with multiple female partners
- Those in relationships with women who are at high risk for HIV (e.g., commercial sex workers, females who inject drugs, and females in defined populations with HIV prevalence of one percent or higher)

MEN WHO HAVE SEX WITH MEN

Providers should inform uncircumcised men who have sex with men (MSM) that data from several observational studies indicate that male circumcision provides partial protection from HIV acquisition for MSM who practice mainly or exclusively insertive anal sex. However, no clinical trials have included large enough numbers of MSM to make a definitive conclusion regarding the usefulness of male circumcision in reducing the risk of HIV acquisition among MSM. Additionally, there is no evidence that male circumcision reduces the risk of acquiring HIV through receptive anal sex.

PARENTS AND GUARDIANS OF MALE NEWBORNS, CHILDREN, AND ADOLESCENTS

Parents should be informed of the medical benefits – including reduced risk of future HIV infection – and the risks of male circumcision and should make decisions in consultation with a healthcare provider. When providing information to parents about male circumcision for an adolescent minor, the adolescent should be included in the decision-making process.

KEY CONSIDERATIONS

The information provided notes a number of key issues that should be considered during the decision-making process:

- **Health benefits**. Male circumcision can reduce a man's risk of acquiring HIV infection by 50–60 percent during sex with HIV-infected female partners, according to data from three clinical trials. Circumcised men compared with uncircumcised men have also been shown in clinical trials to be less likely to acquire new infections with syphilis (by 42 percent), genital ulcer disease (by 48 percent), genital herpes (by 28–45 percent), and high-risk strains of human papillomavirus (HPV) associated with cancer (by 24–47 percent). While male circumcision has not been shown to reduce the risk of HIV transmission to female partners, it does reduce the risk that a female partner will acquire a new syphilis infection by 59 percent. In observational studies, circumcision has been shown to lower the risk of penile cancer, cervical cancer in female sexual partners, and infant urinary tract infections in male infants.
- **Health risks**. The overall risk of adverse events associated with male circumcision is low, with minor bleeding and inflammation cited as the most common complications. A CDC analysis found that the rate of adverse events for medically attended male circumcision is 0.4 percent for infants aged less than

157

one year, about nine percent for children aged one – nine years, and about five percent for males 10 years and older. More severe complications can occur but are exceedingly rare. Adult men who undergo circumcision generally report minimal or no change in sexual satisfaction or function.

- **Stage of life**. Circumcision is simpler, safer and less expensive for newborns and infants than for adult males. Delaying circumcision until adolescence or adulthood enables the male to participate in – or make – the decision, but could diminish the potential benefits related to sexual health and increase the risks.
- **Informed choice**. Male circumcision is a voluntary procedure. The decision regarding circumcision should be made in consultation with a healthcare provider, taking into account personal, cultural, religious and ethical beliefs.

IMPLICATIONS FOR HIV PREVENTION IN THE UNITED STATES

Given the urgency of the HIV epidemic in the United States, the CDC believes it is essential to maximize the impact of all available prevention options and is working to provide clinicians the best possible information on the full range of proven approaches. Male circumcision is one strategy that may help reduce the continued spread of HIV in the United States ultimately, the degree to which male circumcision affects overall HIV transmission in the United States in the future will depend on a number of factors whose impact is not yet known. Those factors include the future contribution of heterosexual transmission to the number of HIV infections that occur each year; future rates of infant male circumcision; the percentage of heterosexual men at high risk who elect to be circumcised; and whether the approach can be effectively integrated with other proven HIV prevention strategies. Data on the cost-effectiveness of male circumcision to prevent HIV in the United States are limited, but suggest that newborn circumcision would offer long-term cost-savings by reducing the lifetime risk of HIV infection.

At an individual level, male circumcision may help reduce the risk of HIV acquisition among men, and may be combined with other proven risk reduction strategies to provide even greater protection. While the benefits of circumcision for uninfected men at risk for HIV infection can be high, the overall public health benefit in the entire U.S. population may be limited due to the lack of definitively proven benefit among people who are infected through the major routes of transmission at a national level (i.e., male-to-male and male-to-female HIV transmission). The greatest benefit will be among uncircumcised heterosexual men living in geographic areas with a high prevalence of HIV.

The CDC is committed to ensuring that healthcare providers have the information they need to make informed decisions about circumcision and other approaches that may reduce the risk of HIV and STIs.

Section 12.3 | Syringe Exchange Programs

This section contains text excerpted from the following sources: Text beginning with the heading "What Is a Syringe Services Program?" is excerpted from "Syringe Services Programs (SSPs) FAQs," Centers for Disease Control and Prevention (CDC), May 23, 2019; Text beginning with the heading "Linkage to Substance-Use Treatment, Naloxone, and Other Healthcare Services" is excerpted from "Summary of Information on the Safety and Effectiveness of Syringe Services Programs (SSPs)," Centers for Disease Control and Prevention (CDC), May 23, 2019.

WHAT IS A SYRINGE SERVICES PROGRAM?

Syringe services programs (SSPs) are also referred to as syringe exchange programs (SEPs) and needle exchange programs (NEPs). Although the services they provide may vary, SSPs are community-based programs that provide access to sterile needles and syringes, facilitate safe disposal of used syringes, and provide and link to other important services and programs such as:

- Referral to substance-use disorder (SUD) treatment programs
- Screening, care, and treatment for viral hepatitis and HIV

159

- Education about overdose prevention and safer injection practices
- Vaccinations, including those for hepatitis A and hepatitis B
- Screening for sexually transmitted diseases
- Abscess and wound care
- Naloxone distribution and education
- Referral to social, mental health, and other medical services

ARE SYRINGE SERVICES PROGRAMS LEGAL?

Some states have passed laws specifically legalizing SSPs because of their life-saving potential. SSPs may also be legal in states where possession and distribution of syringes without a prescription are legal.

Decisions about use of SSPs as part of prevention programs are made at the state and local levels. The Federal Consolidated Appropriations Act of 2016 includes language that gives states and local communities meeting certain criteria the opportunity to use federal funds provided through the U.S. Department of Health and Human Services (HHS) to support certain components of SSPs, with the exception of provision of needles, syringes, or other equipment used solely for the purposes of illicit drug use.

DO SYRINGE SERVICES PROGRAMS HELP PEOPLE TO STOP USING DRUGS?

Yes. When people who inject drugs use an SSP, they are more likely to enter treatment for SUD and stop injecting than those who do not use an SSP. New users of SSPs are five times as likely to enter drug treatment as those who do not use the programs. People who inject drugs and who have used an SSP regularly are nearly three times as likely to report a reduction in injection frequency as those who have never used an SSP.

DO SYRINGE SERVICES PROGRAMS REDUCE INFECTIONS?

Yes. Nonsterile injections can lead to transmission of HIV, viral hepatitis, bacterial, and fungal infections and other complications. By providing access to sterile syringes and other injection equipment,

SSPs help people prevent transmitting bloodborne and other infections when they inject drugs. In addition to being at risk for HIV, viral hepatitis, and other blood-borne and sexually transmitted diseases, people who inject drugs can get other serious, life-threatening, and costly health problems, such as infections of the heart valves (endocarditis), serious skin infections, and deep tissue abscesses. Access to sterile injection equipment can help prevent these infections, and healthcare provided at SSPs can catch these problems early and provide easy-to-access treatment to a population that may be reluctant to go to a hospital or seek other medical care.

DO SYRINGE SERVICES PROGRAMS CAUSE MORE NEEDLES IN PUBLIC PLACES?

No. Studies show that SSPs protect the public and first responders by providing safe needle disposal and reducing the presence of needles in the community.

DO SYRINGE SERVICES PROGRAMS LEAD TO MORE CRIME AND/OR DRUG USE?

No. SSPs do not cause or increase illegal drug use. They do not cause or increase crime.

ARE SYRINGE SERVICES PROGRAMS COST-EFFECTIVE?

Yes. SSPs reduce healthcare costs by preventing HIV, viral hepatitis, and other infections, including endocarditis, a life-threatening heart valve infection. The estimated lifetime cost of treating one person living with HIV is more than $450,000. Hospitalizations in the United States for substance-use-related infections cost over $700 million each year. SSPs reduce these costs and help link people to treatment to stop using drugs.

DO SYRINGE SERVICES PROGRAMS REDUCE DRUG USE AND DRUG OVERDOSES?

Syringe services programs help people overcome substance use disorders. If people who inject drugs use an SSP, they are more likely to enter treatment for substance use disorder and reduce or stop injecting. A Seattle study found that new users of SSPs were five times as likely to enter drug treatment as those who did not use the programs. People who inject drugs and who have used an SSP regularly are nearly three times as likely to report reducing or stopping illicit drug injection as those who have never used an SSP. SSPs play a key role in preventing overdose deaths by training people who inject drugs how to prevent, rapidly recognize, and reverse opioid overdoses. Specifically, many SSPs give clients and community members "overdose rescue kits" and teach them how to identify an overdose, give rescue breathing, and administer naloxone, a medication used to reverse overdose.

LINKAGE TO SUBSTANCE USE TREATMENT, NALOXONE, AND OTHER HEALTHCARE SERVICES

Syringe services programs serve as a bridge to other health services including, hepatitis C virus (HCV) and HIV diagnosis and treatment and medication-assisted treatment (MAT) for substance use. The majority of SSPs offer referrals to MAT, and people who inject drugs who regularly use an SSP are more than five times as likely to enter treatment for a SUD and nearly three times as likely to report reducing or discontinuing injection as those who have never used an SSP. SSPs facilitate entry into treatment for SUD by people who inject drugs. People who use SSPs show high readiness to reduce or stop their drug use. There is also evidence that people who inject drugs who work with a nurse at an SSP or other community-based venue are more likely to access primary care than those who do not, also increasing access to MAT. Many comprehensive community-based SSPs offer a range of preventative services including vaccination, infectious disease testing, and linkage to healthcare services.

Syringe services programs can reduce overdose deaths by teaching people who inject drugs how to prevent and respond to a drug overdose, providing them training on how to use naloxone, a medication used to reverse overdose, and providing naloxone to them. Many SSPs provide "overdose prevention kits" containing naloxone to people who inject drugs. SSPs have partnered with law enforcement, providing naloxone to local police departments to help them keep their communities safer.

PUBLIC SAFETY

Syringe services programs can benefit communities and public safety by reducing needlestick injuries and overdose deaths, without increasing illegal injection of drugs or criminal activity. Studies show that SSPs protect first responders and the public by providing safe needle disposal and reducing community presence of needles. As many as one in every three officers may be stuck by a used needle during her or his career. Needlestick injuries are among the most concerning and stressful events experienced by law officers. A study compared the prevalence of improperly disposed of syringes and self-reported disposal practices in a city with SSPs to a city without SSPs and found eight times as many improperly disposed of syringes in Miami, the city without SSPs. People who inject drugs in San Francisco also reported higher rates of safe disposal practices than those in Miami. Data from the CDC's National HIV Behavioral Surveillance (NHBS) system showed that the more syringes distributed at SSPs per people who inject drugs in a geographic region, the more likely people who inject drugs in that region were to report safe disposal of used syringes.

Evidence demonstrates that SSPs do not increase illegal drug use or crime. Studies in Baltimore and New York City have found no difference in crime rates between areas with and areas without SSPs. In Baltimore, trends in arrests were examined before and after a SSP was opened and found that there was not a significant increase in crime rates. The study in New York City assessed whether proximity to an SSP was associated with experiencing violence in an inner-city neighborhood and found no association.

Chapter 13 | Preventing Mother-to-Child Transmission of HIV

Chapter Contents

Section 13.1 | HIV Medicines during Pregnancy

This section includes text excerpted from "HIV Medicines during Pregnancy and Childbirth," HIVinfo, U.S. Department of Health and Human Services (HHS), August 18, 2021.

SHOULD WOMEN WITH HIV TAKE HIV MEDICINES DURING PREGNANCY?

Yes. All pregnant women with human immunodeficiency virus (HIV) should take HIV medicines throughout pregnancy for their own health and to prevent perinatal transmission of HIV. (HIV medicines are called "antiretrovirals.") Perinatal transmission of HIV is also called "mother-to-child transmission of HIV."

HIV medicines, when taken as prescribed, prevent HIV from multiplying and reduce the amount of HIV in the body (called the "viral load"). An undetectable viral load is when the level of HIV in the blood is too low to be detected by a viral load test. The risk of perinatal transmission of HIV during pregnancy and childbirth is lowest when a woman with HIV has an undetectable viral load. Maintaining an undetectable viral load also helps keep the mother-to-be healthy.

ARE HIV MEDICINES SAFE TO USE DURING PREGNANCY?

Most HIV medicines are safe to use during pregnancy. In general, HIV medicines do not increase the risk of birth defects.

When recommending HIV medicines to use during pregnancy, healthcare providers consider the benefits and risks of specific HIV medicines for women and their unborn babies.

WHEN SHOULD PREGNANT WOMEN WITH HIV START TAKING HIV MEDICINES?

All pregnant women with HIV should start taking HIV medicines as soon as possible during pregnancy. In most cases, women who are already on an effective HIV treatment regimen when they become pregnant should continue using the same regimen throughout their pregnancies.

WHAT HIV MEDICINES SHOULD A PREGNANT WOMAN WITH HIV TAKE?

The choice of an HIV treatment regimen to use during pregnancy depends on several factors, including a woman's current or past use of HIV medicines, other medical conditions she may have, and the results of drug-resistance testing. In general, pregnant women with HIV can use the same HIV treatment regimens recommended for nonpregnant adults – unless the risk of any known side effects to a pregnant woman or her baby outweighs the benefits of a treatment regimen.

Sometimes, a woman's HIV treatment regimen may change during pregnancy. Women and their healthcare providers should discuss whether any changes need to be made to an HIV treatment regimen during pregnancy.

DO WOMEN WITH HIV CONTINUE TO TAKE HIV MEDICINES DURING CHILDBIRTH?

Yes. A baby is exposed to any HIV in the mother's blood and other fluids while passing through the birth canal. During childbirth, HIV medicines that pass from mother to baby across the placenta prevent perinatal transmission of HIV, especially near delivery.

Women who are already taking HIV medicines when they go into labor should continue taking their HIV medicines on schedule as much as possible during childbirth.

CAN A CESAREAN DELIVERY REDUCE THE RISK OF PERINATAL TRANSMISSION OF HIV?

Yes. A scheduled cesarean delivery (sometimes called a "C-section") can reduce the risk of perinatal transmission of HIV in women who have a high viral load (more than 1,000 copies/mL) or an unknown viral load near the time of delivery. A cesarean delivery to reduce the risk of perinatal transmission of HIV is scheduled for the 38th week of pregnancy, 2 weeks before a woman's expected due date.

A scheduled C-section to reduce the risk of perinatal transmission of HIV is not routinely recommended for women who are taking HIV medicines and have a viral load of 1,000 copies/mL or less. Of course, regardless of her viral load, a woman with HIV may have a C-section for other medical reasons.

With the help of their healthcare providers, women can decide which HIV medicines to use during childbirth and whether they should have a scheduled C-section to prevent perinatal transmission of HIV.

DO WOMEN WITH HIV CONTINUE TO TAKE HIV MEDICINES AFTER CHILDBIRTH?

Prenatal care for women with HIV includes counseling on the benefits of continuing HIV medicines after childbirth. HIV medicines help people with HIV live longer, healthier lives and reduce the risk of HIV transmission. Together with their healthcare providers, women with HIV make decisions about continuing or changing their HIV medicines after childbirth.

After birth, babies born to women with HIV receive HIV medicine to reduce the risk of perinatal transmission of HIV. Several factors determine what HIV medicine they receive and how long they receive the medicine.

Section 13.2 | Preventing Mother-to-Child Transmission of HIV during and after Birth

This section includes text excerpted from "Preventing Perinatal Transmission of HIV," HIVinfo, U.S. Department of Health and Human Services (HHS), August 18, 2021.

WHAT IS PERINATAL TRANSMISSION OF HIV?

Perinatal transmission of HIV is when HIV is passed from a woman with HIV to her child during pregnancy, childbirth (also called "labor and delivery"), or breastfeeding (through breast milk). Perinatal transmission of HIV is also called "mother-to-child transmission of HIV."

The use of HIV medicines and other strategies have helped to lower the rate of perinatal transmission of HIV to one percent or less in the United States and Europe. (HIV medicines are called "antiretrovirals.")

IS HIV TESTING RECOMMENDED FOR PREGNANT WOMEN?

The Centers for Disease Control and Prevention (CDC) recommends that all women get tested for HIV before they become pregnant or as early as possible during each pregnancy. The earlier HIV is detected, the sooner HIV medicines can be started.

All women who are pregnant or trying to get pregnant should encourage their partners also to get tested for HIV and, if possible, screened for other sexually transmitted diseases (STDs). STDs can increase viral loads in people with HIV. If any partner has HIV, that partner should take HIV medicine as prescribed to stay healthy and prevent transmission.

HOW DO HIV MEDICINES PREVENT PERINATAL TRANSMISSION OF HIV?

Pregnant women with HIV should take HIV medicines to reduce the risk of perinatal transmission of HIV. When started early, HIV medicines can be more effective at preventing perinatal transmission of HIV. Women with HIV who are trying to conceive should start HIV medicines before they become pregnant to prevent perinatal transmission of HIV. Pregnant women with HIV should take HIV medicines throughout pregnancy and childbirth to prevent perinatal transmission of HIV. HIV medicines also protect the woman's health.

HIV medicines, when taken as prescribed, prevent HIV from multiplying and reduce the amount of HIV in the body (called the "viral load"). An undetectable viral load is when the level of HIV in the blood is too low to be detected by a viral load test. The risk of perinatal transmission of HIV during pregnancy and childbirth is lowest when a woman with HIV has an undetectable viral load. Maintaining an undetectable viral load also helps keep the mother-to-be healthy.

Some HIV medicines used during pregnancy that pass from the pregnant woman to her unborn baby through cesarean delivery (sometimes called a "C-section") can reduce the risk of perinatal transmission of HIV in women who have a high viral load (more than 1,000 copies/mL) or an unknown viral load near the time of delivery.

After birth, babies born to women with HIV receive HIV medicines to reduce the risk of perinatal transmission of HIV. Several factors determine what HIV medicines babies receive and how long they receive the medicines.

ARE THERE OTHER WAYS TO PREVENT PERINATAL TRANSMISSION OF HIV?

Despite ongoing maternal use of HIV medicines after childbirth, a woman with HIV can still pass HIV to her baby while breast-feeding. In the United States, infant formula is a safe and readily available alternative to breast milk. For these reasons, women with HIV who live in the United States should not breastfeed their babies. Women with HIV can talk to their healthcare providers to discuss alternative options for feeding before their babies are born or even if they are already breastfeeding.

Additionally, babies should not eat food that was prechewed by a person with HIV.

Chapter 14 | HIV Vaccines and Microbicides

Chapter Contents

Section 14.1 | **Preventive Vaccines**

This section contains text excerpted from the following sources: Text in this section begins with excerpts from "HIV Vaccines," HIV.gov, U.S. Department of Health and Human Services (HHS), February 1, 2021; Text beginning with the heading "Vaccines Recommendation for People with HIV" is excerpted from "Vaccines and People with HIV," HIV.gov, U.S. Department of Health and Human Services (HHS), November 12, 2021.

Vaccines are products made from very small amounts of weak or dead germs (such as viruses, bacteria, or toxins) that can cause diseases. They help your immune system fight infections faster and more effectively.

When you get a vaccine, it sparks your immune response, helping your body fight off and remember the germ so it can attack it if the germ ever invades again. And since vaccines are made of very small amounts of weak or dead germs, they would not make you sick.

Vaccines are usually administered by a shot, but sometimes can be administered by mouth or nasal spray. They are widely used to prevent diseases such as polio, chickenpox, measles, mumps, rubella, influenza (flu), hepatitis A and B, and human papillomavirus (HPV).

IS THERE A VACCINE TO PREVENT HIV?

No. There is currently no vaccine available that will prevent human immunodeficiency virus (HIV) infection or treat those who have it.

However, scientists are working to develop one. The National Institutes of Health (NIH) is investing in multiple approaches to prevent HIV, including a safe and effective preventive HIV vaccine. These research efforts include two late-stage, multinational vaccine clinical trials called "Imbokodo" and "Mosaico."

IMPORTANCE OF VACCINE TO PREVENT HIV

More people living with HIV than ever before have access to life-saving treatment with HIV medicines (called "antiretroviral therapy" or "ART"), which is good for their health. When people living with HIV achieve and maintain viral suppression by taking HIV medication daily as prescribed, they can stay healthy and have effectively no risk of sexually transmitting HIV to their partners. In addition, others who are at high risk for HIV infection may have access to pre-exposure prophylaxis (PrEP), or ART being used to prevent HIV. Yet, unfortunately, in 2018, 37,968 people were diagnosed with HIV infection in the United States, and in 2019, approximately 1.7 million people newly acquired HIV worldwide. To control and ultimately end HIV globally, we need a powerful array of HIV prevention tools that are widely accessible to all who would benefit from them.

Vaccines historically have been the most effective means to prevent and even eradicate infectious diseases. They safely and cost-effectively prevent illness, disability, and death. Like smallpox and polio vaccines, a preventive HIV vaccine could help save millions of lives.

Developing safe, effective, and affordable vaccines that can prevent HIV infection in uninfected people is the NIH's highest HIV research priority given its game-changing potential for controlling and ultimately ending the HIV/AIDS pandemic.

The long-term goal is to develop a safe and effective vaccine that protects people worldwide from acquiring HIV. However, even if a vaccine only protects some people who get vaccinated, or even if it provides less than total protection by reducing the risk of infection, it could still have a major impact on the rates of transmission and help control the pandemic, particularly for populations at high risk of getting HIV. A partially effective vaccine could decrease the number of people who get infected with HIV, further reducing the number of people who can pass the virus on to others. By substantially reducing the number of new infections, we can stop the epidemic.

VACCINES RECOMMENDATION FOR PEOPLE WITH HIV

The following vaccines are recommended for people with HIV:

- Coronavirus disease (COVID-19)
- Hepatitis B
- Human papillomavirus (for those up to age 26)
- Influenza (flu)
- Meningococcal series which protects against meningococcal disease

- Pneumococcal (pneumonia)
- Tetanus, diphtheria, and pertussis (whooping cough). A single vaccine protects against the three diseases. Every 10 years, a repeat vaccine against tetanus and diphtheria (called "Td") is also recommended

Based on age or other circumstances, your provider may recommend other vaccines as well.

Talk to your healthcare provider about which vaccines are recommended for you.

DO VACCINES CAUSE SIDE EFFECTS?

Any vaccine can cause side effects. Side effects from vaccines are generally minor (e.g., soreness at the location of an injection or a low-grade fever) and go away within a few days.

Severe reactions to vaccines are rare. Before getting a vaccine, talk to your healthcare provider about the benefits and risks of the vaccine and possible side effects.

Section 14.2 | Microbicides

This section includes text excerpted from "Microbicides," HIV.gov, U.S. Department of Health and Human Services (HHS), June 16, 2021.

WHAT ARE MICROBICIDES?

Microbicides are experimental products that could be applied to or inserted into the vagina or rectum to safely prevent human immunodeficiency virus (HIV) acquisition. A microbicide would deliver an anti-HIV drug to the mucus membranes lining the surface of the vagina or rectum through materials such as vaginal rings, gels, films, inserts, suppositories, foams, or enemas. A safe, effective, desirable, and affordable microbicide against HIV would expand the number of biomedical HIV prevention options available. That is why researchers are working to develop them. But, none are on the market yet.

CAN MICROBICIDES PREVENT HIV?

Research studies have shown that some microbicides do offer a modest level of protection against getting HIV.

For example, several large-scale research studies over the past decade have investigated the safety and effectiveness of long-acting vaginal rings that continuously release one or more antiretroviral drugs over time. The ring at the most advanced stage of research is the monthly dapivirine ring, which was tested in two large clinical trials, including the NIH-funded ASPIRE study. This study and another trial called the "Ring Study" found that the dapivirine ring reduced the risk of HIV acquisition by roughly 30 percent overall in women ages 18 to 45 years and was well-tolerated.

The European Medicines Agency (EMA) adopted a positive scientific opinion on the monthly dapivirine vaginal ring in 2020 and the World Health Organization (WHO) subsequently recommended the ring as part of combination prevention approaches for women at substantial risk for acquiring HIV, representing even further progress. If approved by national regulatory agencies, the monthly ring would provide women with a discreet, long-acting HIV prevention option that they can control.

The NIH is also supporting three studies to examine the safety of the monthly dapivirine ring during adolescence and pregnancy, when the risk of HIV acquisition is heightened, and during periods of breastfeeding, when transmission to infants may occur researchers also are evaluating a 90-day dapivirine ring.

Other studies are examining potential rectal microbicide gels to reduce the risk of HIV transmission through anal sex. Some of these studies are testing microbicides originally formulated for vaginal use to determine if they are safe, effective, and acceptable when used in the rectum; others focus on the development of products designed specifically for rectal use.

WHY ARE MICROBICIDES IMPORTANT?

The only currently licensed biomedical HIV prevention method is a daily pill taken orally for pre-exposure prophylaxis (PrEP). Oral PrEP is safe and highly effective when taken daily as prescribed.

However, a daily pill can be challenging for some people to take, so other forms of biomedical HIV prevention such as microbicides are being explored.

For some women, microbicides may offer certain benefits. For example, some women may find microbicides preferable to condoms as an HIV prevention option because women would not have to negotiate their use with a sexual partner. Given that women and girls are at particularly high risk for HIV in many parts of the world, it is especially important to have an effective, desirable, woman-initiated HIV prevention tool. In the future, it may also be possible to formulate products that combine HIV prevention with contraception.

Rectal microbicides would also offer another HIV prevention option for women or men who engage in anal sex.

ARE MICROBICIDES AVAILABLE TO THE PUBLIC?

No microbicide for HIV prevention has received regulatory approval to be marketed yet. However, The International Partnership for Microbicides (IPM), which developed the monthly dapivirine vaginal ring, has applied for regulatory review of the product in countries in eastern and southern Africa, where HIV incidence among women remains high, and in the United States. Meanwhile, research on other formulations and forms of microbicides continues.

For now, available forms of protection against the sexual transmission of HIV continue to be:

- Treatment as prevention (a highly effective strategy in which people with HIV take antiretroviral therapy as prescribed to achieve an undetectable viral load, which prevents the transmission of HIV to their sexual partners)
- Daily oral PrEP
- Voluntary medical male circumcision
- HIV testing – so that you know your and your partner's HIV status
- Using condoms consistently and correctly

- Choosing sexual behaviors that have lower risk of HIV transmission
- Reducing the number of people you have sex with

The more of these actions you take, the safer you will be.

Chapter 15 | **HIV Prophylaxis**

Chapter Contents

Section 15.1 | Pre-exposure Prophylaxis

This section contains text excerpted from the following sources: Text beginning with the heading "What Is Pre-exposure Prophylaxis?" is excerpted from "Pre-exposure Prophylaxis," HIV.gov, U.S. Department of Health and Human Services (HHS), January 7, 2022; Text beginning with the heading "On Demand PrEP" is excerpted from "PrEP (Pre-exposure Prophylaxis)," Centers for Disease Control and Prevention (CDC), May 13, 2021.

WHAT IS PRE-EXPOSURE PROPHYLAXIS?

Pre-exposure prophylaxis, or PrEP, is medicine people at risk for human immunodeficiency virus (HIV) take to prevent getting HIV from sex or injection drug use. PrEP can stop HIV from taking hold and spreading throughout your body.

Currently, there are two U.S. Food and Drug Administration (FDA)-approved daily oral medications for PrEP. A long-acting injectable form of PrEP has also been approved by the FDA.

IS PrEP RIGHT FOR YOU?

Pre-exposure prophylaxis may benefit you if you test negative for HIV and,

- You have had anal or vaginal sex in the past 6 months, and you:
  - Have a sexual partner with HIV (especially if the partner has an unknown or detectable viral load),
  - Have not consistently used a condom, or
  - Have been diagnosed with an sexually transmitted disease (STD) in the past 6 months.

Or

- You inject drugs and:
  - Have an injection partner with HIV, or
  - Share needles, syringes, or other injection equipment.

Or

- You have been prescribed PEP (post-exposure prophylaxis) and you:
  - Report continued risk behavior or
  - Have used multiple courses of PEP

If you are a woman and have a partner with HIV and are considering getting pregnant, talk to your doctor about PrEP. PrEP may be an option to help protect you and your baby from getting HIV while you try to get pregnant, during pregnancy, or while breastfeeding.

WHAT DRUGS ARE APPROVED FOR PrEP?

There are two oral medications approved for daily use as PrEP. They are combinations of two anti-HIV drugs in a single pill:

- Truvada® is for all people at risk for HIV through sex or injection drug use. Generic products are also available.
- Descovy® is for sexually active men and transgender women at risk of getting HIV. Descovy® has not yet been studied for HIV prevention for receptive vaginal sex.

A long-acting injectable form of PrEP, Apretude®, has also been approved by the FDA. It is administered by a healthcare provider every two months instead of daily oral pills.

IS PrEP SAFE?

Pre-exposure prophylaxis is safe. No significant health effects have been seen in people who are HIV-negative and have taken PrEP for up to 5 years.

Some people taking PrEP may have side effects, such as nausea, diarrhea, headache, fatigue, and stomach pain. These side effects are usually not serious and go away over time. If you are taking PrEP, tell your healthcare provider if you have any side effect that bothers you or that does not go away.

And be aware: PrEP protects you against HIV but not against other sexually transmitted infections (STIs) or other types of infections. Combining PrEP with condoms will reduce your risk of getting other STIs.

HOW DO YOU GET PrEP?

If you think PrEP may be right for you, visit your doctor or healthcare provider. PrEP is only available by prescription. Any healthcare provider licensed to write prescriptions can prescribe PrEP; specialization in infectious diseases or HIV medicine is not required.

If you do not have a doctor, you can use the HIV Services Locator (www.locator.hiv.gov) to find a PrEP provider and other HIV services near you. You can visit many community health centers for a PrEP consultation. More than 190 health centers in the 57 jurisdictions prioritized in the Ending the HIV Epidemic initiative are providing PrEP services. Many health centers in other jurisdictions also provide PrEP services.

Because PrEP is for people who are HIV-negative, you will have to get an HIV test before starting PrEP and you may need to get other tests to make sure it is safe for you to use PrEP.

If you take PrEP, you will need to see your healthcare provider every 3 months for repeat HIV tests, prescription refills, and follow-up.

ON DEMAND PrEP
If You Are Not at Ongoing Risk for Getting HIV, Will You Take PrEP Only When You Are at Risk?

Taking PrEP only when you are at risk for getting HIV is known as "on-demand" PrEP.

- It is also known as "intermittent," "nondaily," "event-driven," or "off-label" PrEP use.
- The type of "on-demand" PrEP that has been studied is the "2-1-1" schedule. This means taking 2 pills 2-24 hours before sex, 1 pill 24 hours after the first dose, and 1 pill 24 hours after the second dose.
- There is scientific evidence that the "2-1-1" schedule provides effective protection for gay and bisexual men* when having anal sex without a condom.
- We do not know how "on-demand" PrEP works for heterosexual men and women, people who inject drugs, and transgender persons.

Some health departments in the United States and some health organizations in Europe and Canada are offering guidance for

185

"on-demand" PrEP as an alternative to daily PrEP for gay and bisexual men at risk for HIV.

This type of use is not currently part of the Centers for Disease Control and Prevention's (CDC) guidelines for PrEP use, which still recommends using PrEP as prescribed for those at risk for HIV. Taking PrEP as prescribed is currently the only FDA-approved schedule for taking PrEP to prevent HIV. When taken as prescribed, PrEP is highly effective for preventing HIV.

Anyone considering PrEP should discuss the issue with their healthcare provider.

The term "gay and bisexual men" is used to describe men who identify as gay or bisexual, as well as men who have sex with men who do not identify as gay or bisexual.

EFFECTIVENESS OF PrEP
- PrEP is highly effective for preventing HIV.
- PrEP reduces the risk of getting HIV from sex by about 99 percent when taken as prescribed.
- Although there is less information about how effective PrEP is among people who inject drugs, we do know that PrEP reduces the risk of getting HIV by at least 74 percent when taken as prescribed.
- PrEP is much less effective when it is not taken as prescribed.

How Long Do You Have to Take PrEP before It Is Highly Effective?
- PrEP reaches maximum protection from HIV for receptive anal sex (bottoming) at about 7 days of daily use.
- For receptive vaginal sex and injection drug use, PrEP reaches maximum protection at about 21 days of daily use.
- No data are available for insertive anal sex (topping) or insertive vaginal sex.

Section 15.2 | **Long-Acting PrEP**

This section includes text excerpted from "Long-Acting HIV Prevention Tools," HIV.gov, U.S. Department of Health and Human Services (HHS), December 10, 2020.

WHAT ARE LONG-ACTING HIV PREVENTION TOOLS?

Long-acting human immunodeficiency virus (HIV) prevention tools are new long-lasting forms of HIV prevention being studied by researchers. These are HIV prevention tools that can be inserted, injected, infused, or implanted in a person's body from once a month to once a year to provide sustained protection from acquiring HIV. These products are not available now, but they might be in the not-too-distant future.

WHY ARE LONG-ACTING HIV PREVENTION TOOLS NEEDED?

People who are HIV-negative but at very high risk for HIV can lower their chances of getting HIV by taking a pill that contains two anti-HIV drugs every day. This is called "pre-exposure prophylaxis" (PrEP). When taken daily, PrEP can stop HIV from taking hold and spreading throughout your body.

PrEP is highly effective when taken daily as prescribed. However, studies have shown that PrEP is much less effective if it is not taken consistently, and that taking a daily pill can be challenging for some people.

That is why researchers are working to create new HIV prevention tools that do not require taking a daily pill.

Scientists funded by the National Institutes of Health (NIH) are developing and testing several long-acting forms of HIV prevention that can be inserted, injected, infused, or implanted in a person's body from once a month to once a year. The goal of this research is to provide people with a variety of acceptable, discreet, and convenient choices for highly effective HIV prevention. None of the research on these possible HIV prevention options has been completed, so they are not yet approved by the U.S. Food and Drug Administration (FDA) and are not available for use outside of a clinical trial.

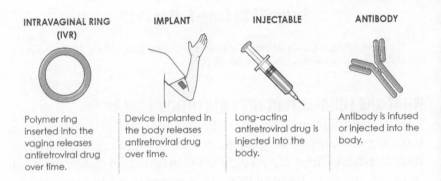

Figure 15.1. The National Institute of Allergy and Infectious Diseases (NIAID) Is Funding Research on Four Types of Long-Acting HIV Prevention

WHAT TYPES OF LONG-ACTING HIV PREVENTION TOOLS ARE UNDER STUDY?

Four types of long-acting HIV prevention are in development and testing in research studies: intravaginal rings, injectable drugs, implants, and antibodies. Figure 15.1 provides information on types of long-acting HIV prevention.

- **Intravaginal rings for women**. Long-acting intravaginal rings are polymer-based products that are inserted into the vagina, where they continuously release one or more antiretroviral drugs over time. The intravaginal ring at the most advanced stage of research is the dapivirine ring, which was tested in two large clinical trials, including the NIH-funded ASPIRE study. This study and another trial called "The Ring Study" found that the dapivirine ring reduced the risk of HIV acquisition by roughly 30 percent in women ages 18 to 45 years and was well-tolerated. If approved by regulatory agencies, the monthly ring would provide women in developing countries with a discreet long-acting HIV prevention option that they control.
- **Injectables**. Injectables are select long-acting antiretroviral drugs that are injected into the body. Injectables are being studied for both HIV prevention

and HIV treatment. Two large-scale clinical trials found that a long-acting form of the investigational antiretroviral drug cabotegravir injected once every eight weeks was safe and more effective than daily oral PrEP at preventing HIV acquisition among both cisgender women and cisgender men and transgender women who have sex with men. These results mark the first time a systemic, long-acting form of HIV prevention has been demonstrated to be highly effective. It is too early to know when long-acting injectable cabotegravir may be available as HIV prevention for individuals outside of these studies.

- **Implants**. Long-acting implants are small devices that are implanted in the body and release an anti-HIV drug at a controlled rate for continuous protection from HIV over time. NIH, among others, is funding the development and testing of several of these implants for HIV prevention. Most of these products are at an early stage of development and have not yet been tested in humans. Studies supported by other funders are exploring an implant for women that protects users from both HIV and unplanned pregnancy.

- **Antibodies**. Scientists have begun to test whether giving people periodic infusions of powerful anti-HIV antibodies can prevent or treat HIV. The antibodies involved can stop a wide variety of HIV strains from infecting human cells in the laboratory and thus are described as "broadly neutralizing antibodies" (bNAbs). Two advanced NIH-funded clinical trials are assessing whether giving infusions of bNAbs to healthy men and women at high risk for HIV protects them from acquiring the virus. Several early-stage clinical trials of other bNAbs for HIV prevention also are underway.

CAN YOU USE LONG-ACTING HIV PREVENTION TOOLS NOW?

No. At this time, some forms of long-acting HIV prevention are being tested in clinical trials. Since their effectiveness has not yet been proven, they have not been considered for approval by the FDA. So, they are not available for your doctor to prescribe yet. However, NIH-supported clinical trials may be seeking volunteers to participate in some studies on long-acting HIV prevention tools. You may be eligible to participate in one of these trials, which are listed in the NIAID's Long-Acting Forms of HIV prevention infographic (www.niaid.nih.gov/diseases-conditions/long-acting-forms-hiv-prevention). Information about these trials can be found at ClinicalTrials.gov or by calling 800-411-1222.

It will probably be several years before long-acting HIV prevention tools are available to the public. In the meantime, the best forms of prevention against sexual transmission of HIV continue to be:

- HIV testing – so that you know your own HIV status and your partner's too.
- Antiretroviral therapy for people who have HIV, to protect their health and prevent transmitting the virus to their sexual partners. People living with HIV who take HIV medication daily as prescribed and get and keep an undetectable viral load have effectively no risk of sexually transmitting HIV to their HIV-negative partners. This is called "treatment as prevention."
- Daily oral PrEP for people who do not have HIV but are at very high risk of getting it.
- Using condoms consistently and correctly.
- Choosing less risky sexual behaviors. HIV is mainly spread by having anal or vaginal sex without a condom or without taking medicines to prevent or treat HIV.
- Reducing the number of people you have sex with.
- Post-exposure prophylaxis, or PEP, meaning taking antiretroviral medicines very soon after being potentially exposed to HIV to prevent becoming infected.

The more of these actions you take, the safer you will be.

Section 15.3 | **Post-exposure Prophylaxis**

This section includes text excerpted from "Post-exposure Prophylaxis," HIV.gov, U.S. Department of Health and Human Services (HHS), April 28, 2021.

WHAT IS POST-EXPOSURE PROPHYLAXIS?

Post-exposure prophylaxis, or PEP, is a short course of HIV medicines taken very soon after a possible exposure to HIV to prevent the virus from taking hold in your body.

You must start it within 72 hours (3 days) after a possible exposure to HIV, or it would not work. Every hour counts!

Post-exposure prophylaxis should be used only in emergency situations. It is not meant for regular use by people who may be exposed to HIV frequently.

HOW DO YOU KNOW IF YOU NEED PEP?

Post-exposure prophylaxis may be right for you if you are HIV-negative or do not know your HIV status, and you think you may have been exposed to HIV in the last 72 hours:

- During sex (e.g., you had a condom break with a partner of unknown HIV status or a partner with HIV who is not virally suppressed)
- Through shared needles, syringes, or other equipment used to inject drugs, or
- Through sexual assault

Contact your healthcare provider immediately or go to an emergency room or urgent care clinic right away.

Your healthcare provider or emergency room doctor will evaluate you, help you decide whether PEP is right for you, and work with you to determine which medicines to take for PEP.

In addition, if you are a healthcare worker, you may be prescribed PEP after a possible exposure to HIV at work, such as from a needlestick injury.

HOW LONG DO YOU NEED TO TAKE PEP?

If you are prescribed PEP, you will need to take the HIV medicines every day for 28 days.

You will also need to return to your healthcare provider at certain times while taking PEP and after you finish taking it for HIV testing and other tests.

HOW WELL DOES PEP WORK?

Post-exposure prophylaxis is effective in preventing HIV infection when it is taken correctly, but it is not 100 percent effective. The sooner you start PEP after a possible HIV exposure, the better.

While taking PEP, it is important to use other HIV prevention methods, such as using condoms the right way, every time you have sex and using only new, sterile needles and works when injecting drugs.

DOES PEP CAUSE SIDE EFFECTS?

Post-exposure prophylaxis is safe, but the HIV medicines used for PEP may cause side effects like nausea in some people. In almost all cases, these side effects can be treated and are not life-threatening.

If you are taking PEP, talk to your healthcare provider if you have any side effect that bothers you or that does not go away.

PEP medicines may also interact with other medicines that a person is taking (called a "drug interaction"). For this reason, it is important to tell your healthcare provider about any other medicines that you take.

CAN YOU TAKE PEP EVERY TIME YOU HAVE A POTENTIAL EXPOSURE TO HIV?

No. PEP should be used only in emergency situations. It is not intended to replace regular use of other HIV prevention methods. If you feel that you might exposed to HIV frequently, talk to your healthcare professional about PrEP (pre-exposure prophylaxis).

CAN YOU GET HELP PAYING FOR PEP?

- If you are prescribed PEP after a sexual assault – You may qualify for partial or total reimbursement for medicines and clinical care costs through the Office for Victims of Crime (OVC), funded by the U.S. Department of Justice (DOJ).
- If you are prescribed PEP for another reason and you cannot get insurance coverage (Medicaid, Medicare, private, or employer-based) – Your healthcare provider can apply for free PEP medicines through the medication assistance programs run by the manufacturers. These requests can be handled urgently in many cases to avoid a delay in getting medicine.
- If you are a healthcare worker who was exposed to HIV on the job – Your workplace health insurance or workers' compensation will usually pay for PEP.

Part 3 | Receiving an HIV/AIDS Diagnosis

Chapter 16 | HIV Testing

Chapter Contents

Section 16.1 | HIV Testing Basics

This section includes text excerpted from "HIV Testing," HIVinfo, U.S. Department of Health and Human Services (HHS), August 16, 2021.

WHAT IS HIV TESTING?

Human immunodeficiency virus (HIV) testing determines if a person is infected with HIV. HIV is the virus that causes acquired immunodeficiency syndrome (AIDS). AIDS is the most advanced stage of HIV infection.

HIV testing can detect HIV infection, but it cannot tell how long a person has had HIV or if the person has AIDS.

WHY IS HIV TESTING IMPORTANT?

Knowing your HIV status can help keep you – and others – safe.

If you are HIV negative:

A negative HIV test result shows that you do not have HIV. Continue taking steps to avoid getting HIV, such as using condoms during sex and, if you are at high risk of getting HIV, taking medicines to prevent HIV (called "pre-exposure prophylaxis" or "PrEP").

If you are HIV positive:

A positive HIV test result shows that you have HIV, but you can still take steps to protect your health. Begin by talking to your healthcare provider about antiretroviral therapy (ART). People on ART take a combination of HIV medicines every day to treat HIV infection. ART is recommended for everyone who has HIV, and people with HIV should start ART as soon as possible. ART cannot cure HIV, but HIV medicines help people with HIV live longer, healthier lives.

A main goal of ART is to reduce a person's viral load to an undetectable level. An undetectable viral load means that the level of HIV in the blood is too low to be detected by a viral load test. People with HIV who maintain an undetectable viral load have effectively no risk of transmitting HIV to their HIV-negative partner through sex.

WHO SHOULD GET TESTED FOR HIV?

The Centers for Disease Control and Prevention (CDC) recommends that everyone 13 to 64 years of age get tested for HIV at least once as part of routine healthcare. As a general rule, people at higher risk for HIV should get tested each year. Sexually active gay and bisexual men may benefit from getting tested more often, such as every three to six months. If you are over 64 years of age and at risk, your healthcare provider may recommend HIV testing.

Factors that increase the risk of HIV include:

- Having vaginal or anal sex with someone who is HIV positive or whose HIV status you do not know.
- Injecting drugs and sharing needles, syringes, or other drug equipment with others.
- Exchanging sex for money or drugs.
- Having a sexually transmitted disease (STD), such as syphilis.
- Having sex with anyone who has any of the HIV risk factors listed above.

Talk to your healthcare provider about your risk for HIV and how often you should get tested for HIV.

SHOULD PREGNANT WOMEN GET TESTED FOR HIV?

The Centers for Disease Control and Prevention (CDC) recommends that all pregnant women get tested for HIV so that they can begin taking HIV medicines if they are HIV positive. Women with HIV take HIV medicines during pregnancy and childbirth to reduce the risk of perinatal transmission of HIV and to protect their own health.

WHAT ARE THE TYPES OF HIV TESTS?

There are three types of tests used to diagnose HIV infection: antibody tests, antigen/antibody tests, and nucleic acid tests (NATs). Your healthcare provider can determine the appropriate HIV test for you. How soon each test can detect HIV infection differs, because each test has a different window period. The window period is the time between when a person may have been exposed to HIV and when a test can accurately detect HIV infection.

- **Antibody tests.** It checks for HIV antibodies in blood or oral fluid. HIV antibodies are disease-fighting proteins that the body produces in response to HIV infection. Most rapid tests and home use tests are antibody tests.
- **Antigen/antibody tests.** This test can detect both HIV antibodies and HIV antigens (a part of the virus) in the blood.
- **NATs.** It look for HIV in the blood.

A person's initial HIV test will usually be either an antibody test or an antigen/antibody test. NATs are very expensive and not routinely used for HIV screening unless the person had a high-risk exposure or a possible exposure with early symptoms of HIV infection.

When an HIV test is positive, a follow-up test will be conducted. Sometimes people will need to visit a healthcare provider to take a follow-up test. Other times, the follow-up test may be performed in a lab using the same blood sample that was provided for the first test. A positive follow-up test confirms that a person has HIV.

Talk to your healthcare provider about your HIV risk factors and the best type of HIV test for you.

IS HIV TESTING CONFIDENTIAL?

HIV testing can be confidential or anonymous.

Confidential testing. It means that your HIV test results will include your name and other identifying information, and the results will be included in your medical record. HIV-positive test results will be reported to local or state health departments to be counted in statistical reports. Health departments remove all personal information (including names and addresses) from HIV test results before sharing the information with CDC. The CDC uses this information for reporting purposes and does not share this information with any other organizations, including insurance companies.

Anonymous testing. It means you do not have to give your name when you take an HIV test. When you take the test, you receive a number. To get your HIV test results, you give the number instead of your name.

WHERE CAN SOMEONE GET TESTED FOR HIV?

Your healthcare provider can give you an HIV test. HIV testing is also available at many hospitals, medical clinics, substance use programs, and community health centers. Use CDC's GetTested (www.gettested.cdc.gov) treatment locator to find an HIV testing location near you. Getting tested through a professional healthcare provider is recommended; however, there are HIV self-testing kits available. Rapid self-test and mail-in self-test are the two types of HIV self-tests, but state laws regarding self-testing may limit their availability in a location.

A rapid self-test is an oral fluid test done entirely at home or in private. There is currently one U.S. Food and Drug Administration (FDA)-approved rapid self-test called "OraQuick In-Home HIV test". A mail-in self-test requires a person to provide a blood sample from a fingerstick, which is then sent to a lab for testing.

Section 16.2 | Frequency of HIV Testing and Time from Infection to Diagnosis Improve

This section includes text excerpted from "Frequency of HIV Testing and Time from Infection to Diagnosis Improve," Centers for Disease Control and Prevention (CDC), November 28, 2017. Reviewed February 2022.

A recent Centers for Disease Control and Prevention (CDC) *Vital Signs* report finds that human immunodeficiency virus (HIV) is being diagnosed sooner after infection than was previously reported. The seven-month improvement is a considerable decrease over a four-year period and reinforces other recent signs that the nation's approach to HIV prevention is paying off.

"These findings are more encouraging signs that the tide continues to turn on your nation's HIV epidemic," said CDC Director Brenda Fitzgerald, M.D. "HIV is being diagnosed more quickly, the number of people who have the virus under control is up, and annual infections are down. So while you celebrate the progress, you pledge to work together to end this epidemic forever."

Getting an HIV test is the first step to learning how to reduce future risk for people who do not have HIV and to starting treatment and getting the virus under control for people living with HIV. Taking HIV medicine as prescribed allows people with the virus to live a long, healthy life and protect their partners from acquiring HIV.

"If you are at risk for HIV, do not guess – get a test," said Jonathan Mermin, M.D., M.P.H, director of CDC's National Center for HIV/AIDS, viral hepatitis, sexually transmitted disease (STD), and tuberculosis (TB) prevention. "The benefits are clear. Prompt diagnosis is prevention. It is the first step to protecting people living with HIV and their partners."

The CDC recommends testing all people ages 13–64 for HIV at least once in their lifetime, and people at higher risk for HIV at least annually. Healthcare providers may find it beneficial to test some sexually active gay and bisexual men more frequently (e.g., every three to six months).

The *Vital Signs* analysis found that the percentage of people at increased risk for HIV who reported getting an HIV test the previous year has increased. Despite that progress, too few are tested.

The *Vital Signs* analysis suggests that, without increased testing, many people living with undiagnosed HIV may not know they have HIV for many years. A quarter of people diagnosed with HIV lived with HIV for seven or more years without knowing it.

In 2015, estimated timing from HIV infection to diagnosis varied by risk group and by race/ethnicity.

- Estimated timing from HIV infection to diagnosis ranged from a median of five years for heterosexual males to two-and-a-half years for heterosexual females and females who inject drugs. The median was three years for gay and bisexual males.

- Estimated timing from HIV infection to diagnosis ranged from a median of four years for Asian Americans to two years for white Americans and about three years for African-Americans and Latinxs.

"Ideally, HIV is diagnosed within months of infection, rather than years later," said Eugene McCray, M.D., director of CDC's Division of HIV/AIDS Prevention. "Further increasing regular HIV testing and closing testing, diagnoses and treatment gaps is essential to stopping HIV in your communities."

The CDC funding supports more than three million tests across the country each year that identify on average more than 12,000 people with HIV who were not previously diagnosed – accounting for one-third of all HIV diagnoses a year in the United States.

VITAL SIGNS ANALYSIS

Estimated diagnosis delays are based on CDC's National HIV Surveillance System data reported from 50 states and Washington, D.C. HIV testing rates are based on data from the CDC's National HIV Behavioral Surveillance System (NHBS), which asks gay and bisexual men, people who inject drugs, and heterosexuals at increased risk for HIV about their HIV risk behaviors and testing. The NHBS data are collected in more than 20 large cities with a high number of HIV cases and are not nationally representative.

VITAL SIGNS

The CDC *Vital Signs* is a report that appears on the first Tuesday of the month as part of the CDC journal Morbidity and Mortality Weekly Report (MMWR) (www.cdc.gov/mmwr). *Vital Signs* is designed to provide the latest data and information on key health indicators – cancer prevention, obesity, tobacco use, alcohol use, HIV/AIDS, motor vehicle safety, healthcare-associated infections, cardiovascular health, teen pregnancy, asthma, and food safety.

Section 16.3 | **HIV Disclosure Policies and Procedures**

This section includes text excerpted from "HIV Disclosure Policies and Procedures," HIV.gov, U.S. Department of Health and Human Services (HHS), May 15, 2017. Reviewed February 2022.

If your human immunodeficiency virus (HIV) test is positive, the clinic or other testing site will report the results to your state health department. They do this so that public health officials can monitor what is happening with the HIV epidemic in your city and state. (It is important for them to know this, because federal and state funding for HIV services is often targeted to areas where the epidemic is strongest.)

Your state health department will then remove all of your personal information (name, address, etc.) from your test results and send the information to the U.S. Centers for Disease Control and Prevention (CDC). The CDC is the federal agency responsible for tracking national public health trends. CDC does not share this information with anyone else, including insurance companies.

Many states and some cities have partner-notification laws – meaning that, if you test positive for HIV, you (or your healthcare provider) may be legally obligated to tell your sex or needle-sharing partner(s). In some states, if you are HIV-positive and do not tell your partner(s), you can be charged with a crime. Some health departments require healthcare providers to report the name of your sex and needle-sharing partner(s) if they know that information–even if you refuse to report that information yourself.

Some states also have laws that require clinic staff to notify a "third party" if they know that person has a significant risk for exposure to HIV from a patient the staff member knows is infected with HIV. This is called "duty to warn." The Ryan White HIV/AIDS Program requires that health departments receiving money from the Ryan White program show "good faith" efforts to notify the marriage partners of a patient with HIV.

DISCLOSURE POLICIES IN CORRECTIONAL FACILITIES

Any individual who believes that her or his employment rights have been violated may file a charge of discrimination with the Federal Equal Employment Opportunity Commission (EEOC). In addition, an individual, an organization, or an agency may file a charge on behalf of another person in order to protect the aggrieved person's identity.

Section 16.4 | An Opt-Out Approach to HIV Screening

This section includes text excerpted from "Opt-Out Screening," Centers for Disease Control and Prevention (CDC), March 4, 2020.

ROUTINE SCREENING SHOULD BE IMPLEMENTED USING AN "OPT-OUT" APPROACH

When an Opt-Out approach is implemented, patients should be informed (e.g., through a patient brochure, practice literature/form, or discussion) that an human immunodeficiency virus (HIV) test will be included in the standard preventive screening tests, and that they may decline the test (opt-out screening). A patient's decision to decline testing should be noted in their medical record. HIV prevention counseling should not be a requirement for HIV testing.

- Risk assessment should be included as part of routine primary care visits for all sexually active patients.
- Individuals at high risk may need to be screened more frequently.
- Prevention counseling also may be needed for patients at high risk for acquiring HIV, but should not be required for general testing.

WHY ROUTINE, OPT-OUT HIV SCREENING
Conducting Risk-Based Screening May Fail to Identify Persons with HIV:

- People <20 years of age
- Women

- Including pregnant women; HIV screening should be included in the routine panel of prenatal screening.
- Members of minority races/ethnicities.
- Nonurban dwellers in low-incidence areas.
- Heterosexual men and women who are unaware of their risk of HIV.

Many people with HIV are not diagnosed until they have advanced HIV or acquired immunodeficiency syndrome (AIDS).

Routine, Opt-Out Screening Has Proved Highly Effective:
- Removes the stigma associated with HIV testing.
- Fosters earlier diagnosis and treatment.
- Reduces risk of transmission
- Is cost-effective

Justification for Routine HIV Screening by Healthcare Providers Includes the Following:
- Serious health disorder that can be detected before symptoms develop.
- Detectable by reliable, inexpensive, acceptable screening tests.
- People diagnosed with HIV have years of life to gain if treatment is started early, before symptoms develop.
- Screening costs are reasonable in relation to anticipated benefits.

Chapter 17 | Types of HIV Diagnostic Tests

Section 17.1 | Types of HIV Tests

This section includes text excerpted from "Types of HIV Tests," Centers for Disease Control and Prevention (CDC), May 13, 2021.

WHAT KINDS OF TESTS ARE AVAILABLE, AND HOW DO THEY WORK?

There are three types of tests available: nucleic acid tests (NAT), antigen/antibody tests, and antibody tests. HIV tests are typically performed on blood or oral fluid. They may also be performed on urine.

- A NAT looks for the actual virus in the blood and involves drawing blood from a vein. The test can either tell if a person has HIV or tell how much virus is present in the blood (known as an "HIV viral load test"). While a NAT can detect HIV sooner than other types of tests, this test is very expensive and not routinely used for screening individuals unless they recently had a high-risk exposure or a possible exposure and have early symptoms of HIV infection.

- An antigen/antibody test looks for both HIV antibodies and antigens. Antibodies are produced by your immune system when you are exposed to viruses such as HIV. Antigens are foreign substances that cause your immune system to activate. If you have HIV, an antigen called "p24" is produced even before antibodies develop. Antigen/antibody tests are recommended for testing done in labs and are now common in the United States. This lab test involves drawing blood from a vein. There is also a rapid antigen/antibody test available that is done with a finger prick.

- HIV antibody tests only look for antibodies to HIV in your blood or oral fluid. In general, antibody tests that use blood from a vein can detect HIV sooner after infection than tests done with blood from a finger

211

prick or with oral fluid. Most rapid tests and the only currently approved HIV self-test are antibody tests.

Talk to your healthcare provider about what type of HIV test is right for you.

HOW LONG DOES IT TAKE TO GET RESULTS?

- Laboratory tests (NAT and antigen/antibody) require blood to be drawn from your vein into a tube and then that blood is sent to a laboratory for testing. The results may take several days to be available.
- With a rapid antibody screening test, usually done with blood from a finger prick or with oral fluid, results are ready in 30 minutes or less.
- The rapid antigen/antibody test is done with a finger prick and takes 30 minutes or less.
- The oral fluid antibody self-test provides results within 20 minutes.

HOW SOON AFTER AN EXPOSURE TO HIV CAN A TEST DETECT IF YOU HAVE THE VIRUS?

No HIV test can detect HIV immediately after infection. If you think you have been exposed to HIV in the last 72 hours, talk to your healthcare provider about post-exposure prophylaxis (PEP), right away.

The time between when a person may have been exposed to HIV and when a test can tell for sure whether they have the virus is called the "window period." The window period varies from person to person and depends on the type of test used to detect HIV. Ask your healthcare provider or test counselor about the window period for the test you are taking.

- A NAT can usually tell you if you have HIV infection 10–33 days after an exposure.
- An antigen/antibody test performed by a laboratory on blood from a vein can usually detect HIV infection 18–45 days after an exposure. Antigen/

antibody tests done with blood from a finger prick can take longer to detect HIV (18–90 days after an exposure).

- Antibody tests can take 23–90 days to detect HIV infection after an exposure. Most rapid tests and self-tests are antibody tests. In general, antibody tests that use blood from a vein can detect HIV sooner after infection than tests done with blood from a finger prick or with oral fluid.

If you get an HIV test after a potential HIV exposure and the result is negative, get tested again after the window period. Remember, you can only be sure you are HIV-negative if:

- Your most recent test is after the window period.
- You have not had a potential HIV exposure during the window period. If you do have a potential exposure, then you will need to be retested.

Section 17.2 | Rapid Oral HIV Tests

This section contains text excerpted from the following sources: Text beginning with the heading "What Is a Rapid Oral HIV Test?" is excerpted from "Rapid Oral HIV Test: Patient Fact Sheet," U.S. Department of Veterans Affairs (VA), March 2017. Reviewed February 2022; Text under the heading "How Accurate Is the Rapid Oral HIV Test?" is excerpted from "Frequently Asked Questions: How Accurate Is the Rapid Oral HIV Test?" U.S. Department of Veterans Affairs (VA), June 13, 2019.

WHAT IS A RAPID ORAL HIV TEST?

This is a test for HIV (human immunodeficiency virus), the virus that causes acquired immunodeficiency syndrome (AIDS). With a rapid oral test, results take about 20 minutes. There are also rapid tests that use a blood sample. Rapid tests are usually used when results need to be delivered within a few minutes, like in an outreach center or homeless clinic; otherwise a traditional blood test is used. The rapid oral test is quite good at detecting chronic (long-standing) HIV infection but not so good at detecting very recent HIV infection.

HOW DOES THE RAPID ORAL HIV TEST WORK?

When HIV enters the body, antibodies are produced. The test looks for HIV antibodies in your oral fluids. The test uses a swab to collect a sample from the inside of your mouth.

WHAT HAPPENS WHEN YOU AGREE TO BE TESTED

- The test is explained to you by a health provider
- A health provider will ask you to swab your gums with a special swab
- Results are ready in about 20 minutes. You will learn your HIV result and discuss what it means
- Your provider will give you information about how to protect yourself and others from HIV
- If your test result is positive, you will do a second, different, test using a blood sample that is sent to the lab
- Your test result will be confidential (results will only be discussed with you). Your test result will not affect your VA benefits

WHAT DOES A NEGATIVE RAPID ORAL HIV TEST RESULT MEAN?

This means that HIV antibodies have not been found in your system. This could mean one of two things:

- You do not have HIV.
- You have HIV but it was not detected by the rapid oral test (this is a false-negative result).

It can take up to 3 months for your system to produce enough antibodies to be detected by the rapid oral test. If you have engaged in activities that might put you at risk of HIV infection in the past 3 months, you should repeat the test in a few weeks, or talk with your VA provider about doing a standard blood test for HIV right away.

WHAT DOES A POSITIVE RAPID ORAL HIV TEST RESULT MEAN?

This means that HIV antibodies may be in your system. Positive results on the rapid test must always be confirmed by doing a second HIV test. This is because sometimes (rarely) the rapid oral test gives a false-positive result. A person is considered to be HIV positive only if two different test results are positive. The second HIV test is a blood test that is sent to the lab; the results may take up to 1–2 weeks to return.

If your positive result is confirmed by a second test, that means:

- You have HIV and should be evaluated right away for treatment.
- Your testing site will refer you to a clinic that has expertise in caring for people with HIV. They may also refer you for counseling and other support services.
- HIV treatment (medication) greatly improves health, and can prevent transmission (infection) to others.

WHY SHOULD YOU GET TESTED?

- Many HIV-positive people do not know they are infected with HIV, because they have never been tested.
- Knowing your HIV status helps you protect yourself and others.
- Getting diagnosed early can greatly improve your health. Although there is no cure for HIV, there are many effective medicines that can control it. Most people with HIV who take their medication every day can live long, healthy lives.
- If you test negative, you may feel less anxious after testing, and you may be more committed to preventing yourself from becoming infected.
- An HIV test is part of routine medical care.

HOW ACCURATE IS THE RAPID ORAL HIV TEST?

The rapid oral HIV test detects antibodies made by the immune system in response to HIV infection, just like the standard blood antibody test. The rapid oral test, however, detects these antibodies in oral fluid, and does not require a blood sample.

The rapid oral HIV test is quite accurate (similar to the standard blood antibody test) for persons with chronic, or longstanding, HIV infection, but it is not as accurate for people with new or recent HIV infection. Like any antibody test for HIV, the rapid oral HIV test is not reliable during the "window period" (lasting several weeks to months) between the time a person is infected and the time the body has made enough antibodies for the test to detect. During this window period, someone who is infected might test negative for antibodies (a false-negative result). The "window period" for the rapid oral test is longer than it is for some HIV blood tests, meaning that for someone with acute or new HIV infection certain blood tests can detect HIV earlier than the oral rapid tests.

It also is possible to have false-positive results (a person may have a positive rapid oral HIV test result but not actually be infected with HIV). That is why anyone who has a positive result with a rapid oral HIV test must have a more specific "confirmatory" blood test before a diagnosis of HIV infection can be made.

Section 17.3 | HIV Self-Testing (Home Testing)

This section contains text excerpted from the following sources: Text under the heading "Home Access Human Immunodeficiency Virus Infection (HIV)-1 Test System" is excerpted from "Information Regarding the Home Access HIV-1 Test System," U.S. Food and Drug Administration (FDA), March 7, 2018. Reviewed February 2022; Text under the heading "OraQuick In-Home HIV Test" is excerpted from "Information Regarding the OraQuick In-Home HIV Test," U.S. Food and Drug Administration (FDA), June 3, 2020; Text beginning with the heading "Can You Get an HIV Test to Use at Home or in a Private Location?" is excerpted from "Self-Testing: A Convenient and Private Option," Centers for Disease Control and Prevention (CDC), July 16, 2021.

HOME ACCESS HUMAN IMMUNODEFICIENCY VIRUS (HIV)-1 TEST SYSTEM
What Is the Home Access HIV-1 Test System?

The Home Access HIV-1 Test System is a laboratory test sold over-the-counter (OTC) that uses fingerstick blood mailed to the testing laboratory. The test kit consists of multiple components, including materials for specimen self-collection, prepaid materials for mailing the specimen to a laboratory for testing, testing directions, an information booklet, an anonymous registration system and a call center to receive your test results and follow-up counseling by telephone.

This approved system uses a finger prick process for home blood collection which results in dried blood spots on special paper. The dried blood spots are mailed to a laboratory with a confidential and anonymous unique personal identification number (PIN) and are analyzed by trained clinicians in a laboratory using the same tests that are used for samples taken in a doctor's office or clinic. Test results are obtained through a toll-free telephone number using the PIN, and posttest counseling is provided by telephone when results are obtained.

When Should You Take a Test for HIV?

If you actively engage in behavior that puts you at risk for HIV infection, or your partner engages in such behavior, then you should consider testing on a regular basis. It may take some time for the immune system to produce sufficient antibodies for the test to detect, and this time period can vary from person to person. This time-frame is commonly referred to as the "window period," when a person is infected with HIV but antibodies to the virus cannot be detected, however, the person may be able to infect others. According to the Centers for Disease Control and Prevention (CDC), it can take up to 6 months to develop antibodies to HIV, although most people (97 percent) will develop detectable antibodies in the first 3 months following the time of their infection.

How Reliable Is the Home Access HIV-1 Test System?

Clinical studies reported to the FDA showed that the sensitivity (i.e., the percentage of results that will be positive when HIV is present) was estimated to be greater than 99.9 percent. The specificity (i.e., the percentage of results that will be negative when HIV is not present) was also estimated to be greater than 99.9 percent. Results reported as positive have undergone testing using both a screening test and another test to confirm the positive result.

What about Counseling

The Home Access HIV-1 Test System has a built-in mechanism for pretest and posttest counseling provided by the manufacturer. This counseling is anonymous and confidential. Counseling, which uses both printed material and telephone interaction, provides the user with an interpretation of the test result. Counseling also provides information on how to keep from getting infected if you are negative, and how to prevent further transmission of disease if you are infected. Counseling provides you with information about treatment options if you are infected, and can even provide referrals to doctors who treat HIV-infected individuals in your area.

If the Test Results Are Positive, What Should You Do?

The counselors can provide you with information about treatment options and referrals to doctors who treat HIV-infected individuals in your area.

Do You Need a Confirmatory Test?

No, a positive result from the Home Access HIV-1 Test System means that antibodies to the HIV-1 virus are present in the blood sample submitted to the testing laboratory. The Home Access HIV-1 Test System includes confirmatory testing for HIV-1, and all confirmation testing is completed before the results are released and available to users of the test system.

How Quickly Will You Get the Results of the Home Access HIV-1 Test System?

You can anonymously call for the results approximately 7 business days (3 business days for the Express System) after shipping your specimen to the laboratory by using the unique PIN on the tear-off label included with your test kit. This label includes both the unique PIN and the toll-free number for the counseling center.

How Are Unapproved Test Systems Different?

The manufacturers of unapproved test systems have not submitted data to FDA to review to determine whether or not their test systems can reliably detect HIV infection. Therefore, FDA cannot give the public any assurance that the results obtained using an unapproved test system are accurate.

ORAQUICK IN-HOME HIV TEST
What Is the OraQuick In-Home HIV Test and How Does It Work?

The OraQuick In-Home HIV Test is a rapid self-administered over-the-counter (OTC) test. The OraQuick In-Home HIV Test kit consists of a test stick (device) to collect the specimen, a test tube (vial) to insert the test stick (device) and complete the test, testing directions, two information booklets ("HIV, Testing and Me" and "What your results mean to you"), a disposal bag and phone numbers for consumer support.

This approved test uses oral fluid to check for antibodies to HIV Type 1 and HIV Type 2, the viruses that cause AIDS. The kit is designed to allow you to take the HIV test anonymously and in private with the collection of an oral fluid sample by swabbing your upper and lower gums with the test device. After collecting the sample you insert the device into the kit's vial which contains a developer solution, wait 20–40 minutes, and read the test result. A positive result with this test does not mean that an individual is definitely infected with HIV but rather that additional testing should be done in a medical setting to confirm the test result. Additionally, a negative test result does not mean that an individual is definitely not infected with HIV, particularly when exposure may have been within the previous three months. Again an individual should obtain a confirmatory test in a medical setting.

When Should You Take a Test for HIV?

If you actively engage in behavior that puts you at risk for HIV infection, or your partner engages in such behavior, then you should consider testing on a regular basis. It can take some time for the immune system to produce enough antibodies for the test to detect, and this time period can vary from person to person. This timeframe is commonly referred to as the "window period," when a person is infected with HIV but antibodies to the virus can not be detected, however, the person may be able to infect others. According to the

CDC, although it can take up to 6 months to develop antibodies for HIV, most people (97 percent) will develop detectable antibodies in the first 3 months following the time of their infection.

How Reliable Is the OraQuick In-Home HIV Test?

As noted in the package insert, clinical studies have shown that the OraQuick In-Home HIV Test has an expected performance of approximately 92 percent for test sensitivity (i.e., the percentage of results that will be positive when HIV is present). This means that one false negative result would be expected out of every 12 test results in HIV-infected individuals. The clinical studies also showed that the OraQuick In-Home HIV Test has an expected performance of 99.98 percent for test specificity (i.e., the percentage of results that will be negative when HIV is not present). This means that one false positive result would be expected out of every 5,000 test results in uninfected individuals.

It is extremely important for those who self-test using the OraQuick In-Home HIV Test to carefully read and follow all labeled directions. Even when used according to the labeled directions, there will be some false negative results and a small number of false positive results. The OraQuick test package contains step-by-step instructions, and there is also an OraQuick Consumer Support Center to assist users in the testing process.

If the Test Says You Are HIV Positive, What Should You Do?

A positive test result does not necessarily mean that you are infected with HIV. If you test positive for HIV using the OraQuick In-Home Test, you should see your healthcare provider or call the OraQuick Consumer Support Center, which has support center representatives available 24 hours a day/7 days a week to answer your questions and provide referrals to local healthcare providers for follow-up care. You will be advised to obtain confirmatory testing to confirm a positive result or inform you that the initial result was a false positive result. The test kit also contains an information booklet, "What your results mean to You," which is designed to instruct individuals on what to do once they have obtained their test results.

Do You Need a Confirmatory Test?

A positive test result on the OraQuick In-Home HIV Test indicates that you may be infected with HIV. Additional testing in a medical setting will either confirm a positive test result or inform you that the initial result was a false positive result.

What Is a "False Positive" Result?

A "false positive" result occurs when an individual not infected with the HIV virus receives a test result that indicates that she or he is infected with HIV.

If the Test Says You Are HIV Negative, What Should You Do?

A negative result on this test does not necessarily mean that you are not infected with HIV. The OraQuick test kit contains an information booklet, "What your results mean to You," which is designed to instruct individuals on what to do once they have obtained their test results. The test is relatively reliable if there has been sufficient time for HIV antibodies to develop in the infected person. For the OraQuick In-Home HIV Test, that period of time, called the "window period," is about three months. If you have recently been engaging in behavior that puts you at high risk for HIV infection, you should take the test again at a later time. Alternatively, you should see your healthcare provider who can discuss other options for HIV testing.

What Is a "False Negative" Result?

A "false negative" result occurs when an HIV-infected individual receives a test result that incorrectly indicates that she or he is not infected with HIV.

How Quickly Will You Get the Results of the OraQuick Test?

You can read the results of the OraQuick In-Home HIV Test within 20–40 minutes.

How Are Unapproved Test Systems Different?

The manufacturers of unapproved test systems have not submitted data to FDA in order for FDA to review and determine whether their test systems can reliably detect HIV infection. Therefore, FDA cannot give the public any assurance that the results obtained using an unapproved test system are accurate.

CAN YOU GET AN HIV TEST TO USE AT HOME OR IN A PRIVATE LOCATION?

Yes. These are known as "HIV self-tests." There are two kinds:

- A Rapid Self-Test is done entirely at home or in a private location and can produce results within 20 minutes. You can buy a rapid self-test kit at a pharmacy or online. The only rapid self-test available in the United States is an oral fluid test.
- A Mail-In Self-Test includes a specimen collection kit that contains supplies to collect dried blood from a finger stick at home. The sample is then sent to a lab for testing and the results are provided by a healthcare provider. Mail-in self-tests can be ordered through various online merchant sites. Your healthcare provider can also order a mail-in self-test for you.

Check to see if the health department or other organization near you is providing a rapid self-test for a reduced cost or for free. Directly purchased self-tests may not be covered by private health insurance or Medicaid. Be sure to check with your insurance provider and your healthcare provider about reimbursement for tests that are self-purchased.

WHAT SHOULD YOU EXPECT WHEN YOU USE A RAPID HIV SELF-TEST?

There is one FDA-approved rapid self-test (OraQuick). For this test, you must swab your gums to collect an oral fluid sample and use the materials in the kit to test your oral fluid sample. You will be able to get a result within 20 minutes. It is important to follow the directions as described in the instructions or the test will not work. There is a phone number included with the HIV self-test for anyone to call to get help with conducting the test.

You should always interpret the rapid self-test according to the test manufacturer's instructions.

- If the test result is negative, and you have not had a possible exposure during the previous 3 months, you can be confident you do not have HIV
- If your test result is positive, go to a healthcare provider for follow-up testing

Some people have difficulty in conducting a rapid self-test and the test does not perform as it should. If a rapid HIV self-test is invalid as described in the instructions, then the test has not worked. In this case, you will need to use another rapid self-test, a mail-in self-test, or seek testing at a healthcare provider or testing center.

WHAT SHOULD YOU EXPECT WHEN YOU USE A MAIL-IN HIV SELF-TEST?

There are many mail-in self-testing services available through online merchants. The kit you receive provides the tools you will need to safely prick your finger and collect a very small sample of blood on a card. The sample is then mailed to a laboratory for testing. When the testing is completed a healthcare provider will contact you with the results.

You should always follow the manufacturer's instructions carefully to ensure you collect a good sample.

- If the test result is negative, and you have not had a possible exposure during the previous 3 months, you can be confident you do not have HIV
- If your test result is positive, go to a healthcare provider for follow-up testing

Directly purchased self-tests (purchased online) may not be covered by private health insurance or Medicaid. Check with your insurance provider and your healthcare provider about reimbursement for mail-in self-tests that are self-purchased. Some mail-in self-test providers can bill your insurance for you.

Chapter 18 | **Understanding Your Test Results**

WHAT IF YOUR TEST RESULT IS NEGATIVE?

Great news! If your test result is negative, it means you do not have human immunodeficiency virus (HIV), unless you had a recent exposure. If you did have a recent exposure, then ask your health-care provider if you need a follow-up test.

After exposure to HIV, it takes time for enough HIV to grow inside of you for a test to be able to detect it; this is called the "window period."

Depending on when you were tested for HIV, you may need another test to be sure that you were not in the window period during the first test. If you test again after the window period, have no possible HIV exposure during the window period, and the result comes back negative, you do not have HIV.

If you are sexually active or use needles to inject drugs, continue to take actions to prevent HIV, like taking HIV medicine ("pre-exposure prophylaxis," or PrEP) if you are at risk.

Call your healthcare provider right away if you feel sick or have common HIV symptoms, such as:
- Flu-like symptoms
- Swollen lymph nodes (swelling in the neck, groin, or armpit)
- Extreme tiredness
- Rash
- Sores in your mouth

This chapter includes text excerpted from "Understanding Your HIV Test Results," Centers for Disease Control and Prevention (CDC), March 2021.

WHEN DO YOU NEED ANOTHER HIV TEST?

Some people should get tested more often. If you were HIV negative the last time you were tested, the test was more than 1 year ago, and you can answer yes to any of the following questions, then you should get an HIV test as soon as possible:

- Are you a man who has had sex with another man?
- Have you had sex – anal or vaginal – with a partner who has HIV?
- Have you had more than one sex partner since your last HIV test?
- Have you injected drugs and shared needles, syringes, or other drug injection equipment (e.g., cookers) with others?
- Have you exchanged sex for drugs or money?
- Have you been diagnosed with or treated for another sexually transmitted disease (STD)?
- Have you been diagnosed with or treated for hepatitis or tuberculosis?
- Have you had sex with someone who could answer yes to any of the above questions or someone whose sexual history you do not know?

You should be tested at least once a year if you keep doing any of these things. Sexually active gay and bisexual men may benefit from more frequent testing (e.g., every 3 to 6 months).

WHAT STEPS YOU CAN TAKE TO PREVENT GETTING HIV?

You should continue to take care of yourself, even if you do not have HIV

- See your healthcare provider regularly.
- Discuss your HIV risk behaviors honestly with your healthcare provider.
- Your healthcare provider can provide information on steps you can take to lower your risk of getting HIV and direct you to HIV prevention counseling services. If you are sexually active, get tested for other STDs and

have your partner get tested too. Having another STD increases the chances of getting or transmitting HIV.

- Use condoms the right way every time you have sex. Condoms can protect against other STDs.
- Consider taking PrEP, a medication that can help you stay HIV negative, even if your partner might have HIV.
- If you inject drugs, the best way to protect yourself is to stop injecting drugs. If you continue to inject drugs, use new, sterile needles and other tools every time and never share them.
- Call your healthcare provider immediately if you think you may have been exposed to HIV and ask them about medicine that may help prevent HIV infection within 72 hours of exposure (called "post-exposure prophylaxis," or PEP).
- If your partner has HIV, encourage them to stay on treatment. People with HIV who take their medicine as prescribed and maintain an undetectable viral load have effectively no risk of transmitting HIV to their HIV-negative sexual partners.

IF YOU GET A NEGATIVE RESULT, DOES THAT MEAN YOUR PARTNER IS ALSO HIV NEGATIVE?

No. Your HIV test result reveals only your HIV status.

- HIV is not necessarily transmitted every time you have sex or share needles, syringes, or other drug injection equipment. And the risk of getting HIV varies depending on the type of exposure or behavior. It is important to remember that taking an HIV test is not a way to find out if your partner has HIV.
- It is important to be open with your partners and ask them to tell you their HIV status. But keep in mind that your partners may not know or may be wrong about their status, and some may not tell you if they have HIV, even if they are aware of their status.

- Consider getting tested together so you can both know your HIV status and take steps to keep yourselves healthy.

WHAT IF YOUR TEST RESULT IS POSITIVE?

This is not the result you wanted. You may feel overwhelmed and worried but do not panic.

- If you use any type of antibody test and have a positive result, you will need another (follow-up) test to confirm your results.
- If you test in a community testing program or take a self-test, and it is positive, you should go to a healthcare provider to get follow-up testing.
- If your test is done in a healthcare setting or a lab, and it is positive, the lab will conduct the follow-up testing.

If your follow-up test is also positive, it means you have HIV (or are HIV positive).

IF YOU TEST POSITIVE FOR HIV, DOES THAT MEAN YOU HAVE AIDS?

No. Testing positive for HIV does not mean you have AIDS. AIDS is the most advanced stage of HIV disease. HIV can lead to AIDS if a person does not get treatment or take care of their health. But if a person with HIV takes their HIV medicine as prescribed, they may stay healthy for many years and may never be diagnosed with AIDS.

WILL OTHER PEOPLE KNOW YOUR TEST RESULT?

HIV tests may be "anonymous" or "confidential," depending on the reporting requirements in the state where you are tested.

- If you take an anonymous test, your name will not appear on the test results, and only you will see them.
- If you take a confidential test, your test results will go in your medical record like any other medical test results (e.g., blood pressure or cholesterol) and may be shared

with your primary healthcare provider and health insurance company.

- Otherwise, your HIV test results are protected by the same privacy laws that protect the rest of your health information.
- In other words, your information remains private and confidential.

SHOULD YOU TALK TO YOUR PARTNER ABOUT YOUR POSITIVE TEST RESULT?

You should tell any sex partners and anyone with whom you share needles or injection equipment that you have HIV, even if you are uncomfortable talking about it.

Communicating with each other about your HIV test result means you can take steps to protect both of you.

HOW DOES HIV AFFECT YOUR HEALTH?

HIV damages the body's ability to fight infections. It destroys CD4 cells, which are important infection-fighting cells in the body.

It is important that you start medical care and begin HIV treatment as soon as you are diagnosed with HIV. Antiretroviral therapy (taking medicine to treat HIV infection) is recommended for all people with HIV, regardless of how long they have had the virus or how healthy they are.

- HIV medicine works by lowering the amount of virus in your body to very low levels. HIV medicine can make the viral load so low that a test cannot detect it. This is called an "undetectable viral load."
- HIV medicine slows the progression of HIV and helps protect your immune system. If you take HIV medicine as prescribed and get and keep an undetectable viral load, you can stay healthy for many years.
- Having an undetectable viral load also helps prevent transmitting the virus to others. For example, if you have an undetectable viral load, you have effectively no

risk of transmitting HIV to an HIV-negative partner through sex.

Your healthcare provider will help:
- Decide which HIV medicines you should take based on how well your CD4 cells are working and how fast HIV is growing in your body.
- Assess your overall health and whether you have other diseases that need to be treated along with HIV.

Chapter 19 | You and Your HIV/AIDS Healthcare Provider: First Steps

Chapter Contents

Section 19.1 | Choosing a Healthcare Provider

This section includes text excerpted from "Locate an HIV Care Provider," HIV.gov, U.S. Department of Health and Human Services (HHS), February 10, 2022.

HOW DO YOU FIND AN HIV HEALTHCARE PROVIDER?

You can find an human immunodeficiency virus (HIV) healthcare provider by using your HIV Testing Sites and Care Services Locator (www.locator.hiv.gov). Just enter your zipcode to be connected to HIV medical care and other services such as HIV testing locations, housing assistance, and substance abuse and mental-health services.

There are other ways to find HIV providers and services too:

- **Ask your primary care provider**. If you have a primary care provider (someone who manages your regular medical care), that person may have the medical knowledge to treat your HIV. If not, she or he can refer you to a provider who specializes in providing HIV care and treatment.
- **Call your state HIV/AIDS hotline**. State HIV/AIDS toll-free hotlines (www.hab.hrsa.gov/get-care/state-hivaids-hotlines) are available to help connect you to agencies that can help determine what services you are eligible for and help you get them.
- **Search the Referral Link directory**. The American Academy of HIV Medicine's (AAHIVM) Referral Link (providers.aahivm.org/referral-link-search) is a directory of healthcare providers specializing in HIV management and prevention across the country. The doctors and clinicians represented in this database practice in a variety of care settings including health centers, Ryan White clinics, and private practices.
- **Use your home HIV test hotline**. If you received an HIV diagnosis by using an HIV home test kit, it is important that you take the next steps to make sure your test result is correct. Home test manufacturers

provide confidential counseling to answer questions and provide local referrals for follow-up testing and care.

WHY DO YOU NEED TO FIND AN HIV HEALTHCARE PROVIDER?

After you are diagnosed with HIV, it is important to see a healthcare provider who can help you start HIV medication (called "antiretroviral therapy" or "ART") as soon as possible. Treatment with HIV medicine is recommended for all people with HIV, regardless of how long they have had the virus or how healthy they are.

HIV medicine can reduce the amount of HIV in your blood (also called "your viral load") to an undetectable level – a level so low that a standard lab test can't detect it. People with HIV who take HIV medicine exactly as prescribed and get and keep an undetectable viral load can stay healthy and have effectively no risk of transmitting HIV to their HIV-negative sexual partners. This is often referred to as treatment as prevention or "undetectable = untransmittable" (U=U).

HOW SOON DO YOU NEED TO FIND AN HIV HEALTHCARE PROVIDER?

The U.S. Department of Health and Human Services (HHS) guidelines on the use of HIV medicines in adults and adolescents recommend that people with HIV start medical care and begin HIV treatment as soon as possible. If you have the following conditions, it is especially important to start ART right away: pregnancy, AIDS, certain HIV-related illnesses and coinfections, and early HIV infection. (Early HIV infection is the period up to six months after infection with HIV.)

Section 19.2 | Types of Healthcare Providers

This section contains text excerpted from the following sources: Text under the heading "Who Should Be on Your Healthcare Team?" is excerpted from "Types of Providers," HIV.gov, U.S. Department of Health and Human Services (HHS), May 21, 2018. Reviewed February 2022; Text under the heading "How Can You Work Best with Your Healthcare Team?" is excerpted from "Take Charge of Your Care," HIV.gov, U.S. Department of Health and Human Services (HHS), May 15, 2017. Reviewed February 2022.

WHO SHOULD BE ON YOUR HEALTHCARE TEAM?

Finding a healthcare team that is knowledgeable about HIV care is an important step in managing your care and treatment. If you are able to choose your provider, you should look for someone who has a great deal of experience treating HIV. This matters because the more HIV experience your provider has, the more familiar she or he will be with the full range of treatment options that exist today, as well as the unique issues that can come up in HIV care over time.

Who is on your HIV healthcare team will depend on your healthcare needs and the way that the healthcare system, clinic, or office you will get your care from is set up. It should also be based on your preferences and what will work best for you. Do not get hung up on finding the perfect provider the first week after you are diagnosed. The most important thing you can do now for your health is to meet with an HIV provider who can order your first lab tests and start HIV treatment as soon as possible. Do not let the search for the perfect doctor slow you down on this. You can change doctors later if you need to.

Your HIV healthcare provider should lead your healthcare team. That person will help you determine which HIV medicines are best for you, prescribe antiretroviral therapy (ART), monitor your progress, and partner with you in managing your health. She or he can also help put you in touch with other types of providers who can address your needs. Your primary HIV healthcare provider may be a doctor of medicine (MD) or doctor of osteopathic medicine (DO), nurse practitioner (NP), or a physician assistant (PA). Some women may prefer to see an obstetrics and gynaecology (OB-GYN) provider who has expertise in HIV/AIDS. On the whole, the patients of providers with more experience in HIV care tend to do better than those who see a provider who only has limited HIV care experience.

In addition to your HIV healthcare provider, your healthcare team may include other healthcare providers, allied healthcare professionals, and social service providers who are experts in taking care of people living with HIV.

The types of professionals who may be involved in your HIV care include:

Healthcare Providers

- **Medical doctors (MD or DO).** Healthcare professionals who are licensed to practice medicine.
- **Nurse practitioners (NP).** Registered nurses, with specialized graduate education, who can diagnose and treat illnesses independently, or as part of a healthcare team.
- **Physician assistants (PA).** Healthcare professionals who are trained to examine patients, diagnose injuries and illnesses, and provide treatment to patients under the supervision of physicians and surgeons.

Allied Healthcare Professionals

- **Nurses.** Healthcare professionals who provide and coordinate patient care as part of a healthcare team.
- **Mental-health providers.** Professionals, such as a counselor, psychologist, or psychiatrist, who provide mental healthcare in the form of counselling or other types of therapy.
- **Pharmacists.** Healthcare professionals who provide prescription medicines to patients and offer expertise in the safe use of prescriptions. Pharmacists may also provide advice on how to lead a healthy life; conduct health and wellness screenings; provide immunizations; and oversee medicines given to patients.
- **Nutritionists/dietitians.** Experts in food and nutrition who advise people on what to eat in order to lead a healthy lifestyle or achieve a specific health-related goal.

- **Dentists.** Healthcare professionals who diagnose and treat problems with a person's teeth, gums, and related parts of the mouth. Dentists also provide advice and instruction on taking care of teeth and gums and on diet choices that affect oral health.

Social Service Providers

- **Social workers.** Professionals who help people solve and cope with problems in their everyday lives.
- **Case managers.** Professionals who help people find the support and services they need, develop a services plan, and follow up to make sure that services are provided.
- **Substance use/abuse specialists.** Counselors who provide advice, treatment, and support to people who have problems with substance use.

Patient navigators. There are a number of different types of navigators who are trained and culturally sensitive workers who provide support and guidance to people by helping them "navigate" through the healthcare system. For example, navigators could be healthcare workers, social workers, those who work for community-based organizations, or peers.

HOW CAN YOU WORK BEST WITH YOUR HEALTHCARE TEAM?

Human immunodeficiency virus treatment is most successful when you actively take part in your medical care. That means taking your HIV medications every time, at the right time, and in the right way; keeping your medical appointments, and communicating honestly with your healthcare provider. This can be achieved when you:

- **Keep all of your medical appointments.** There are many tools you can use to help you remember and prepare for your appointments. You can:
  - Use a calendar to mark your appointment days
  - Set reminders on your phone
  - Download a free app from the Internet to your computer or smartphone that can help remind you

of your medical appointments. Search for "reminder apps" and you will find many choices.

- Keep your appointment card reminder in a place where you will see it often, such as on a mirror, or on your refrigerator
- Ask a family member or friend to help you remember your appointment
- **Be prepared for your medical appointments**. Before an appointment, write down questions or concerns you want to discuss with your healthcare provider. Be prepared to write down the answers you receive during your visit.
  - If you cannot keep a scheduled appointment, contact your provider to let them know, and make a new appointment as soon as possible.
- **Communicate openly and honestly with your healthcare providers**. Your healthcare provider needs to have the most accurate information to manage your care and treatment.
- **Keep track of your medical services**. You may have multiple healthcare providers working on your healthcare team. Keep records of your lab results, medical visits, appointment dates and times, medicines and medicine schedules, and care and treatment plans.
- **Update your contact information**. Make sure your healthcare providers have your correct contact information (telephone number, address, and e-mail address) and let them know if any contact information changes.

Chapter 20 | Laboratory Tests after an HIV Diagnosis

Laboratory tests can help keep tabs on your health. Some of these tests will be done soon after you learn you are HIV positive. Then depending on your immune status, whether you are on medication or not, and a variety of other factors, your provider will set up a schedule for you.

The lab tests look at:

- How well your immune system is functioning cluster of differentiation 4 (CD4 count)
- How rapidly HIV is replicating, or multiplying (viral load)
- How well your body is functioning (tests to look at your kidneys, liver, cholesterol, and blood cells)
- Whether you have other diseases that are associated with HIV (tests for certain infections)

The first set of lab tests ideally is done shortly after you find out you have HIV, and the results establish a starting point or "baseline." Future tests will let you know how far from this baseline you have moved. This can help you tell how fast or slow the disease is moving and indicate whether treatments are working.

Most labs include a "normal" range (high and low values) when they report test results. The most important results are the ones

This chapter includes text excerpted from "Understanding Laboratory Tests," U.S. Department of Veterans Affairs (VA), October 17, 2019.

that fall outside these normal ranges. Test results often go up and down over time so do not worry about small changes. Instead, look for overall trends.

CD4 COUNT (OR T-CELL COUNT)

The CD4 cells (also known as "CD4+ T cells") are white blood cells (WBCs) that fight infection. CD4 cell count is an indicator of immune function in patients living with HIV and one of the key determinants for the need of opportunistic infection (OI) prophylaxis. CD4 cell counts are obtained from bloodwork as part of laboratory monitoring for HIV infection.

The CD4+ cell counts are usually measured when you are diagnosed with HIV (at baseline), every 3 to 6 months during first 2 years or until your CD4 count increases above 300 cells/mm3. Otherwise, your CD4+ cell count may be measured every 12 months. Most people who are on HIV treatment can expect an average increase of about 50–100 cells/mm3 a year. Patients who initiate therapy with a low CD4 count or at an older age may not have the same increase in their CD4 count despite virologic suppression.

There are multiple factors that affect your CD4 count. Taking your medication is one way to keep your count high, but medications or acute infections are among the things that could affect the CD4 count. If you are responding well to your medications, you may need less frequent testing going forward.

HIV VIRAL LOAD (OR HIV RNA)

Human immunodeficiency virus (HIV) viral load tests measure the amount of HIV in the blood. Lower levels are better than higher levels. The main goal of HIV drugs is to reduce the HIV viral load to an "undetectable" level, meaning that the HIV ribonucleic acid (RNA) is below the level that the test is able to count.

The lower limit of HIV RNA detection depends on the test used – some go down to 50 copies/ml, while other go as low as 20. High viral loads are linked to faster disease progression. Reducing the viral load to "undetectable" levels slows or stops disease progression and prevents HIV transmission to sex partners. Treatment for HIV suppresses the virus but does not eliminate it. Even if HIV levels are not detectable in the bloodstream, HIV is still in the body and will rebound to detectable if the HIV medicines are stopped.

CD4 counts and HIV viral load tests are usually done when you first see a medical provider and about every 3 months afterward. Results tell whether the HIV medications are working well; and for people who have chosen to delay taking medicines, they can help you and your provider monitor your health and decide how urgent it is for you to start taking HIV drugs or medicines to prevent infections (more on this in Treatment Decisions).

RESISTANCE TEST (HIV GENOTYPE)

This test determines whether the particular virus in your body is resistant to HIV medications.

HIV reproduces rapidly and, as the virus makes copies of itself, small changes (or mutations) sometimes result. These changes can lead to different HIV strains, particularly if the person is taking (or has taken) HIV medicines but the HIV virus is not completely controlled or suppressed. If a strain that is resistant to your HIV drugs develops, the virus will be able to grow even though you are on medication. Your viral load will start to rise. The resistant virus soon will become the most common strain in your body. If this occurs, your provider may order a resistance test to check for mutations in the HIV virus.

A person can be infected with a drug resistant strain of HIV if the infection was from an individual with resistant virus. For this reason, an HIV resistance test is recommended for all people as soon as they are diagnosed with HIV.

Therefore, resistance testing is performed upon diagnosis of HIV and if a medication regimen is no longer keeping the viral load suppressed.

COMPLETE BLOOD COUNT

This test looks at the different cells in your blood, including red blood cells (RBCs), WBCs, and platelets.

- The RBCs cells carry oxygen to other cells in your body. If the level of your RBCs is too low, you have anemia.

Anemia can cause fatigue. Tests that look at your red blood cells include hemoglobin and hematocrit. Hematocrit refers to the percentage of your blood that consists of RBCs. A normal hematocrit is about 37–47 percent in females and 40–54 percent in males.

- WBCs come in many types, and all are involved in your immune system's effort to keep you healthy (the CD4 cell is a type of WBC). High WBC counts may indicate that you are fighting an infection. Low counts may put you at risk of getting an infection.
- Platelets help with clotting, so if your platelets fall too low, your blood may not clot well. You may bleed more than usual, for example, when you brush your teeth or shave your skin. As the platelet count falls, the chance of internal bleeding rises.

These tests are usually done every 3 to 6 months, unless your lab values are fluctuating a lot, or you have symptoms of HIV disease. Then the tests may be done more often.

BLOOD CHEMISTRY TESTS

Chemistry tests examine the levels of different elements and waste products in the blood and help determine how well different organs are functioning. Usually, the tests are divided into two panels:

- **Electrolyte tests (sometimes called "lytes") and kidney function.** These tests help measure how well your kidneys are working, and measure the balance of fluids, acids, and sugar in your body. They include tests for sodium, potassium, chloride, blood urea nitrogen (BUN), creatinine, and glucose.
- **Liver function tests (LFTs).** These tests measure whether your liver is being damaged. (Things that can damage the liver include viral hepatitis, alcohol, street drugs, and certain medications.) These tests measure alkaline phosphatase, alanine aminotransferase (ALT), aspartate aminotransferase (AST), albumin, and bilirubin.

Blood chemistry tests are usually done every 3 to 6 months. It is important to have these done at baseline and while you are on HIV medications to make sure the medications are safe for your kidneys and liver.

LIPID PROFILE

The level of certain fats in the blood can give clues to your risk of heart disease. Cholesterol and triglycerides are important for health, but too much of them in the blood can cause fatty deposits to form in the arteries. This increases the chances of a heart attack. Too much triglyceride can also lead to pancreatitis, a serious inflammation of the pancreas. High cholesterol and high triglycerides can occur in people living with HIV. They can also be a side effect of some of the older HIV medications.

Cholesterol is measured by three different tests:

- Total cholesterol
- High-density lipoprotein (HDL), often referred to as "good" cholesterol because high levels lower your risk of heart disease
- Low-density lipoprotein (LDL), often referred to as "bad" cholesterol because high levels raise your risk of heart disease

These tests are usually done at least once a year, and more often if your levels are high or you require medication to control triglyceride and cholesterol levels. Your provider may want the lipid panel to be done while you are fasting, which means nothing to eat or drink (except water) after midnight the night before the test. This gives the most accurate evaluation of the cholesterol and triglycerides in the blood. Be sure to ask your provider if the blood tests are recommended to be done fasting.

TUBERCULOSIS TEST

Tuberculosis test (TB) is short for tuberculosis, an infection usually spread by breathing in air that has been contaminated by someone with TB of the lungs. Most people who are exposed to TB do not get sick from it, the bacteria can live in the body for a long time without causing disease. But, some people who carry the bacteria develop tuberculosis disease, and this is more likely if the immune system is weakened.

There are two types of tests to determine whether people are carrying the TB bacteria. One is the TB skin test (also known as "Pharmaceutical Product Development" (PPD), which requires the person to return to the clinic 2–3 days after the skin test is placed for the test to be interpreted. The other is a blood test called an "interferon-gamma release assay" (IGRA) (QuantiFERON and TSpotTB are two examples of IGRA blood tests).

If a person tests positive for carrying the TB bacteria in their body, tests are done to determine whether it is currently causing infection of the lungs (which is contagious). Anyone with active TB should get an effective combination of medications to be cured. If, however, there is no active infection, antibiotics can be used to prevent trouble in the future. In this setting antibiotics are given for 3–9 months.

SEXUALLY TRANSMITTED DISEASES SCREENING

If you got infected with HIV from unprotected sex, there is a chance you may have become infected with other sexually transmitted diseases, too. These include syphilis, gonorrhea, and chlamydia. Hepatitis B and hepatitis C can be sexually transmitted as well, particularly among men who have sex with men.

Infections of syphilis, gonorrhea, and chlamydia can occur in the throat, penis, vagina, and rectum. The bacteria that cause syphilis and gonorrhea can also spread through the blood to other parts of your body. Having one of these other diseases can make your HIV worse. They can also make you 2 to 5 times more likely to pass HIV along to a sexual partner. Syphilis, for example, can cause open sores on your genitals, which allows easy passage of HIV from you to your partner.

Tests for sexually transmitted diseases (STDs), hepatitis B, and hepatitis C should be done at baseline. STD tests should be repeated at least once a year if you are sexually active and have had more than one sex partner since your last clinic visit. Men who have sex with men who have multiple or anonymous sex partners are rec-ommended to be screened every 3 to 6 months, and this is a good idea for anyone with new partners.

HEPATITIS A, B, AND C

Your liver is an organ that processes almost everything you put into your body, including medications. Viruses can infect and irritate the liver causing damage, scarring, and possibly liver failure. The three most common viruses that can infect the liver are hepatitis A, hepatitis B, and hepatitis C.

- **Hepatitis A virus (HAV).** This virus is transmitted through contaminated food, water, or through the feces of someone who is infected. When you are diagnosed with HIV, your providers will check your blood to see whether you have protection from HAV either from previous infection or previous vaccination. If you have protection, great! There is nothing more to do. But if you do not, you may be offered the vaccine to prevent future infection.
- **Hepatitis B virus (HBV).** This virus is easily spread through contaminated blood and body fluids. When you are diagnosed with HIV, your providers will check your blood to see if you have either active infection, protection from infection, or no protection from HBV. If you have protection from infection, great! There is nothing else to do. If you do not have protection, you will be offered the HBV vaccine to protect from future infection. If HBV is found in your bloodstream (i.e., active infection), you will be offered medication that can kill both HBV and HIV.
- **Hepatitis C virus (HCV).** This virus is transmitted through contaminated blood. When you are diagnosed with HIV, your providers will check your blood to see if you have HCV. If so, you will be offered medication to cure your HCV. There is always risk of reinfection if re-exposed to the virus. Unfortunately, there is no vaccine for protection against HCV.

Part 4 | Treatments and Therapies for HIV/AIDS

Chapter 21 | Treatment Overview

WHAT IS HIV TREATMENT?

Human immunodeficiency virus (HIV) treatment involves taking medicines that slow the progression of the virus in your body. HIV is a type of virus called a "retrovirus," and the combination of drugs used to treat it is called "antiretroviral therapy" (ART). ART is recommended for all people living with HIV, regardless of how long they have had the virus or how healthy they are. ART must be taken every day, exactly as your healthcare provider prescribes.

WHY IS HIV TREATMENT IMPORTANT?

Getting and staying on HIV treatment because it reduces the amount of HIV in your blood (also called the "viral load") to a very low level. This keeps you healthy and prevents illness. There is also a major prevention benefit. People living with HIV who take HIV medication daily as prescribed and get and keep an undetectable viral load have effectively no risk of sexually transmitting HIV to their HIV-negative partners. This is called "treatment as prevention."

If left untreated, HIV attacks your immune system and can allow different types of life-threatening infections and cancers to develop. If your CD4 cell count falls below a certain level, you are at risk of getting an opportunistic infection. These are infections that do not normally affect people with healthy immune systems but that can infect people with immune systems weakened by HIV infection.

This chapter includes text excerpted from "HIV Treatment Overview," HIV.gov, U.S. Department of Health and Human Services (HHS), March 29, 2019.

Your healthcare provider may prescribe medicines to prevent certain infections.

HIV treatment is most likely to be successful when you know what to expect and are committed to taking your medicines exactly as prescribed. Working with your healthcare provider to develop a treatment plan will help you learn more about HIV and manage it effectively.

WHEN SHOULD YOU START HIV TREATMENT?

Treatment guidelines from the U.S. Department of Health and Human Services (HHS) recommend that a person living with HIV begin ART as soon as possible after diagnosis. Starting ART slows the progression of HIV and can keep you healthy for many years.

If you delay treatment, the virus will continue to harm your immune system and put you at higher risk for developing opportunistic infections that can be life-threatening.

DOES ANTIRETROVIRAL THERAPY CAUSE SIDE EFFECTS?

Like most medicines, antiretroviral therapy can cause side effects. However, not everyone experiences side effects from ART. The HIV medications used today have fewer side effects, fewer people experience them, and they are less severe than in the past. Side effects can differ for each type of ART medicine and from person to person. Some side effects can occur once you start medicine and may only last a few days or weeks. Other side effects can start later and last longer.

If you experience side effects that are severe or make you want to stop taking your HIV medication, talk to your healthcare provider or pharmacist before you miss any doses or stop taking the medication. Skipping doses or starting and stopping medication can lead to drug resistance, which can harm your health and limit your future treatment options.

Some side effects of ART that are most commonly reported include:
- Nausea and vomiting
- Diarrhea

- Difficulty sleeping
- Dry mouth
- Headache
- Rash
- Dizziness
- Fatigue and
- Pain

And be aware; HIV medicines also may cause different side effects in women than men.

Contact your healthcare provider or pharmacist immediately if you begin to experience problems or if your treatment makes you sick. If side effects make you want to skip taking your medications sometimes or stop taking them altogether, talk to your healthcare provider or pharmacist right away to find solutions that work for you. Your healthcare provider may prescribe medicines to reduce or eliminate side effects or may recommend changing your medication to another type of ART that might work better for you.

HIV DRUG RESISTANCE?

Drug resistance can be a cause of treatment failure for people living with HIV. As HIV multiplies in the body, it sometimes mutates (changes form) and produces variations of itself. Variations of HIV that develop while a person is taking ART can lead to drug-resistant strains of HIV.

With drug resistance, HIV medicines that previously controlled a person's HIV are not effective against new, drug-resistant HIV. In other words, the HIV medicines cannot prevent the drug-resistant HIV from multiplying. Drug resistance can cause HIV treatment to fail.

A person can initially be infected with drug-resistant HIV or develop drug-resistant HIV after starting HIV medicines. Drug-resistant HIV also can spread from person to person. Drug-resistance testing identifies which, if any, HIV medicines would not be effective against your specific strain of HIV. Drug-resistance testing results help determine which HIV medicines to include in an HIV treatment regimen.

Taking HIV medication every day, exactly as prescribed helps prevent drug resistance.

Chapter 22 | Decision Making: To Start Therapy or Not

Human immunodeficiency virus (HIV) is a virus that can multiply quickly in your body and damage your immune system. Your immune system is what allows your body to fight off infections and cancers. Without treatment, HIV can make your immune system very weak. When it is weakened, you will have a hard time staying well.

Even though we do not yet have a cure for HIV, there are many different drugs that can shut down the HIV virus, greatly slow down the damage it does, and allow the immune system to recover. Effective treatment allows most people to live long and healthy lives, and essentially prevents transmission of HIV to sex partners.

It is important to talk through treatment decisions with your provider.

STARTING THERAPY

HIV drugs are essential in keeping people healthy over the years. Effective treatment stops or slows the progression of HIV and has important benefits, even for persons whose immune systems appear to be functioning well. HIV drugs are recommended for all people with HIV infection. Starting treatment as soon as possible

This chapter includes text excerpted from "Treatment Decisions for HIV," U.S. Department of Veterans Affairs (VA), August 1, 2019.

after someone is diagnosed with HIV is better than delaying, so long as you are ready to start.

Studies show that starting treatment early is the most effective way to prevent long-term consequences of HIV. And, treatment that suppresses the HIV virus can prevent transmission (spread) of HIV to sex partners (or injection drug use partners); for pregnant women, it can prevent infection of the baby in the womb or at birth.

There are a few things to know about as you think about starting treatment. First, the current drug regimens usually are very simple (between 1 and 3 pills per day), and they work very well, so long as you take them every day. Second, it is really important to take the medicines correctly every day or the virus may become resistant to the drugs. That means the virus may change in a way that makes the drugs no longer work. The most common cause of drug resistance is not taking medications correctly every day. So, people need to be ready to commit to taking the medications every day (we call this "adherence"). And third, HIV medicines, like any other drugs, may cause side effects in some people. But, people who take the newer HIV drugs usually do not have any problems with them. If you do have side effects, let your providers know so that they can work with you to solve this problem.

So, as we said earlier, treatment is recommended for all people with HIV. Experts generally advise starting treatment soon after you are diagnosed with HIV, and your provider may even offer you treatment on the same day you receive your diagnosis. Here are some things your provider may consider in advising you about when to start:

- Symptoms of HIV disease (also called your clinical status, or how well you feel)
- Your CD4 count and HIV viral load
- Whether you have certain other medical conditions that may be helped by HIV treatment
- Whether you can and will stick to your treatment plan (adherence)
- Whether you have sex partner(s) who are HIV-negative and may be at risk of becoming infected through you

- Whether you are pregnant or wish to become pregnant soon

Symptoms (Clinical Status)

"Clinical status" refers to how well you are doing in general, including how well you feel. Your provider will look at whether you have symptoms of HIV disease. These symptoms are signs that HIV is weakening your immune system, and include things such as weight loss, chronic fevers, and opportunistic infections. (Opportunistic infections – also called "OIs" – are infections that can happen in someone with a damaged immune system.)

CD4 Count and Viral Load

Even though you may not feel it, when you have HIV, the virus and your immune system are at war with each other. The virus is trying to multiply as fast as it can, and your body is trying to stop it. Two tests, the CD4 count and the HIV viral load, help you and your provider know how strong your immune system is, and whether it is keeping HIV under control.

CD4 cells play a major role in helping your immune system work properly. HIV causes disease by killing off CD4 cells. It does this by infecting the cells and turning them into virus factories. The CD4 count tells us how many CD4 cells you have. The higher the number, the better.

The HIV viral load test indicates how much of the HIV virus is present in your blood, and how fast it is multiplying. The higher the viral load, the faster HIV is infecting and killing your CD4 cells. The lower the viral load, the better.

Your provider will look at these two things carefully. People whose CD4 count is low, and people whose viral load is high, are more likely to get sick sooner than people with a high CD4 count and low viral load.

CD4 count and viral load tests usually are done before treatment is started and then regularly while someone is on treatment. As we said earlier, HIV medicines are recommended for everyone, no matter how high or low their CD4 count is. And HIV treatment is especially urgent if your CD4 count is lower, or if you have symptoms.

Whether You Have Certain Other Medical Conditions That May Be Helped by HIV Treatment

Starting HIV drugs may be particularly important for people with certain other medical conditions. For example, your provider will recommend HIV treatment if you are pregnant or plan to become pregnant, if you have kidney disease that is caused by HIV, or if you have hepatitis B or hepatitis C.

Whether You Can and Will Stick to Your Treatment Plan (Adherence)

Before you start medications for HIV, it is very important to make a strong commitment to sticking to a drug treatment plan (or regimen). With an HIV drug regimen, you need to take medicines every day!

In order for the drugs to work and keep working, you must carefully follow the directions for taking them. If you are not sure you can do this, you might need help in finding ways to stick to the plan.

If you are wondering whether you should start taking treatment for HIV, talk with your provider as soon as possible. Depending on your specific needs, your provider can come up with a personal treatment plan for you.

Risk of Transmitting HIV: To Sex Partners or during Pregnancy

HIV treatment has been shown to greatly reduce the risk of transmitting HIV to uninfected sex partners. In fact, if you take your medicines every day and your HIV treatment is working well, there is almost no risk of transmitting HIV to a sex partner. Thus, if you have a sex partner who is HIV negative, you may consider starting HIV treatment both to protect and improve your own health and to prevent transmission to your partners. Similarly, if you are pregnant or intend to become pregnant, it is important to start HIV treatment right away both to protect your own health and to reduce the risk of passing HIV to the baby during pregnancy or at the time of birth.

WHAT DRUGS TO TAKE

Your provider will talk with you and together you will come up with a personal treatment plan. You may find it easier to understand your plan if you learn about the different drugs available and what they do.

What Kinds of Drugs Are Available?

HIV drugs are also called "antiretroviral drugs" or "antiretrovirals" (ARVs). A whole treatment regimen is called "antiretroviral therapy," or "ART." The ARVs work because they attack the HIV virus directly – they cripple the ability of the virus to make copies of itself. Usually, an ART regimen consists of 3 different medicines from at least 2 classes (types) of drugs. This is because it takes a powerful combination of medicines to suppress the HIV virus.

There are 5 main classes of HIV drugs:

- Nucleoside reverse transcriptase inhibitors (NRTIs or "nukes")
- Nonnucleoside reverse transcriptase inhibitors (NNRTIs or "nonnukes")
- Integrase inhibitors
- Protease inhibitors (PIs)
- Entry inhibitors

Each group attacks HIV in its own way and helps your body fight the infection. Most of these drugs come as tablets or capsules. Several of these drugs may be combined into one tablet to make it easier to take your medications. These are known as "fixed-dose combinations" or "single tablet regimens."

The following is a short description of how each group of drugs works.

Nucleoside Reverse Transcriptase Inhibitors (Nucleoside Analogues, NRTIs, or Nukes)

When the HIV virus enters a healthy cell, it attempts to make copies of itself. It does this by using an enzyme called "reverse transcriptase." The NRTIs work because they block that enzyme. Without reverse transcriptase, HIV cannot make new virus copies of itself.

Nonnucleoside Reverse Transcriptase Inhibitors (NNRTIs, Nonnukes, or Nonnucleosides)

These drugs also prevent HIV from using reverse transcriptase to make copies of itself, but in a different way.

Protease Inhibitors

Once HIV has infected a cell and made copies of itself, it uses an enzyme called "protease" to process itself correctly so it can be released from the cell to infect other cells. These medicines work by blocking protease.

Integrase Inhibitors

This class of anti-HIV drugs works by blocking an enzyme (HIV integrase) that the virus needs in order to insert copies of itself into human deoxyribonucleic acid (DNA).

Chemokine Coreceptor Antagonists

To infect a cell, HIV must bind to two types of molecules on the cell's surface. One of these is called a "chemokine coreceptor." Drugs known as "chemokine coreceptor antagonists" (CCR5) block the virus from binding to the coreceptor.

Entry Inhibitors

The entry inhibitors that are currently available work in different ways, by preventing HIV from entering the CD4 T cell, blocking HIV from binding to the CD4 receptor, or blocking HIV from binding to a coreceptor.

Multi-Class Drug Combinations

There are a number of combination tablets that include drugs from two different groups in a complete HIV drug regimen. A patient prescribed one of these combinations typically takes only one tablet, once a day. You and your provider can decide whether these drug combinations are right for you.

Which Drugs Should You Take?

Now that you have learned a little about the types of drugs that are available and how they work, you may be wondering how your provider will know which treatment you should take.

HIV drugs are used in combination with one another in order to get the best results. The goal is to get the viral load as low as possible (to levels that are undetectable by standard laboratory tests) for as long as possible.

HIV drugs do different things to the virus – they attack it in different ways – so using combinations works better than using just one by itself. Combinations usually include three antiretroviral drugs. Except in very special circumstances, anti-HIV drugs should never be used one or two at a time. Using only one or two drugs at a time can fail to control the viral load and let the virus adapt (or become resistant) to the drug. Once the virus adapts to a drug, the drug would not work as well against the virus, and maybe it would not work at all.

There is no one combination of HIV drugs that works best for everyone. Each combination has its pluses and minuses.

So, how will your provider know which combination to choose? You and your provider can consider the options, keeping certain things in mind, such as possible side effects, the number of pills you will need to take, and how the drugs interact with each other and with other medications you may take.

Print out these questions to ask your healthcare provider so that you will be ready to discuss combination therapy.

Combination Therapy

So, how will your health provider know which combination to choose? You and your provider can consider the options, keeping certain things in mind, such as possible side effects, the number of pills you will need to take, and how the drugs interact with each other and with other medications you may take.

Print out these questions to ask your healthcare provider if you are considering combination therapy.

Sticking to Your Medicines (Adherence)

"Adherence" refers to how well you stay on your treatment plan – whether you take your medications exactly as your provider tells you.

If you follow your provider's instructions, the HIV drugs will work well to lower the amount of virus in your blood. Taking your drugs correctly increases your likelihood of success.

But, if you miss doses, or do not follow a regular schedule, your treatment may not work, and the HIV virus may become resistant to the medicines.

Before you start a treatment plan, you should:
- Get your provider to write everything down for you. names of the drugs, what they look like, how to take them (e.g., with food or not, with other medications or not), and how often to take them. This way, you will have something to look at in case you forget what you are supposed to do.
- With your provider's help, develop a plan that works for you.
- Pop question. True or false. Missing doses and not following a regular schedule can lessen the effect of your HIV medication.
- Answer. TRUE. Missing doses and not following a regular schedule can lessen the effect of your HIV medication. It is very important that you stay on your treatment plan and follow your provider's instructions for taking your medicine.

Questions to Ask about Each Drug

One of the most important things you can do to make sure you take your medicine correctly is to talk with your medical provider about your lifestyle, such as your sleeping and eating schedule. If your provider prescribes a drug, be sure and ask the following questions (and make sure you understand the answers):
- What dose of the drug should be taken? How many pills does this mean?
- How often should the drug be taken?

- Does it matter if it is taken with food, or on an empty stomach?
- Does the drug have to be kept in a refrigerator?
- What are the possible side effects of the drug?
- What should be done to deal with the side effects?
- How severe do side effects have to be before a provider is called?

During every medical visit you should talk about whether you are having trouble staying on your treatment plan. Studies show that people who take their medicine in the right way get the best results, their viral loads stay down, their CD4 counts stay up, and they feel healthier.

Tips for Staying on Your Treatment Plan

Before you start a treatment plan, you should:
- Get your healthcare provider to write everything down for you. Names of the drugs, what they look like, how to take them (e.g., with food or not, with other medications or not), and how often to take them. This way, you will have something to look at in case you forget what you are supposed to do.
- With your provider's help, develop a plan that works for you.

WHETHER TO CONTINUE THERAPY
Other Challenges You Might Have While on HIV Therapy

Now that you have thought about adherence and some of the other factors you should consider before starting HIV drug therapy, let us look at some of the other things you will need to know once you are taking the medicine. These involve drug interactions and drug side effects.

What Are Drug Interactions?

Your HIV medications can be affected by other medicines, including other prescription drugs you are taking and drugs you buy over the counter at a pharmacy. Even herbal therapies, nutritional supplements, and some things found in common foods can affect your HIV medicines.

When one drug affects how another drug behaves, this is called a "drug-drug interaction." For example, some drugs become less effective or cause side effects when they are taken with certain other drugs.

When something in food affects how a drug behaves, it is called a "drug-food interaction." For example, grapefruit juice, taken at the same time as certain drugs, can boost the amount of these drugs in your bloodstream to an undesirable level. Everyone taking HIV drugs needs to be very careful about these interactions. Luckily, many of these interactions are well known to your provider and can be managed.

Your provider can give you a list of drugs and foods to avoid, depending on what treatment you are taking. Ask for this information for each drug that you are taking.

Also, be sure that you tell your provider about every single medication, drug, supplement, and herb you are taking – whether you got them by prescription or not.

How Do You Deal with Side Effects?

Some side effects can be hard to deal with. One way to cope with them is to know what to watch out for and have a plan to deal with problems that come up.

That is why you need to talk to your provider about the risk of side effects from different drugs, before you start therapy.

At the beginning of any treatment, you go through a period of adjustment – a time when your body has to get used to the new drugs you are taking. Sometimes you will have headaches, an upset stomach, fatigue, or aches and pains. These side effects may go away after a few days or a few weeks.

If you notice any unusual or severe reactions after starting or changing a drug, report the side effects to your provider immediately.

How Do You Know If the Drugs Are Working?

After you have started taking drugs for HIV, your provider will look at how much HIV virus is in your bloodstream (your viral load) to see how well the drug therapy is working. If the drugs are working, your viral load goes down. You will have less of the virus in your bloodstream. A very important goal of treatment is to reduce the viral load to below the level that can be counted by laboratory tests, and to keep it there. This sometimes is called an "undetectable" level of HIV.

Other ways you and your provider can see if the drugs are working are:

- Your CD4 count. This number should stay the same or go up if your drugs are working.
- Your health checkups. Your treatment should help keep you healthy and help you fight off infections and diseases.

Should You Ever Take a 'Holiday' from the Drugs?

Taking a "drug holiday" from your HIV treatments for reasons other than a severe reaction to medications may be harmful to your health. Having said that, your provider may suggest that you temporarily stop your antiretroviral drugs for certain specific reasons. Be sure to talk with your provider about this issue if you have questions about it. How you stop taking your HIV drugs safely can be a complicated process.

Remember, just skipping doses without your provider's instruction is dangerous; you should never change your treatment plan without talking with your provider.

Should You Ever Switch the Drugs You Are Taking?

You should never change the drug plan you are on without talking with your provider. This is a very important decision and one that must be made with your provider.

There are a few reasons that your provider may suggest you change your medicines. There may be a fixed-dose combination pill that could simplify your therapy. Or your treatment may not be working well enough and you may need different medicines. Or you may have side effects that are bothering you, or lab tests that show signs of ill effects from the HIV drugs (this is called "drug toxicity").

Before changing medicines, you and your provider should talk about:

- All the HIV drugs you have taken before and the ones you have not taken
- Any drug resistance your HIV virus may have
- Possible side effects of the new medicines
- How well you will be able to follow the new drug treatment plan
- Always be sure to talk with your provider about any changes in your drug treatment

If the Viral Load Is Undetectable, Can You Stop Treatment?

No! Having a viral load below levels that laboratory tests can measure (an "undetectable" viral load) tells us that the HIV drugs are working. An undetectable viral load does not mean the HIV virus is gone from your body, though. Even though the virus is not detected in the blood, it is still present in other parts of your body, such as the lymph nodes, brain, and reproductive organs. If you stop treatment, the virus will start reproducing again and your viral load will increase, putting your health at risk.

What If Your Treatment Is Not Working?

Sometimes the HIV medications do not work. This may occur because the drugs do not completely stop the virus from reproducing. As the virus makes copies of itself, changes (or mutations) sometimes occur. These changes may result in a new strain of the virus that is resistant to the action of the drugs. If your providers think this has happened, they will do a blood test (called a "resistance test," "genotype," or "phenotype") that can help show which drugs the virus has become resistant to. This can help identify other drugs that might still work against your virus.

If a person has a strain of HIV that is resistant to most or all available drugs, that person may want to consider joining a clinical trial that is testing new drugs that have not yet been approved by the U.S. Food and Drug Administration (FDA).

Chapter 23 | How to Find HIV Treatment Services

WHERE CAN PEOPLE WITH HIV FIND A HEALTHCARE PROVIDER?

Healthcare providers are an essential part of successful human immunodeficiency virus (HIV) treatment. They prescribe HIV medicines and order tests to monitor their patients' health. People with HIV work with their healthcare providers to select an HIV treatment regimen that works best for their needs.

The following resources can help you find a healthcare provider:

- **State human immunodeficiency virus (HIV)/ acquired immunodeficiency syndrome (AIDS) Hotlines, from Health Resources and Services Administration (HRSA).** If you need help finding a healthcare provider or HIV/AIDS-related services in your area, call your state's HIV/AIDS hotline. The HRSA maintains a list of HIV/AIDS hotlines for the United States, the U.S. Virgin Islands, and Puerto Rico.
- **Find a Ryan White HIV/AIDS Program Medical Provider, from HRSA.** The Ryan White HIV/AIDS Program provides HIV treatment services to people with HIV who have no health insurance or who are underinsured. Use findhivcare.hrsa.gov to find a Ryan White HIV/AIDS Program Medical Provider search tool from HRSA to find medical providers in your area that participate in the Ryan White HIV/AIDS Program.
- **Find HIV Services Near You, from HIV.gov.** This search tool from HIV.gov can help you locate services

This chapter includes text excerpted from "How to Find HIV Treatment Services," HIVinfo, U.S. Department of Health and Human Services (HHS), August 23, 2021.

in your area, including HIV testing centers, sexually transmitted infections (STI) testing centers, pre-exposure prophylaxis (PrEP) services, mental-health services, family planning services, medical centers that participate in the Ryan White HIV/AIDS Program, housing assistance programs, and substance abuse treatment facilities.

WHERE CAN PEOPLE WITH HIV GET HELP PAYING FOR HIV MEDICINES?

There are several resources that can help people with HIV get the medicines they need:

- **AIDS Drug Assistance Programs (ADAPs) Directory, from the Advocacy Association**. ADAP makes HIV medicines and other services available to people who are living with HIV and who do not have sufficient health insurance or who need financial assistance. The ADAP Directory is an online resource that includes current ADAP-related information from the United States and several U.S. territories.
- **National Alliance of State and Territorial AIDS Directors' (NASTAD) Membership Directory**. Use the NASTAD directory to find healthcare specialists who administer HIV healthcare programs in your state.
- **Ready, Set, PrEP, from U.S. Department of Health and Human Services (HHS)**. The Ready, Set, PrEP program from HHS provides the HIV medicines that are used for PrEP at no cost for qualified applicants.
- **Drug Companies**. Some companies that make HIV medicines also have drug-assistance programs. To find the contact information for the manufacturer of an HIV medicine, search for the drug in the Clinical Info Drug Database (clinicalinfo.hiv.gov/en/drugs) and then scroll down the drug fact sheet to the section titled "Manufacturer Information."

WHERE CAN PEOPLE WITH HIV FIND HOUSING ASSISTANCE?

A stable living situation makes it easier for people with HIV to keep appointments with their healthcare provider and stick to an HIV treatment regimen.

- **Housing Opportunities for Persons with AIDS Program, from Housing and Urban Development (HUD).** The U.S. Department of HUD manages the Housing Opportunities for Persons with AIDS (HOPWA) program, which is designed to provide housing assistance to people living with HIV/AIDS and their families.

HOW CAN PEOPLE WITH HIV GET HELP WITH MENTAL-HEALTH ISSUES?

Anyone can have problems with mental health, but people with HIV are more likely to experience some mental-health conditions, such as depression, than people without HIV.

Below are some places to find mental health treatment services:

- **Substance Abuse and Mental Health Services Administration (SAMHSA).** SAMHSA is a U.S. government agency that offers resources for those looking for help with mental health problems or substance abuse. SAMHSA's treatment locator allows people to search for mental health and substance use treatment facilities in the United States. SAMHSA also operates a 24-hour National Suicide Prevention Lifeline.

- **Help for Mental Illnesses, from the National Institute of Mental Health (NIMH).** As part of HHS, the NIMH funds research on ways to prevent and treat mental health disorders. Their website includes a resources page to help people find healthcare providers and treatment services, locate clinical trials, and learn more about mental health.

Chapter 24 | Antiretroviral Treatment

Chapter Contents

Section 24.1 | **Antiretroviral Drug Discovery and Development**

This section includes text excerpted from "Antiretroviral Drug Discovery and Development," National Institute of Allergy and Infectious Diseases (NIAID), November 26, 2018. Reviewed February 2022.

For more than three decades, the National Institute of Allergy and Infectious Diseases (NIAID) has fostered and promoted development of antiretroviral therapies that have transformed human immunodeficiency virus (HIV) infection from an almost uniformly fatal infection into a manageable chronic condition. In the 1980s, the average life expectancy following an acquired immunodeficiency syndrome (AIDS) diagnosis was approximately one year. Nowadays, with combination antiretroviral drug treatments started early in the course of HIV infection, people living with HIV can expect a near-normal lifespan.

The NIAID plays a role in many stages of the antiretroviral drug discovery and development process. The search for new drugs remains a priority due to the development of resistance against existing drugs and the unwanted side effects associated with some current drugs. NIAID supports basic research to identify novel strategies to prevent HIV from taking hold and replicating in the body, as well as preclinical research to formulate antiretroviral drugs that can be tested in people.

The NIAID also helps advance clinical drug development. NIAID nowadays supports the largest networks of HIV therapeutic clinical trial units in the world, including the AIDS Clinical Trials Group (ACTG), the International Network for Strategic Initiatives in Global HIV Trials (INSIGHT), and the International Maternal Pediatric Adolescent AIDS Clinical Trials (IMPAACT) network.

In addition to drug discovery, NIAID-supported research has contributed to optimizing antiretroviral therapy by reducing the number of pills needed, decreasing side effects, and determining the best drug combinations. NIAID-supported research also has provided clear-cut scientific evidence supporting current recommendations that all people diagnosed with HIV begin treatment immediately.

AZIDOTHYMIDINE: THE FIRST DRUG TO TREAT HIV INFECTION

Scientists funded by the National Institutes of Health (NIH), National Cancer Institute (NCI) first developed azidothymidine (AZT) in 1964 as a potential cancer therapy. AZT proved ineffective against cancer and was shelved, but in the 1980s, it was included in an NCI screening program to identify drugs to treat HIV/AIDS. In the laboratory, AZT suppressed HIV replication without damaging normal cells, and the British pharmaceutical company Burroughs Wellcome funded a clinical trial to evaluate the drug in people with AIDS. Used alone, AZT decreased deaths and opportunistic infections, albeit with serious adverse effects. In March 1987, AZT became the first drug to gain approval from the U.S. Food and Drug Administration (FDA) for treating AIDS. AZT, also referred to as zidovudine, belongs to a class of drugs known as "nucleoside reverse transcriptase inhibitors," or "NRTIs."

The ACTG, established in 1987, quickly began work to build on this discovery. The ACTG 016 clinical trial established a lower therapeutic dosage of AZT, helping to reduce some of the drug's serious side effects. The pivotal ACTG 019 trial investigated whether it was beneficial to put people living with HIV on AZT before their infections progressed to AIDS. ACTG 019 showed that AZT effectively delayed the onset of AIDS in asymptomatic people with HIV, marking the first demonstration of a treatment for HIV infection.

ACCELERATING ANTIRETROVIRAL DRUG DEVELOPMENT

Established in the early years of the HIV/AIDS pandemic, the NIAID-supported National Cooperative Drug Discovery Group Program for the Treatment of AIDS (NCDDG-AIDS) provided a framework for scientists from academia, industry, and government to collaborate on research related to the identification and development of new drugs. NIAID-supported researchers developed cell culture and biochemical test systems that allowed researchers to more easily screen drug candidates, and NIAID also played a key role in the development of animal models for preclinical testing.

In the early 1990s, additional NRTI drugs gained FDA approval. The development of AZT and other NRTI showed that treating

HIV was possible, and these drugs paved the way for discovery and development of new generations of antiretroviral drugs.

While the earliest antiretroviral agents were developed before many HIV diagnostics were available in the clinic, the development of laboratory tests to measure viral load and CD4+ cell count greatly accelerated progress in drug development. Viral load describes the amount of HIV in the blood. Typically, the higher the viral load, the faster the CD4+ cell count – an indicator of how well the immune system is working – will fall. These advances made it possible for researchers to use lab test results, viral load measurements in particular, to assess how well an investigational antiretroviral agent worked. This approach required drug trials to last roughly 6 months, whereas relying solely on clinical indicators, such as progression to AIDS or death, ordinarily required trials to last years before a result was available.

THE ADVENT OF COMBINATION THERAPY

The limitations of single-drug treatment regimens quickly became apparent. HIV replicates swiftly and is prone to errors each time it does. These errors, or mutations, cause small changes in the virus. HIV variants with mutations that confer resistance to an antiretroviral drug can evolve rapidly. In some people taking AZT alone, drug resistance developed in a matter of days. Scientists thus tested whether combining drugs would make it difficult for the virus to become resistant to all the drugs simultaneously.

The data from an NIAID-funded study of AZT in combination with another NRTI drug called "dideoxycytidine" (ddC), or "zalcitabine," showed that this two-drug therapy was more effective than AZT alone, raising hopes about the use of combination therapy in treating HIV/AIDS.

Results from the ACTG 175 trial, announced in 1995, showed that two-drug combinations were superior to AZT alone in preventing decline in CD4+ cell count or death. The trial also showed that antiretroviral therapy reduced the risk of death in people with asymptomatic, intermediate-stage disease.

Around the same time, another NIAID-supported trial called "CPCRA 007" assessed combination therapy for people with more advanced HIV, the majority of whom had previously been treated with AZT. This study was conducted by the NIAID-supported Terry Beirn Community Programs for Clinical Research on AIDS (CPRCA), a network of community-based healthcare providers who integrated scientific research into primary care that later became part of the INSIGHT network.

CPCRA investigators found that two-drug therapy had no significant benefit over AZT alone in slowing disease progression or death in this patient group. However, among CPCRA 007 participants with little or no prior AZT use, combination therapy was more effective than AZT alone.

The results of ACTG 175 and CPCRA 007, as well as other studies, indicated that prior antiretroviral experience can profoundly influence the effectiveness of some treatments, underscoring the importance of careful planning in the use of antiretroviral drugs.

DURABLE HIV SUPPRESSION WITH TRIPLE-DRUG THERAPY

While the effects of two-NRTI therapy were better than those of single-drug therapy for many people with HIV, they were of limited duration. A major advance came in 1996, when researchers found that triple-drug therapy could durably suppress HIV replication to minimal levels, while creating a high genetic barrier against development of drug resistance.

The possibility and success of triple-drug therapy, also called "highly active antiretroviral therapy," or "HAART," was partially due to the appearance of a new antiretroviral drug class – the protease inhibitors. In December 1995, saquinavir became the first protease inhibitor to receive FDA approval. In 1996, results from an NIAID-sponsored trial showed that a three-drug regimen of saquinavir, ddC, and AZT was more effective than two-drug therapy with ddC and AZT.

One of the key studies demonstrating the efficacy of triple-drug therapy was ACTG 320, also supported by NIAID. This study found that a three-drug combination of the protease inhibitor indinavir and two NRTIs reduced viral loads to very low levels for up to one year in people who had previously been taking single-drug therapy.

ACTG 320 also showed that adding at least two new drugs when switching therapy is more effective than adding a single new drug.

With highly active antiretroviral therapy (HAART), which combines drugs from at least two different classes, many patients saw the amount of HIV in their blood drop to undetectable levels. But while HAART was lifesaving, the early regimens were far from perfect. The side effects were burdensome, and the daily dosing was complex. Certain drugs had to be taken in combination at different intervals throughout the day, some with food and some without. The complexity made it difficult for people to adhere to the regimens long-term.

IDENTIFYING NEW CLASSES OF ANTIRETROVIRAL DRUGS

To address the complexity of antiretroviral regimens, drug toxicities, and the issue of drug resistance, NIAID supports research aimed at novel formulations and development of drugs that work by different mechanisms and target various steps in the HIV replication process. Currently, more than 30 antiretroviral drugs are available, including several fixed-dose combinations, which contain two or more medications from one or more drug classes in a single tablet. Today, many people control their HIV by taking as little as one pill once a day. Access an infographic comparing antiretroviral therapy in the 1990s and today

The mid-1990s marked the emergence of another new class of antiretroviral drugs called "nonnucleoside reverse transcriptase inhibitors" or "NNRTIs." Because they are cheaper and easier to produce than protease inhibitors, they helped scale up antiretroviral therapy in resource-limited settings.

Identification of novel drug targets has played a key role in discovery and development of new antiretroviral drug classes. For example, since the 1980s, scientists have known that a molecule called "CD4" is the primary receptor for HIV on immune cells. In the mid-1990s, NIAID scientists reported the discovery of a co-receptor called "CXCR4," which is required for entry of certain HIV strains into immune cells. This discovery inspired researchers to look for other co-receptors. A number of research groups, including NIAID scientists, determined that a different receptor called "CCR5" is actually the primary co-receptor used by HIV to infect immune cells. This work laid the foundation for the development of the CCR5-blocking drug maraviroc, which received FDA approval in 2007.

Another major antiretroviral drug class emerged in 2007, with FDA approval of the integrase inhibitor raltegravir. Raltegravir quickly became a valued component for combination antiretroviral therapy, but HIV can follow several pathways to develop resistance to the drug. HIV variants resistant to raltegravir may also be resistant to elvitegravir, another first-generation integrase inhibitor.

Dolutegravir, which received FDA approval in 2013, is a second-generation integrase inhibitor that appears to have a high barrier to the development of HIV drug resistance. In clinical trials, dolutegravir was effective both for people living with HIV who had not previously taken HIV therapy and for people who were treatment-experienced, including those for whom first-generation integrase inhibitors were ineffective. Additional advantages of dolutegravir include convenient once-daily dosing, a good safety profile, and a relatively low production cost. Dolutegravir now is included in two of the first-line regimens that the HHS medical practice guidelines recommend for adults with HIV, and it was added to World Health Organization (WHO) guidelines as an alternative first-line agent for adults.

The NIAID continues to support work to develop new antiretroviral drugs and new tools to improve HIV treatment, such as long-acting therapies that may serve as alternatives to daily antiretroviral therapy.

Section 24.2 | **Choosing an HIV Treatment Regimen**

This section includes text excerpted from "What to Start: Choosing an HIV Treatment Regimen," HIVinfo, U.S. Department of Health and Human Services (HHS), August 16, 2021.

WHAT IS AN HIV TREATMENT REGIMEN?

A human immunodeficiency virus (HIV) treatment regimen is a combination of HIV medicines used to treat HIV infection. HIV treatment (also called "antiretroviral therapy" or "ART") begins with choosing a regimen. People on ART take the HIV medicines in their HIV regimens every day. ART helps people with HIV live longer, healthier lives and reduces the risk of HIV transmission.

The U.S. Food and Drug Administration (FDA) has approved more than 30 HIV medicines to treat HIV infection. Some HIV medicines are available in combination (in other words, two or more different HIV medicines combined in one pill).

HIV medicines are grouped into seven drug classes according to how they fight HIV.

WHAT ARE THE HIV DRUG CLASSES?

The seven HIV drug classes are:
- Nonnucleoside reverse transcriptase inhibitors (NNRTIs)
- Nucleoside reverse transcriptase inhibitors (NRTIs)
- Protease inhibitors (PIs)
- Fusion inhibitors
- CCR5 antagonists
- Integrase strand transfer inhibitors (INSTIs)
- Postattachment inhibitors

The choice of HIV medicines to include in a treatment regimen depends on a person's individual needs.

WHAT FACTORS ARE CONSIDERED WHEN CHOOSING AN HIV TREATMENT REGIMEN?

When choosing an HIV treatment regimen, people with HIV and their healthcare providers consider the following factors:

- Other diseases or conditions that the person with HIV may have, such as heart disease or pregnancy.
- Possible side effects of HIV medicines.
- Potential interactions between HIV medicines or between HIV medicines and other medicines the person with HIV is taking.
- Results of drug-resistance testing (and other tests). Drug-resistance testing identifies which, if any, HIV medicines will not be effective against a person's HIV.
- Convenience of the treatment regimen. For example, a regimen that includes two or more HIV medicines combined in one pill is convenient to follow.
- Any issues that can make it difficult to follow an HIV treatment regimen. For example, a lack of health insurance or an inability to pay for HIV medicines can make it hard to take HIV medicines consistently every day.

The best HIV treatment regimen for a person depends on their individual needs.

HOW LONG DOES IT TAKE FOR HIV MEDICINES TO WORK?

Viral load is the amount of HIV in a person's blood. A main goal of HIV treatment is to reduce a person's viral load to an undetectable level. An undetectable viral load means that the level of HIV in the blood is too low to be detected by a viral load test.

Once HIV treatment is started, it usually takes 3 to 6 months for a person's viral load to reach an undetectable level. Although HIV medicines cannot cure HIV, having an undetectable viral load shows that the medicines are controlling a person's HIV. Maintaining an undetectable viral load helps people with HIV live longer, healthier lives. In addition, people with HIV who maintain an undetectable viral load have effectively no risk of transmitting HIV to their HIV-negative partners through sex.

Section 24.3 | Following an HIV Treatment Regimen and Use

This section contains text excerpted from the following sources: Text beginning with the heading "Before Starting an HIV Treatment Regimen, Talk to Your Healthcare Provider about Medication Adherence" is excerpted from "Following an HIV Treatment Regimen: Steps to Take before and after Starting HIV Medicines," HIVinfo, U.S. Department of Health and Human Services (HHS), August 4, 2021; Text under the heading "FDA-Approved HIV Medicines" is excerpted from "FDA-Approved HIV Medicines," HIVinfo, U.S. Department of Health and Human Services (HHS), August 24, 2021; Text beginning with the heading "Why Should You Take Your HIV Medication Every Day?" is excerpted from "Taking Your HIV Medication Every Day," HIV.gov, U.S. Department of Health and Human Services (HHS), January 9, 2019.

BEFORE STARTING AN HIV TREATMENT REGIMEN, TALK TO YOUR HEALTHCARE PROVIDER ABOUT MEDICATION ADHERENCE

Before starting an HIV treatment regimen, talk to your healthcare provider about medication adherence.

Talking with your healthcare provider will help you understand why you are starting HIV treatment and why medication adherence is important. Medication adherence means sticking to an HIV treatment regimen – taking HIV medicines every day and exactly as prescribed.

Treatment with HIV medicines (called "antiretroviral therapy" or "ART") is recommended for everyone with HIV. HIV medicines help people with HIV live longer, healthier lives. Adherence to an HIV treatment regimen reduces the risk of drug resistance and HIV transmission, among other benefits as listed in Figure 24.1.

WHAT SHOULD YOU TELL YOUR HEALTHCARE PROVIDER BEFORE STARTING AN HIV TREATMENT REGIMEN?

Tell your healthcare provider about other prescription and non-prescription medicines, vitamins, nutritional supplements, and herbal products you are taking or plan to take. Other medicines or products you take may interact with HIV medicines. A drug interaction may affect how an HIV medicine works or cause side effects.

Tell your healthcare provider about any issues that might make adherence difficult. For example, people who have difficulty swallowing pills or people who do not have health insurance may find it hard to stick to an HIV treatment regimen.

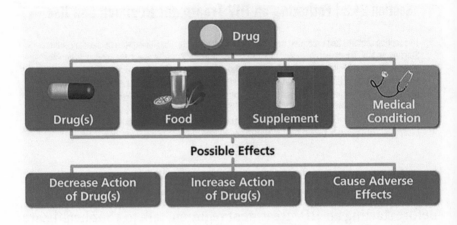

Figure 24.1. Benefits of Adherence

Describe your daily schedule to your healthcare provider. You and your healthcare provider can work together to design an HIV medication schedule that fits in with your day-to-day routine.

Ask your healthcare provider for written instructions on how to follow your HIV treatment regimen. The instructions should include the following details:
- How much of each medicine to take
- When to take each medicine
- How to take each medicine (e.g., with or without food)

USE A VARIETY OF STRATEGIES TO STICK TO YOUR HIV TREATMENT REGIMEN
To maintain adherence, try some of the following strategies:
- Use a 7-day pill box. Once a week, fill the pill box with your HIV medicines for the entire week.
- Take your HIV medicines at the same time every day.
- Set an alarm on your cell phone to remind you to take your medicines.
- Ask a family member or friend to remind you to take your medicines.

- Plan and prepare for changes in your daily routine, including weekends and holidays. If you are going away, pack enough medicine to last the entire trip.
- Use an app or an online or paper medicine diary to record each medicine as you take it. Reviewing your diary will help you identify the times that you are most likely to forget to take your medicines.
- Keep all your medical appointments. Be sure to refill your prescriptions before you run out of HIV medicines.

WHAT SHOULD YOU DO IF YOU FORGET TO TAKE YOUR HIV MEDICINES?

Unless your healthcare provider tells you otherwise, take the medicine you missed as soon as you realize you skipped it. But if it is almost time for the next dose, do not take the missed dose; just take your next dose at the usual time. Do not take a double dose of a medicine to make up for a missed dose.

DISCUSS MEDICATION ADHERENCE AT EACH APPOINTMENT WITH YOUR HEALTHCARE PROVIDER

Tell your healthcare provider if you are having difficulty following your treatment regimen. Do not forget to mention any side effects you are having. Side effects from HIV medicines (or from other medicines that you are taking) can interfere with medication adherence.

Let your healthcare provider know if your treatment regimen is too complicated to follow. Your healthcare provider may recommend that you switch to a simpler HIV treatment regimen.

FDA-APPROVED HIV MEDICINES

Treatment with HIV medicines is called "antiretroviral therapy" (ART). ART is recommended for everyone with HIV, and people with HIV should start ART as soon as possible. People on ART take a combination of HIV medicines (called an "HIV treatment regimen") every day. A person's initial HIV treatment regimen generally includes three HIV medicines from at least two different HIV drug classes.

Figure 24.2 shows HIV medicines recommended for the treatment of HIV infection in the United States, based on the U.S. Department of Health and Human Services (HHS) HIV/AIDS medical practice guidelines. All of these drugs are approved by the U.S. Food and Drug Administration (FDA).

A timeline with all the FDA approval dates for HIV medicines, categorized by drug class.

WHY SHOULD YOU TAKE YOUR HIV MEDICATION EVERY DAY?

Taking your HIV medication daily as prescribed provides many benefits. Among them, it:

- Allows the HIV medication to reduce the amount of HIV in your body (also called the "viral load") to a very low level. This is called "viral suppression." If the viral load is so low that it does not show up in a standard lab test, this is called "having an undetectable viral load." Getting and keeping an undetectable viral load is the best thing you can do to stay healthy.
- Helps protect your partners. If you take HIV medication every day, exactly as prescribed and get and keep an undetectable viral load, you have effectively no risk of transmitting HIV to an HIV-negative partner through sex. This is called "Treatment as Prevention"

Taking your HIV medication daily is also important because skipping doses makes it easier for HIV to change form, causing your medication to stop working. This is called "drug resistance." HIV can become resistant to your medication and to similar medications that you have not yet taken. This limits your options for successful HIV treatment. Drug-resistant strains of HIV can be transmitted to others, too.

WHAT SHOULD YOU DO IF YOU MISS A DOSE?

Taking your HIV medication every day, exactly the way your healthcare provider tells you to will help keep your viral load low

1981: First AIDS cases are reported in the United States.

'85-'89

1987
Zidovudine (NRTI)

'90-'94

1991
Didanosine* (NRTI)

1992
Zalcitabine* (NRTI)

1994
Stavudine* (NRTI)

'95-'99

1995
Lamivudine (NRTI)
Saquinavir (PI)

1996
Indinavir* (PI)
Nevirapine (NNRTI)
Ritonavir (PI)

1997
Combivir (FDC)
Delavirdine* (NNRTI)
Nelfinavir* (PI)

1998
Abacavir (NRTI)
Efavirenz (NNRTI)

1999
Amprenavir* (PI)

'00-'04

2000
Didanosine EC* (NRTI)
Kaletra (FDC)
Trizivir (FDC)

2001
Tenofovir DF (NRTI)

2003
Atazanavir (PI)
Emtricitabine (NRTI)
Enfuvirtide (FI)
Fosamprenavir (PI)

2004
Epzicom (FDC)
Truvada (FDC)

'05-'09

2005
Tipranavir (PI)

2006
Atripla (FDC)
Darunavir (PI)

2007
Maraviroc (CA)
Raltegravir (INSTI)

2008
Etravirine (NNRTI)

'10-'14

2011
Complera (FDC)
Nevirapine XR (NNRTI)
Rilpivirine (NNRTI)

2012
Stribild (FDC)

2013
Dolutegravir (INSTI)

2014
Cobicistat (PE)
Elvitegravir* (INSTI)
Triumeq (FDC)

'15-'19

2015
Evotaz (FDC)
Genvoya (FDC)
Prezcobix (FDC)

2016
Descovy (FDC)
Odefsey (FDC)

2017
Juluca (FDC)

2018
Biktarvy (FDC)
Cimduo (FDC)
Delstrigo (FDC)
Doravirine (NNRTI)
Ibalizumab-uiyk (PAI)
Symfi (FDC)
Symfi Lo (FDC)
Symtuza (FDC)
Temixys (FDC)

2019
Dovato (FDC)

'20-'24

2020
Fostemsavir (AI)

2021
Cabenuva (FDC)
Cabotegravir (INSTI)

Figure 24.2. FDA Approval of HIV Medicines

Drug Class Abbreviations

AI: Attachment Inhibitor; CA: CCR5 Antagonist; FDC: Fixed Dose Combination; FI: Fusion Inhibitor; INSTI: Integrase Inhibitor; NNRTI: Nonnucleoside ReverseTranscriptase Inhibitor; NRTI: Nonnucleoside ReverseTranscriptase Inhibitor; PE: Pharmacokinetic Enhancer; PI: Protease Inhibitor; PAI: Postattachment Inhibitor.

*Drugs with an asterisk are no longer available and/ or no longer recommended for use in the United States by the HHS HIV/AIDS medical practice guidelines. These drugs may still be used in fixed dose combination formulations.

and your CD4 cell count high. If you skip doses, even now and then, you are giving HIV the chance to multiply rapidly. This could weaken your immune system, and you could become sick.

Talk to your healthcare provider if you miss a dose. In most cases, if you realize you missed a dose, take the medicines as soon as you can, then take the next dose at your usual scheduled time (unless your pharmacist or healthcare provider has told you something different).

If you find you miss a lot of doses, talk to your healthcare provider or pharmacist about ways to help you remember your medicines. You and your healthcare provider may even decide to change your treatment regimen to fit your healthcare needs and life situation, which may change over time.

Section 24.4 | Antiretroviral Treatment Failure and Its Management

This section includes text excerpted from "Virologic Failure," ClinicalInfo, U.S. Department of Health and Human Services (HHS), June 3, 2021.

VIROLOGIC FAILURE

Antiretroviral (ARV) regimens that are currently recommended for initial therapy in patients with human immunodeficiency virus (HIV) have a high likelihood of achieving and maintaining plasma HIV Ribonucleic acid (RNA) levels that are below the lower limits of detection (LLOD) of currently used assays. Patients on antiretroviral therapy (ART) who do not achieve this treatment goal or who experience virologic rebound can develop resistance mutations to one or more components of their regimen. Adherence to ARV regimens can be challenging for some patients, and poor adherence can result in detectable viral loads. Depending on their treatment histories, some of these patients may have minimal or no drug resistance, and others may have extensive resistance. Managing patients with extensive resistance is complex and usually requires consultation with an HIV expert. This section defines virologic failure in patients on ART and discusses strategies to manage ART in these individuals.

ANTIRETROVIRAL THERAPY GOALS AND PRESENCE OF VIREMIA WHILE ON ANTIRETROVIRAL THERAPY

The goal of ART is to suppress HIV replication to a level below which drug-resistance mutations do not emerge. Although not conclusive, the evidence suggests that selection of drug-resistance mutations does not occur in patients with HIV RNA levels that are persistently suppressed below the LLOD of current assays.

Virologic blips are not usually associated with subsequent virologic failure. In contrast, there is controversy regarding the clinical implications of persistently low HIV RNA levels that are between the LLOD and <200 copies/mL in patients on ART. Viremia at this threshold is detected with some frequency by commonly used real-time polymerase chain reaction (PCR) assays, which are more sensitive than the PCR-based viral load platforms used in the past. Several retrospective studies support the supposition that virologic failure is more likely to occur in patients with viral loads ≥200 copies/mL than in those with low-level viremia between 50 copies/mL and 199 copies/mL. However, other studies have suggested that detectable viremia at this low level (<200 copies/mL) can be predictive of virologic failure and can be associated with the evolution of drug resistance.

Persistent HIV RNA levels ≥200 copies/mL are often associated with evidence of viral evolution and accumulation of drug-resistance mutations. This association is particularly common when HIV RNA levels are >500 copies/mL. Therefore, patients who have persistent HIV RNA levels ≥200 copies/mL are considered to be experiencing virologic failure.

CAUSES OF VIROLOGIC FAILURE

Virologic failure can occur for many reasons. Data from patient cohorts in the earlier era of combination ART suggested that suboptimal adherence and drug intolerance/toxicity are key contributors to virologic failure and regimen discontinuations. The presence of preexisting (transmitted) drug resistance also may lead to virologic failure.

Virologic failure may be associated with a variety of factors, including the following:

- **Patient/adherence-related factors**
  - Comorbidities that may affect adherence (e.g., active substance abuse, mental-health disorders, neurocognitive impairment)
  - Unstable housing and other psychosocial factors
  - Missed clinic appointments
  - Interruption of, or intermittent access to, ART
  - Cost and affordability of ARV drugs (i.e., these factors may affect the ability to access or continue therapy)
  - Adverse drug effects
  - High pill burden and/or dosing frequency
- **HIV-related factors**
  - Presence of transmitted or acquired drug-resistant virus documented by current or past resistance test results
  - Prior treatment failure
  - Innate resistance to prescribed ARV drugs
  - Higher pretreatment HIV RNA level (some regimens may be less effective at higher levels)
- **Antiretroviral regimen-related factors**
  - Suboptimal pharmacokinetics (PKs) (e.g., variable absorption, metabolism, or penetration into reservoirs)
  - Suboptimal virologic potency
  - Low barrier to resistance
  - Reduced efficacy due to prior exposure to suboptimal regimens (e.g., monotherapy, dual-nucleoside reverse transcriptase inhibitor (NRTI) therapy, or the sequential introduction of drugs)
  - Food requirements

- Drug-drug interactions with concomitant medications, which may reduce concentrations of the ARV drugs
- Prescription (prescribing or dispensing) errors

MANAGING PATIENTS WITH VIROLOGIC FAILURE

If virologic failure is suspected or confirmed, a thorough assessment of whether one or more of the above factors could have been the cause(s) of failure is indicated. Often, the causes of virologic failure can be identified, but in some cases, they are not obvious. Distinguishing among the causes of virologic failure is important, because the approaches to subsequent therapy may differ, depending on the cause. Potential causes of virologic failure should be explored in depth. Once virologic failure is confirmed, steps should be taken to improve virologic outcomes.

MANAGING VIROLOGIC FAILURE IN DIFFERENT CLINICAL SCENARIOS
Virologic Failure on the First Antiretroviral Regimen

- **NNRTI plus NRTI regimen failure.** These patients often have viral resistance to the NNRTI, with or without the M184V/I mutation, which confers high-level resistance to lamivudine (3TC) and FTC. Additional NRTI mutations may also be present. Below are some switch options.
  - **DTG plus one or two fully active NRTIs.** In the dawning trial, patients who experienced virologic failure while on a first-line, NNRTI-based regimen were randomized to receive either LPV/r or DTG; each of these drugs was given with two NRTIs, one of which had to be fully active based on real-time resistance testing. The study was stopped early after an interim analysis showed that the DTG arm was superior to the LPV/r arm. Thus, DTG plus two NRTIs (at least one of which is fully active) can be an option after failure of a first-line, NNRTI-based therapy. BIC may have activity that is similar to that of DTG in this setting; however,

no data currently support its use. Not enough data exist on the efficacy of elvitegravir (EVG) or raltegravir (RAL) to recommend the use of these INSTIs in the setting of first-line, NNRTI-based therapy failure.

- **Boosted PI plus two NRTIs.** Three large randomized controlled trials (primarily conducted in resource-limited settings where NNRTI-based regimens have been used as first-line therapy) have explored different second-line regimen options. The studies found that regimens that contained LPV/r plus two NRTIs were as effective as regimens that contained LPV/r plus RAL. However, LPV/r alone, and probably other ritonavir-boosted PIs (PI/r) as monotherapy, cannot be recommended (AI). Participants in some of these studies did not undergo resistance testing before randomization. Thus, based on these data and those of the prior section, the Panel recommends that a boosted PI plus two NRTIs can be an option after failure of a first-line NNRTI-based regimen in settings with no access to second-generation INSTIs or to genotypic resistance testing (AI). However, in settings where second-generation INSTIs are not available, but genotypic resistance tests can be conducted, the Panel favors using a boosted PI plus two NRTIs with at least one being fully active. Even though LPV/r was the PI used in these studies, other boosted PIs (e.g., DRV) would likely have similar activities and may be better tolerated.

- **Boosted PI plus an INSTI.** As noted earlier, a regimen that consisted of LPV/r plus RAL was found to be as effective as LPV/r plus two NRTIs. Thus, LPV/r plus RAL can be a treatment option for those who experienced virologic failure on an NNRTI-based regimen. Although data are limited, another boosted PI (e.g., DRV) combined with RAL or an alternative INSTI (e.g., DTG) may also be an option in this setting. BIC (which is only available in a combination pill with

FTC/TAF) combined with a boosted PI in the setting of first-line, NNRTI-based therapy failure may have activity that is similar to DTG; however, there are currently no data to support its use in this situation.

- **Boosted PI plus NRTI regimen failure.** In this scenario, most patients will have either no resistance or resistance that is limited to 3TC and FTC. Failure in this setting is often attributed to poor adherence, drug-drug interactions, or drug-food interactions. Below are some management options.
  - **Maintain on the same regimen.** A systematic review of multiple randomized trials that investigated the failures of first-line, PI/r-based regimens showed that maintaining the same regimen while making efforts to enhance adherence is as effective as changing to new regimens with or without drugs from new classes. If the regimen is well tolerated with no concerns about drug-drug or drug-food interactions or drug resistance, then the regimen can be continued with adherence support and viral monitoring.
  - **Switch to another regimen.** If poor tolerability, drug interactions, or drug resistance may be contributing to virologic failure, then the regimen can be modified to one of the following:
    - A different boosted PI (with no evidence for cross-resistance) plus two NRTIs (at least one of which is fully active); or
    - DTG, or possibly BIC plus two NRTIs (at least one of which is fully active). As noted above, if only one of the NRTIs is fully active or if adherence is a concern, DTG is currently preferred over BIC. There are limited to no data on the efficacy of BIC or EVG in this setting. However, considering the high resistance barrier of BIC, it might also be considered a viable option in this setting, despite limited supportive data; or

- A different boosted PI (with no evidence for cross-resistance) plus an INSTI.
- **INSTI plus NRTI Regimen failure**. Virologic failure in patients on a regimen that consists of RAL or EVG plus two NRTIs may be associated with emergent resistance to 3TC or FTC and, possibly, the INSTI. Viruses with EVG or RAL resistance often remain susceptible to DTG and BIC. In contrast, in clinical trials, persons who experienced virologic failure while receiving DTG or BIC plus two NRTIs as first-line therapy were unlikely to develop resistance to DTG or BIC. No existing clinical trial data guide therapy for first-line INSTI failures; therefore, treatment strategy should be based on resistance test results and the potential potency of the next regimen. Below are some treatment options, based on resistance pattern considerations.
  - **Virologic failure without any resistance mutations**. The patient should be managed as outlined above in the section on virologic failure without resistance.
  - **Virologic failure without INSTI resistance**. The regimen can be modified to one of the following:
    - A boosted PI plus two NRTIs (at least one of which is fully active); or
    - DTG, or possibly BIC plus two NRTIs (at least one of which is fully active); or
    - A boosted PI plus an INSTI.
  - **Virologic failure with resistance to RAL and/or EVG, but susceptibility to DTG**. The regimen can be modified to one of the following:
    - A boosted PI plus two NRTIs (at least one of which is fully active); or
    - DTG, (twice daily) or possibly BIC plus two NRTIs (at least one of which is fully active); or
    - DTG, (twice daily) or possibly BIC plus a boosted PI.

Currently no data exist on the efficacy of BIC in patients who experience virologic failure while on an EVG- or RAL-based regimen. Considering the high resistance barrier of BIC, it might be considered a viable option, although its use cannot be formally recommended in these settings currently.

Second-Line Regimen Failure and Beyond

- **Drug resistance with fully active antiretroviral therapy (AART) options**. Using a patient's treatment history and drug-resistance data, a clinician can decide whether to include a fully active, boosted PI or INSTI in future regimens. For example, those who have no documented PI resistance and who have never been treated with an unboosted PI likely harbor virus that is fully susceptible to PIs. Similarly, patients who have no documented INSTI resistance and who have never been treated with an INSTI, or even those who have been treated with only RAL or EVG, may have virus susceptible to DTG or BIC. In this setting, viral suppression should be achievable using a boosted PI combined with either two NRTIs (at least one of which is fully active), a boosted PI combined with an INSTI, or DTG or BIC combined with two NRTIs (at least one of which is fully active) – provided the virus is susceptible to these drugs. If a fully active, boosted PI or DTG or BIC is not an option, the new regimen should include at least two, and preferably three, fully active agents. Drugs should be selected based on the likelihood that they will be fully active, as determined by the patient's treatment history, past and present drug-resistance testing, and tropism testing if a CCR5 antagonist is being considered.
- **Multidrug resistance without fully active antiretroviral therapy options**. Use of currently available ARV drugs has resulted in a dramatic decline in the number of patients who have few treatment options because of multiclass drug-resistance. Despite this progress, some patients remain who have experienced toxicities with and/ or developed resistance to most currently available drugs. Maximal virologic suppression should remain the goal;

however, if it cannot be achieved, the goals of ART will be to preserve immunologic function, prevent clinical progression, and minimize the development of further resistance that may compromise future regimens.

- Consensus on the optimal management of these patients is lacking. If resistance to NNRTIs, T-20, MVC, BIC, DTG, EVG, or RAL are identified, there is rarely a reason to continue using these drugs, because there is little evidence that keeping them in the regimen helps delay disease progression. Moreover, continuing these drugs (in particular, early-generation INSTIs) may allow selection of additional resistance mutations and development of within-class cross-resistance that may limit future treatment options. It should be noted that even partial virologic suppression of HIV RNA to >0.5 log10 copies/mL from baseline correlates with clinical benefit. Cohort studies provide evidence that continuing ART even in the presence of viremia and the absence of CD4 count increases reduces the risk of disease progression. Other cohort studies suggest that even modest reductions in HIV RNA levels continue to confer immunologic and clinical benefits. However, these potential benefits must be balanced with the ongoing risk of accumulating additional resistance mutations. In general, adding a single, fully active ARV drug to the regimen is not recommended because of the risk of rapid development of resistance.

- Patients with ongoing detectable viremia who lack sufficient treatment options to construct a fully suppressive regimen may be candidates for the first-in-class CD4 post-attachment inhibitor IBA62 and/or the gp120-directed attachment inhibitor FTR.

  - **IBA.** A single-arm, multicenter clinical trial enrolled 40 heavily ART-experienced participants who had multidrug-resistant HIV-1 and who were experiencing virologic failure on an ARV regimen. Subjects received intravenous infusions of IBA every two weeks, in addition to an optimized background regimen that included at least one additional agent to which the subject's virus was susceptible. At Week 24, 43 percent of participants achieved HIV RNA <50 copies/mL, and 50 percent of participants achieved HIV RNA <200 copies/mL.63 Of the 27 participants who continued to the 48-week follow-up study, 59 percent and 63 percent had HIV RNA <50 copies/mL and <200 copies/mL, respectively. All 15 patients who had HIV RNA <50 copies/mL at Week 24 maintained viral suppression up to Week 48.

- **FTR.** A Phase 3 multicenter trial enrolled 371 heavily ART-experienced participants who had multidrug-resistant HIV-1 and who were experiencing virologic failure. Participants were enrolled into two cohorts, according to their remaining treatment options. The randomized cohort (n = 272) included those with at least one fully active, approved ARV drug in at least one, but no more than two classes. These individuals were randomized to FTR (oral 600 mg twice daily) or placebo for 8 days, followed by open-label FTR plus optimized background ART. In the nonrandomized cohort (n = 99), participants with no remaining ARV options were started on open-label FTR (oral 600 mg twice daily) plus optimized background ART on Day 1. The primary endpoint for the randomized cohort was change in viral load from baseline at Day 8. In the FTR group, the mean viral load decrease was 0.79 log10 copies/mL versus 0.17 log10 copies/mL in the placebo group (P < 0.001). At Week 96, 60 percent of participants in the randomized cohort and 37 percent of those in the nonrandomized cohort had viral load <40 copies/mL, with mean CD4 increases of 205 cells/ mm and 119 cells/mm, respectively. In this study, 15 individuals in the nonrandomized cohort used the CD4 post-attachment inhibitor IBA in combination with FTR and other ARVs. The virological response rate for these participants by snapshot analysis was 53 percent at Week 48 and 33 percent at Week 96.

Patients who continue to have detectable viremia and who lack sufficient treatment options to construct a fully suppressive regimen may also be candidates for research studies or expanded access programs, or they may qualify for single-patient access to an investigational new drug as specified in the U.S. Food and Drug Administration (FDA) regulations.

Chapter 25 | HIV/AIDS Treatment Adherence

WHAT IS HIV TREATMENT ADHERENCE?

For people with HIV, treatment adherence means:

- Starting HIV treatment
- Taking HIV medicines every day and exactly as prescribed (also called "medication adherence")
- Keeping all medical appointments

Adherence to treatment is a key part of staying healthy with HIV.

HOW SOON SHOULD A PERSON START TREATMENT AFTER TESTING POSITIVE FOR HIV?

It is best to see a healthcare provider as soon as possible after testing positive for HIV. Once in medical care, people with HIV should start taking HIV medicines as soon as possible. Treatment with HIV medicines (called "antiretroviral therapy" or "ART") is recommended for everyone with HIV. HIV medicines help people with HIV live longer, healthier lives. HIV medicines also reduce the risk of HIV transmission.

Because HIV requires lifelong treatment, it is important for people with HIV to regularly visit their healthcare provider. Ongoing medical care includes monitoring to make sure a person's HIV treatment regimen is keeping the virus under control. During regular medical appointments, healthcare providers can

This chapter includes text excerpted from "HIV Treatment Adherence," HIVinfo, U.S. Department of Health and Human Services (HHS), August 12, 2021.

also recommend resources to help people deal with any issues that may interfere with medication adherence.

WHY IS MEDICATION ADHERENCE IMPORTANT?

Taking HIV medicines every day prevents HIV from multiplying, which reduces the risk that HIV will mutate and produce drug-resistant HIV. Skipping HIV medicines allows HIV to multiply, which increases the risk of drug resistance and HIV treatment failure.

Poor adherence to an HIV treatment regimen also allows HIV to destroy the immune system. A damaged immune system makes it hard for the body to fight off infections and certain cancers.

Chapter 26 | Treatment Recommendations for Pediatric HIV Infection

Human immunodeficiency virus (HIV) infection is a persistent viral infection that can cause acquired immunodeficiency syndrome (AIDS) if left untreated. Since the first cases of HIV infection were discovered, the number of youngsters infected with the virus has increased. Infants born to HIV-positive mothers are now deemed at considerable risk of infection if their mother's viral load is 50 copies/ml or above.

MOTHER-TO-CHILD-TRANSMISSION (MTCT)

More than 95 percent of HIV-infected children in the United States acquired the virus from their mothers who were carriers of HIV. This is known as "vertical transmission" which has fallen in the United States from 25 percent in 1991 to almost 1 percent in 2018. The transmission to newborn babies has been reduced with the help of extensive serologic screening, treating infected pregnant women during both pregnancy and delivery, and offering short-term antiretroviral prophylaxis to neonates who have been exposed.

TREATING HIV IN CHILDREN

Conventional HIV treatment involves the combination of medications and therapies, together, known as "antiretroviral therapy"

(ART). ART medications slow the rate at which the virus replicates in the body and can help keep the child healthy. These medications are available in powders and flavored syrups.

All HIV-infected children older than six weeks, but less than 12 weeks should begin treatment within 1–2 weeks after diagnosis. This quickstart must include a talk about the necessity of adherence.

PRACTICAL RECOMMENDATIONS IN PEDIATRIC HIV TREATMENT
Adherence
Antiretroviral medication therapies are most successful when the family of an HIV-infected child is willing to follow a strict medical regimen. Nonadherence however can lead to treatment failure, resulting in limited future therapy options. Though it can be tough to stick to a tight treatment plan, associating with the kid's daily routine, such as having the child take medicine with breakfast or before brushing their teeth, can assist. Using a pillbox, noting it down on calendars, sticky notes, and setting alarms can help a family follow and stick to the routine.

Monitoring
Clinical and laboratory testing are critical for detecting therapy failure and drug toxicity. At the time of admission, a physical examination, complete blood count, serum chemistry values including electrolytes, liver and kidney tests, HIV plasma viral load, and CD4 positive lymphocyte counts are required. This should be done every 3–4 months, with lipid profiles and urinalysis added every 6–12 months.

Valuing Privacy of HIV-infected Children
When a child becomes infected with HIV, the entire family is affected. They may be hesitant to communicate the diagnosis with others since it might lead to social isolation. Only with the informed consent of the parents or legal guardians and the child's age-appropriate consent should the information be disclosed if deemed necessary.

Vaccination

Routine pediatric vaccination procedures are advised for HIV-infected children, except for live-virus and live-bacteria vaccinations, which should be avoided or administered only in limited circumstances. Though inactivated polio vaccine should be administered regularly, and inactivated influenza vaccination should be administered once a year, live oral poliovirus vaccine and live-attenuated influenza vaccine are not suggested. Similarly, children with significant immunosuppression should not be administered the live measles-mumps-rubella (MMR) vaccine or varicella vaccine.

SIGNIFICANCE OF PEDIATRIC HIV TREATMENT

Historically, some older drugs were more toxic and were linked to faster resistance development. As a result, withholding therapy was once widely suggested in various age groups and early-stage HIV infection. However, this is no longer the case. All children with HIV should be treated to prevent disease progression, infections, neurocognitive implications of HIV infection, reaching a normal expected lifetime, and eventually avoiding additional HIV transmission.

The long-term future of HIV-positive youngsters is unknown. HIV-infected children today have a high chance of living as long as anyone else with the disease, which can be decades, if they receive proper care.

As a result, ART has become the gold standard in HIV treatment. HIV-affected children ought to take the medications exactly as prescribed by the doctor, with no missed doses. If the medications are not taken as directed, the HIV can become drug-resistant, making the illness more difficult to cure. Early intervention may help protect the immune system and slow the spread of infection.

References

"Care and Treatment for Children Living with HIV," The Well Project, October 28, 2021.

"HIV Treatment in Children," Healthwise, February 13, 2012.

Rivera, Delia M. "Pediatric HIV Infection Treatment &
Management," WebMD LLC., November 11, 2020.

Secord, Elizabeth A. "HIV Treatment Regimens CDC
Guidelines, Pediatric," WebMD LLC., July 26, 2021.

Weinberg, Geoffrey A. "Human Immunodeficiency Virus
(HIV) Infection in Infants and Children," Merck Manuals,
July 15, 2020.

"When to Initiate Therapy in Antiretroviral-Naive Children,"
ClinicalInfo, April 7, 2021.

Chapter 27 | **HIV and AIDS Treatment for Pregnant Women**

The human immunodeficiency virus (HIV) attacks the immune system of the body and is usually transmitted when a person comes into contact with infected blood or other infected bodily fluids such as semen or vaginal fluids. Once an individual is diagnosed with HIV and starts regular treatment, she or he will be required to have regular medical checkups to ensure that the treatment is working, and the HIV is under control.

HIV AND PREGNANCY

Around 5,000 women affected with HIV give birth every year in the United States, according to 2018 estimates. Women's fertility is not affected by HIV, and many of the latest advances in HIV treatments make it safe for them to conceive and give birth to a child. In fact, every woman in the United States who becomes pregnant is required to get tested for HIV. However, women planning to have babies should be aware that it is still possible to pass the HIV infection on to the baby during the period of pregnancy, during delivery, and in some cases, through breastfeeding. The good news is that the use of certain HIV antiretroviral drugs during pregnancy and delivery can reduce this risk dramatically.

CARE BEFORE PREGNANCY

As a precaution, HIV-positive women should consult their obstetrician or an HIV specialist before they start trying to conceive. They should also be taking HIV antiretroviral drugs for some time and should have an undetectable viral load in the blood. (The viral load is the quantity of virus in a person's blood at the time of testing.) Most HIV medications are safe even during pregnancy and should be taken regularly as per the doctors' instructions. Women who have no virus detected in their blood (complete viral suppression) during their pregnancy will have a reduced risk of transmitting HIV to their babies.

Pregnant women with HIV can go through the same HIV treatment regimens recommended for nonpregnant women – unless the risk of any side effects to a pregnant woman or her infant outweighs the benefits of the treatment regimen. HIV medications, such as Zidovudine or ZDV (Retrovir), have been shown to significantly reduce the risk of HIV infection to the baby when the medication is given during pregnancy and labor, and also given to the baby following delivery. HIV-affected pregnant women should talk to their healthcare provider about the benefits and risks of taking HIV medications during pregnancy.

CARE DURING PREGNANCY

Once the pregnancy is confirmed, the expectant mother should meet with her obstetrical provider and HIV specialist to discuss the treatment of HIV during pregnancy and minimize the risk of HIV transmission to the baby. Blood tests will be taken to determine the amount of HIV viral load in the blood and the strength of the immune system as measured by the number of CD4 T cells that play a significant role in the immune system. If the patient is not taking HIV medications, the doctor will test the blood to look for mutations in the HIV virus. The doctor may also have the patient start taking HIV medication even before test results are known.

Pregnant women with HIV will be put under a combination of three or more antiretroviral medicines (triple antiretroviral therapy or anti-HIV "cocktail") that are regarded as more effective than using just a single medicine (monotherapy), such as Zidovudine.

Starting HIV drugs earlier in pregnancy is thought to increase the chance of having a low viral load in the blood by the time of delivery. HIV medications will be given throughout pregnancy to prevent infecting the baby with HIV and will also be given orally to the baby for 4–6 weeks following birth in order to reduce the risk of the baby contracting HIV. However, some women may prefer to begin taking the medication after the first trimester due to pregnancy-related nausea making it difficult to take the drugs.

DURING LABOR AND DELIVERY

If the "viral load" in the mother's blood is above ≥1,000 copies/mL during labor, she will be given the HIV drug zidovudine intravenously in order to lower the risk of passing on HIV to the baby. Those taking an anti-HIV "cocktail" will be told to continue them on schedule during labor to provide maximum protection to mother and baby. Safe delivery of the baby, either through vaginal or cesarean delivery (C-section) will depend on the mother's HIV viral load during pregnancy. Vaginal delivery will be scheduled if the HIV viral load is low (HIV viral load <1,000 copies/mL within four to six weeks of due date), that is if the transmission risk is low. Cesarean delivery may be recommended if the mother's viral load is high (≥1,000 copies/mL within four to six weeks of due date) or for other reasons, such as the position of the baby in the womb.

AFTER DELIVERY CARE

Mothers should continue to take HIV medications after delivery. Postdelivery care for HIV-positive mothers includes screening for postpartum depression, help with medication adherence, counseling, and information and resources regarding birth control and family planning. Highly developed countries such as the United States have baby formulas and clean water readily available as a safe and viable alternative to breastfeeding. As it is possible to pass HIV onto the infant while breastfeeding, the United States Public Health Service (USPHS) strongly recommends American mothers who have HIV not to breastfeed their babies, even if they are following an antiretroviral HIV medication regimen.

CARE FOR NEWBORNS AND BABIES

Babies born to HIV-affected women are treated with HIV drugs for four to six weeks after delivery to prevent the baby from getting infected after being exposed to the mother's blood during delivery. The normal HIV "antibody testing" used to determine whether an adult or child is infected with HIV may not give accurate results in the case of newborn babies. As HIV antibodies can be transmitted from mother to baby, the test could show a positive HIV antibody result for the baby which does not necessarily mean that the baby is infected with HIV.

So, a special test called an "HIV PCR" test is taken which will give accurate results as to whether the baby is infected or not. The chances of a baby having HIV is small if the HIV-positive mother has followed the treatment/medication regimen throughout her pregnancy. If unfortunately, the baby does test positive for HIV after birth, the family need not lose hope. With the right type of treatment, the baby can still grow and develop to live a healthy and normal life in the future.

References

Choudhary, Madhu Chhanda. "Antiretroviral Therapy (ART) in Pregnant Women with HIV Infection Overview of HIV Antiretroviral Therapy (ART) in Pregnancy," Medscape, July 26, 2021.

"HIV and Pregnancy," HIVinfo, U.S. Department of Health and Human Services (HHS), August 18, 2021.

Hughes, Brenna L; Cu-Uvin, Susan. "Patient Education: HIV and Pregnancy (Beyond the Basics)," UpToDate.com, July 14, 2020.

Iftikhar, Noreen. "What You Need to Know about HIV and Pregnancy," Healthline, April 29, 2021.

Chapter 28 | **HIV/AIDS Treatment Interruptions**

The treatment for human immunodeficiency virus (HIV) primarily comprises an antiretroviral therapy (ART) that involves a combination of HIV medicines. HIV-affected patients are placed under an HIV treatment regimen that includes such combinations of medicines. Treatment interruptions are known as "structured treatment interruptions" or "analytical treatment interruptions."

An analytical treatment interruption (ATI) is a temporary pause in the standard HIV treatment procedure. As an assessment tool, ATI is preferred among scientists working on clinical trials to test the efficacy of alternative therapies for HIV.

A treatment interruption may become necessary if the patient experiences severe side effects, the onset of an illness, oral surgery, or the unavailability of medicines. The goal of any HIV treatment is to reduce the viral load of HIV in the blood. In such cases, ATI helps researchers observe how and whether a particular treatment approach improves the condition. However, ATI also poses certain risks to HIV patients. Discontinuation of ART can lead to viral rebound, clinical progression of the disease, or immunity decompensation, which is why they are not recommended outside of a clinical trial. Circumstances where an unplanned interruption in ART can occur include:

- **Sudden interruptions in taking oral antiretroviral drugs**. Short-term interruptions in ART could be due to intercurrent illnesses before the oral intake of drugs and drug toxicity.

- **Interrupting long-acting antiretroviral drugs**. Certain drugs for HIV are long-acting and have extended half-lives. These medicines are given as intramuscular (IM) injections. Discontinuing these medicines without a bridge regimen, such as oral medication can put the patient at an increased risk for virologic failure and drug resistance.

TYPES OF ANALYTICAL TREATMENT INTERRUPTIONS

Two types of ATIs are generally mediated during HIV treatment regimens, and they include:

- **Fixed period ATIs**. This is an interruption in treatment for a predefined set duration lasting between 1–24 weeks. The interruption is focused on measuring the viral load in the blood after the virus has decreased to a steady level. This level is often termed as a "viral set point." Viral set points are instrumental in assessing the potency of immunity-related interventions that boost immunity after an ART interruption.
- **Monitored ART pause ATIs**. Considered to be one of the safest strategies in managing HIV, this ATI does not last for a set period of weeks and requires frequent monitoring. The ATI is mediated as soon as the first sign of viral rebound is detected. This is when the virus is detected in the blood after being undetected for a certain period.

Monitored ART pause ATIs effectively assess interventions that aim to decrease the number of viral cells in the blood. This refers to the groups of cells in the body affected by HIV having not produced new HIV for a long duration but can potentially restart production.

RISKS OF TREATMENT INTERRUPTIONS

Though discontinuing ART for HIV patients has shown considerable benefits, it also comes with significant risks and side-effects such as:

- Causing viremia (an increased presence of viruses in the blood) in patients

- Causing a reduction of CD4 count in patients that can lead to infections and illness.
- Increasing the risk for heart, kidney, and liver disease
- Developing drug resistance
- Platelet deficiency
- Higher risk of transmitting HIV to partners
- Increased chances of systemic inflammation of the body

Since the most apparent side effect of stopping ART for HIV patients is viremia, it can also lead to a condition known as "acute retroviral syndrome" or "ARS" whose symptoms include:
- Rashes
- Muscle pain
- Fever
- Headache
- Swollen lymph nodes
- Sore throat

Once ART treatment resumes, these symptoms diminish.

HIV/AIDS treatment interruptions can be considered safe if ART interruptions are followed by stopping all drugs simultaneously. In cases requiring interruptions due to drug toxicity, once the cause of toxicity is determined, most medications can be restarted safely as monotherapy for a few days.

References

Cachay, Edward R. "Drug Treatment of HIV Infection," MSD Manual, January 2021.

"Guidelines for the Use of Antiretroviral Agents in Adults and Adolescents Living with HIV," ClinicalInfo, U.S. Department of Health and Human Services (HHS), January 20, 2022.

Spach, David H. "Antiretroviral Medications and Initial Therapy," National HIV Curriculum, U.S. Department of Health and Human Services (HHS), June 4, 2021.

West, Mary. "What to Know about ATI for HIV," *Medical News Today*, October 28, 2021.

Chapter 29 | **HIV/AIDS Treatment Side Effects**

Chapter Contents

Section 29.1 | Understanding HIV Treatment Side Effects

This section includes text excerpted from "HIV Medicines and Side Effects," HIVinfo, U.S. Department of Health and Human Services (HHS), October 17, 2018. Reviewed February 2022.

CAN HIV MEDICINES CAUSE SIDE EFFECTS?

HIV medicines help people with HIV live longer, healthier lives. Sometimes HIV medicines can also cause side effects. Most side effects from HIV medicines are manageable, but a few can be serious. Overall, the benefits of HIV medicines far outweigh the risk of side effects. In addition, newer HIV regimens cause fewer side effects than regimens used in the past. As HIV treatment options continue to improve, people are less likely to experience side effects from their HIV medicines.

Before starting HIV medicines, people with HIV discuss possible side effects from HIV medicines with their healthcare providers. They work together to select an HIV regimen based on the person's individual needs.

DO HIV MEDICINES CAUSE THE SAME SIDE EFFECTS?

Different HIV medicines can cause different side effects. In addition, people taking the same HIV medicine can have different side effects.

Side effects from HIV medicines can last only a few days or weeks or continue for much longer. Some side effects may not appear until many months or even years after starting an HIV medicine.

If you are taking HIV medicines, tell your healthcare provider about any side effects that you are having. Some side effects, like headaches or occasional dizziness, may not be serious. Other side effects, such as swelling of the throat and tongue or damage to the liver, can be life-threatening.

WHAT ARE SOME SHORT-TERM SIDE EFFECTS FROM HIV MEDICINES?

People starting an HIV medicine for the first time may have side effects that last a couple of weeks.

These short-term side effects can include:

- Feeling tired
- Nausea (upset stomach)
- Vomiting
- Diarrhea
- Headache
- Fever
- Muscle pain
- Occasional dizziness
- Insomnia

Sometimes, side effects that may not seem serious, such as fever, rash, nausea, or fatigue, can be a sign of a life-threatening condition. Any swelling of the face, eyes, lips, throat, or tongue is considered a life-threatening side effect that requires immediate medical attention.

HIV infection itself, another medical condition, or other medicines a person is taking can also cause side effects. Drug interactions between HIV medicines or with other medicines a person is taking can also cause side effects.

Always tell your healthcare provider about any side effects that you are having. Your healthcare provider can determine the cause of the side effect and recommend ways to treat or manage the side effect.

If you are taking HIV medicines and have any side effects, do not cut down on, skip, or stop taking your HIV medicines unless your healthcare provider tells you to. Stopping HIV medicines allows HIV to multiply and damage the immune system. A damaged immune system makes it harder for the body to fight off infections and certain HIV-related cancers. Stopping HIV medicines also increases the risk of drug resistance.

WHAT ARE SOME LONG-TERM SIDE EFFECTS FROM HIV MEDICINES?

Some side effects from HIV medicines can appear months or even years after starting a medicine and can continue for a long time. Examples of long-term side effects include:

- Kidney problems, including kidney failure
- Liver damage (hepatotoxicity)
- Heart disease
- Diabetes or insulin resistance
- An increase in fat levels in the blood (hyperlipidemia)
- Changes in how the body uses and stores fat (lipodystrophy)
- Weakening of the bones (osteoporosis)
- Nerve damage (peripheral neuropathy)
- Mental health-related effects, including insomnia, depression, and thoughts of suicide

WHAT ARE WAYS TO MANAGE SIDE EFFECTS FROM HIV MEDICINES?

When taking HIV medicines, it helps to plan ahead. Before starting HIV medicines, talk to your healthcare provider about possible side effects. Tell your healthcare provider about your lifestyle and point out any possible side effects that would be especially hard for you to manage. The information will help your healthcare provider recommend medicines best suited to your needs.

Depending on the HIV medicines you take, your healthcare provider will:

- Tell you which specific side effects to look out for
- Offer you suggestions on how to deal with those side effects. For example, to manage nausea and vomiting, eat smaller meals more often and avoid spicy foods.
- Tell you about the signs of life-threatening side effects that require immediate medical attention. One example is swelling of the mouth and tongue.

Tell your healthcare provider if you have any side effect that bothers you or that does not go away. Your healthcare provider may recommend that you change HIV medicines. Fortunately, there are many HIV medicines available to include in an HIV regimen. The choice of HIV medicines to replace those causing side effects will depend on a person's individual needs.

Section 29.2 | **Diabetes and HIV**

This section includes text excerpted from "HIV and Diabetes," HIVinfo, U.S. Department of Health and Human Services (HHS), August 10, 2021.

WHAT IS DIABETES?

Diabetes is a disease that develops when levels of glucose in the blood (also called "blood sugar") are too high. Glucose comes from the breakdown of the foods we eat and is our main source of energy.

Over time, diabetes can cause serious health problems, including heart disease, stroke, kidney disease, eye problems, and nerve damage.

There are different types of diabetes, including type 1 diabetes, type 2 diabetes, and gestational diabetes. This section discusses type 2 diabetes, which is the most common type of diabetes.

RISK FACTORS FOR TYPE 2 DIABETES

Risk factors for type 2 diabetes include being 45 years of age or older, having a family history of diabetes, being overweight or obese, and lack of physical activity. People whose family background is African American, Alaska Native, American Indian, Asian American, Hispanic/Latinx, Native Hawaiian, or Pacific Islander American are at greater risk of type 2 diabetes.

People with HIV are more likely to have type 2 diabetes than people without HIV. Additionally, some HIV medicines may increase the risk of type 2 diabetes in people with HIV.

SYMPTOMS OF DIABETES

The symptoms of diabetes can include:
- Increased thirst
- Frequent urination
- Increased hunger
- Unusual weight loss
- Fatigue
- Blurred vision
- Tingling or numbness in the hands or feet
- Sores that do not heal

People who have symptoms of diabetes should get tested for the disease. Testing is also recommended for people with certain risk factors for diabetes. Blood tests are used to measure blood glucose levels and diagnose diabetes.

SHOULD PEOPLE WITH HIV GET TESTED FOR DIABETES?

People with HIV should have their blood glucose levels checked before starting treatment with HIV medicines. People with higher-than-normal glucose levels may need to avoid taking some HIV medicines.

Blood glucose testing is also important after starting HIV medicines. If testing shows high glucose levels, a change in HIV medicines may be necessary.

HOW CAN A PERSON PREVENT, DELAY, OR MANAGE TYPE 2 DIABETES?

You can take the following steps to lower your risk of developing type 2 diabetes:

- **Maintain a healthy weight**. If you are overweight, lose weight and keep it off.
- **Eat healthy**. Eat a variety of healthy foods and limit foods high in fat, sugar, and salt.
- **Keep moving**. Aim for 30 minutes of physical activity on most days of the week.

People who have type 2 diabetes can also follow these steps to manage the disease. In addition, some people may take medicine to manage their type 2 diabetes.

If you have HIV, talk to your healthcare provider about your risk for diabetes.

Section 29.3 | Hepatotoxicity and Lactic Acidosis

This section contains text excerpted from the following sources: Text beginning with the heading "What Is Hepatotoxicity?" is excerpted from "HIV and Hepatotoxicity," HIVinfo, U.S. Department of Health and Human Services (HHS), August 19, 2021; Text beginning with the heading "What Is Lactic Acidosis?" is excerpted from "HIV and Lactic Acidosis," HIVinfo, U.S. Department of Health and Human Services (HHS), August 10, 2021.

WHAT IS HEPATOTOXICITY?

Hepatotoxicity is the medical term for damage to the liver caused by a medicine, chemical, or herbal or dietary supplement. Hepatotoxicity can be a side effect of some HIV medicines.

ARE THERE OTHER FACTORS THAT CAN INCREASE THE RISK OF HEPATOTOXICITY?

The following factors may increase the risk of hepatotoxicity due to HIV medicines:
- Having hepatitis B virus (HBV) infection and/or hepatitis C virus (HCV) infection
- Taking other medicines that can cause liver damage
- Alcohol use, which can cause liver damage
- Preexisting liver damage

SYMPTOMS OF HEPATOTOXICITY

Symptoms of hepatotoxicity include the following:
- Rash
- Stomach pain
- Nausea and vomiting
- Fatigue
- Dark-colored urine
- Light-colored bowel movements
- Jaundice (yellow skin and eyes)
- Loss of appetite
- Fever

People taking HIV medicines that may cause hepatotoxicity should know about these symptoms. In some cases, hepatotoxicity can be life-threatening. If you have any of these symptoms, contact your healthcare provider immediately.

ARE THERE TESTS TO DETERMINE WHETHER I AM AT RISK FOR DEVELOPING HEPATOTOXICITY FROM HIV MEDICINES?

Before starting HIV medicines, people with HIV have several lab tests done. These include blood tests to check for liver damage and for HBV and HCV infection. If the test results and other information shows that the person is at risk for developing hepatotoxicity, they can avoid HIV medicines that may cause hepatotoxicity.

TREATMENT OF HEPATOTOXICITY

Once a person starts taking HIV medicines, they are monitored for signs of hepatotoxicity. HIV medicines that are causing serious, life-threatening hepatotoxicity must be stopped immediately. However, a person should never stop taking an HIV medicine unless their healthcare provider tells them to.

Choosing an HIV medicine to replace one that is causing hepatotoxicity will depend on a person's individual needs. Fortunately, there are many HIV medicines available to include in an HIV treatment regimen.

If you are taking or plan to take HIV medicines, talk to your healthcare provider about the risk of hepatotoxicity.

WHAT IS LACTIC ACIDOSIS?

Lactic acidosis is a condition caused by the buildup of lactic acid in the blood. The condition is a rare, but serious side effect of some HIV medicines in the nucleoside reverse transcriptase inhibitor (NRTI) drug class.

Women and people who are obese may have an increased risk of developing lactic acidosis if they are taking NRTIs.

Although lactic acidosis is a rare side effect of NRTIs, the condition can be life-threatening. Fortunately, lactic acidosis is less likely to occur with newer NRTIs than with NRTIs used in the past.

SYMPTOMS OF LACTIC ACIDOSIS

Lactic acidosis often develops gradually. Early signs of lactic acidosis can include fatigue, nausea, vomiting, and weight loss. These symptoms may not seem serious, but they can be the first signs of life-threatening lactic acidosis. If you are taking HIV medicines, always tell your healthcare provider about any symptoms that you are having – even symptoms that may not seem serious.

Lactic acidosis can advance rapidly. Signs of life-threatening lactic acidosis include the following:

- Above-normal heart rate
- Rapid breathing
- Yellowing of the skin and the whites of the eyes (jaundice)
- Weakness

If you are taking HIV medicines and have any of these symptoms, get medical help immediately.

TREATMENT OF LACTIC ACIDOSIS

Healthcare providers monitor people taking HIV medicines for side effects, such as lactic acidosis. If an HIV medicine is causing lactic acidosis, the HIV medicine should be stopped immediately. However, stopping an HIV medicine because of lactic acidosis does not mean stopping HIV treatment. Choosing an HIV medicine to replace one that is causing lactic acidosis will depend on a person's individual needs. Fortunately, there are many HIV medicines that can be included in an HIV treatment regimen.

Section 29.4 | Hyperlipidemia and HIV

This section includes text excerpted from "HIV and High Cholesterol," HIVinfo, U.S. Department of Health and Human Services (HHS), August 20, 2021.

WHAT IS HIGH CHOLESTEROL?

High cholesterol (also called "hyperlipidemia") refers to high levels of cholesterol in the blood. Cholesterol is a waxy, fat-like substance made by the body. Cholesterol is also found in foods from animal sources, including egg yolks, meat, and cheese.

The body needs cholesterol to function properly, but having too much can cause problems. High cholesterol increases the risk of heart disease.

RISK FACTORS OF HIGH CHOLESTEROL

The most common causes of high cholesterol are unhealthy lifestyle habits, including the following:

- Eating foods high in saturated fat, trans fat, and cholesterol
- Lack of physical activity
- Smoking

The following are additional risk factors for high cholesterol:

- Age – as people get older, their cholesterol levels tend to rise
- A family history of high cholesterol
- Other medical conditions, such as diabetes
- Being overweight or obese
- Certain medicines

Some HIV medicines may also increase the risk of high cholesterol in people with HIV.

SYMPTOMS OF HIGH CHOLESTEROL

Usually, high cholesterol has no symptoms. A blood test is used to measure cholesterol levels.

Cholesterol testing is recommended before and after a person starts taking HIV medicines. If cholesterol levels are normal, testing is recommended once a year. If cholesterol levels are too high, more frequent testing is recommended.

PREVENTION OF HIGH CHOLESTEROL

People can take these steps to prevent high cholesterol or lower cholesterol levels.

- **Eat a healthy diet**. Eat foods low in saturated fat, trans fat, and cholesterol. Choose low-fat or fat-free dairy products, eat more foods that are high in fiber, and eat more vegetables and fruits.
- **Get active**. Try to get at least 30 minutes of physical activity on most days of the week.
- **Maintain a healthy weight**. If you are overweight or obese, losing weight can improve cholesterol levels.
- Quit smoking

TREATMENT OF HIGH CHOLESTEROL

Treatment for high cholesterol begins with lifestyle changes. Sometimes cholesterol-lowering medicine is also needed. The most common medicines used to reduce cholesterol levels are called "statins."

In people with HIV, treatment for high cholesterol may include changing an HIV treatment regimen to avoid taking HIV medicines that can increase cholesterol levels.

Some HIV medicines can interact with medicines that lower cholesterol levels. Healthcare providers carefully consider potential drug-drug interactions between HIV medicines and any other medicines a person may be taking.

Section 29.5 | **Lipodystrophy**

This section includes text excerpted from "HIV and Lipodystrophy," HIVinfo, U.S. Department of Health and Human Services (HHS), August 19, 2021.

WHAT IS LIPODYSTROPHY?

Lipodystrophy refers to the changes in body fat that can affect some people with HIV. Lipodystrophy can include buildup of body fat, loss of body fat, or both.

Fat buildup (also called "lipohypertrophy") can occur:
- Around the organs in the abdomen
- On the back of the neck between the shoulders (called a "buffalo hump")
- In the breasts

Fat loss (also called "lipoatrophy") tends to occur:
- In the arms and legs
- In the buttocks
- In the face

CAUSES OF LIPODYSTROPHY

Lipodystrophy may be due to HIV infection or medicines used to treat HIV, but its actual cause is not understood. Newer HIV medicines are less likely to cause lipodystrophy than HIV medicines developed in the past.

Lipodystrophy is not a concern for most people who start HIV treatment now, because newer HIV medicines are less likely to cause lipodystrophy.

TREATMENT OF LIPODYSTROPHY

If you have lipodystrophy, talk to your healthcare provider about treatment options. Your healthcare provider may recommend that you switch to another HIV medicine.

There are ways to manage lipodystrophy. Making dietary changes and getting regular exercise may help to build muscle and reduce abdominal fat.

Liposuction (surgical removal of fat) and injectable facial fillers are sometimes used to treat lipodystrophy. There are also medicines that may help lessen the effects of lipodystrophy.

Section 29.6 | Osteoporosis

This section includes text excerpted from "HIV and Osteoporosis," HIVinfo, U.S. Department of Health and Human Services (HHS), August 20, 2021.

WHAT IS OSTEOPOROSIS?

Osteoporosis is a disease that develops due to bone loss. The bones of people with osteoporosis become weak and are more likely to break. Osteoporosis increases the risk of broken bones of the hip, spine, and wrist.

The risk of osteoporosis increases as people age. Anyone can get osteoporosis, but it is most common in older women.

HIV infection and some HIV medicines may increase the risk of osteoporosis in people with HIV.

RISK FACTORS OF OSTEOPOROSIS

There are many risk factors for osteoporosis. Some risk factors cannot be changed, while other risk factors can be managed with lifestyle choices.

Risk factors for osteoporosis that cannot be changed include:

- **Age.** The risk of osteoporosis increases as people get older.
- **Gender.** Compared to men, women have smaller bones and lose bone faster due to hormonal changes after menopause.
- **Race/ethnicity.** The risk of osteoporosis is greatest for White and Asian women.
- **Family history.** Osteoporosis tends to run in families.

The following risk factors for osteoporosis can be controlled by lifestyle choices:

- **Poor diet**. A diet low in calcium and vitamin D increases the risk of osteoporosis.
- **Physical inactivity**. Physical inactivity tends to weaken bones.
- **Smoking**. Smoking increases the risk of osteoporosis.
- **Alcohol**. Too much alcohol can cause bone loss and broken bones.

SYMPTOMS OF OSTEOPOROSIS

Bone loss that leads to osteoporosis occurs without symptoms. The first sign of osteoporosis is often a broken bone.

A bone mineral density test (also called "dual energy x-ray absorptiometry") is used to measure bone health. The test, which is painless, is used to diagnose osteoporosis.

People with HIV may wish to discuss bone mineral density testing with their healthcare providers.

PREVENTION OF OSTEOPOROSIS

People can take the following steps to prevent osteoporosis.

- **Eat a healthy diet rich in calcium and vitamin D**. Foods high in calcium include milk and other dairy products, broccoli, sardines, tofu, and almonds. Milk is fortified with vitamin D. Egg yolks, saltwater fish, and liver are also high in vitamin D. People can also take calcium and vitamin D supplements.
- **Stay active**. Physical activities, such as walking and lifting weights, can make bones stronger and help slow down bone loss.
- Do not smoke.
- **Cut down on alcohol**. If you drink alcohol, drink in moderation.

TREATMENT OF OSTEOPOROSIS

Treatment for osteoporosis includes eating a healthy diet rich in calcium and vitamin D and getting regular exercise to improve bone health. There are also medicines to help prevent and treat osteoporosis.

People with osteoporosis also need to avoid falls that can lead to broken bones. For example, they may use a cane or walker to help prevent falls.

Section 29.7 | Skin Rash

This section includes text excerpted from "HIV and Rash," HIVinfo, U.S. Department of Health and Human Services (HHS), August 10, 2021.

WHY DO PEOPLE WITH HIV DEVELOP A RASH?

A rash is an irritated area of the skin that is sometimes itchy, red, and painful. Possible causes of a rash in people with HIV include:

- **Acute HIV infection**. It is the earliest stage of HIV infection. Symptoms of acute HIV infection may include a rash.
- **Other infections**. Without treatment, HIV gradually destroys the immune system. Damage to the immune system puts people with HIV at risk of infections, and a rash is a symptom of many infections.
- **Medicines**. Many medicines, including some HIV medicines, can cause a rash. A rash due to an HIV medicine is often not serious and goes away in several days to weeks without treatment. But, sometimes, when an HIV medicine is causing a rash, it may be necessary to switch to another HIV medicine. If you are taking HIV medicines, tell your healthcare provider if you have a rash. In rare cases, a rash caused by an HIV medicine can be a sign of a serious, life-threatening condition.

WHAT ARE SERIOUS RASH-RELATED CONDITIONS?

A rash can be a sign of a hypersensitivity reaction. A hypersensitivity reaction is a potentially serious allergic reaction to a medicine. In addition to a rash, signs of a hypersensitivity reaction can include difficulty breathing, dizziness, or lightheadedness. A severe hypersensitivity reaction can be life-threatening and requires immediate medical attention.

Stevens-Johnson syndrome (SJS) is a rare, but life-threatening hypersensitivity reaction reported with the use of some HIV medicines. People taking HIV medicines need to know about this condition. It rarely occurs, but when it does, it can cause death.

Symptoms of SJS include fever, flu-like symptoms, rash, and painful blisters that may spread throughout the body.

If you have symptoms of SJS, get medical help immediately. SJS can be life-threatening.

Chapter 30 | Other HIV/AIDS Treatment Complications

Section 30.1 | Drug Interactions

This section includes text excerpted from "What Is a Drug Interaction?" HIVinfo, U.S. Department of Health and Human Services (HHS), August 4, 2021.

WHAT IS A DRUG INTERACTION?

Medicines help us feel better and stay healthy. But sometimes drug interactions can cause problems. There are three types of drug interactions:

- **Drug-drug interaction.** A reaction between two (or more) drugs.
- **Drug-food interaction.** A reaction between a drug and a food or beverage.
- **Drug-condition interaction.** A reaction that occurs when taking a drug while having a certain medical condition. For example, taking a nasal decongestant if you have high blood pressure may cause an unwanted reaction. A drug interaction can affect how a drug works or cause unwanted side effects.

DO HIV MEDICINES EVER CAUSE DRUG INTERACTIONS?

Treatment with human immunodeficiency virus (HIV) medicines (called "antiretroviral therapy" or "ART") helps people with HIV live longer, healthier lives and reduces the risk of HIV transmission. But drug interactions, especially drug-drug interactions, can complicate HIV treatment.

Drug-drug interactions between different HIV medicines and between HIV medicines and other medicines are common. Before recommending an HIV treatment regimen, healthcare providers carefully consider potential drug-drug interactions between HIV medicines. They also ask about other medicines a person may be taking. For example, some HIV medicines may make hormonal birth control less effective, so women using hormonal contraceptives may need to use an additional or different method of birth control to prevent pregnancy. Figure 30.1 shows drug interaction factors and possible side effects.

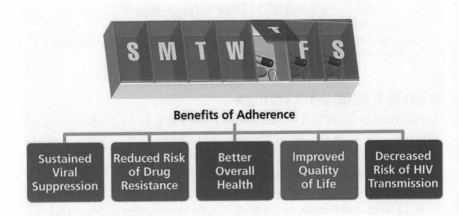

Figure 30.1. Drug Interaction

CAN DRUG-FOOD INTERACTIONS AND DRUG-CONDITION INTERACTIONS AFFECT PEOPLE TAKING HIV MEDICINES?

Yes, the use of HIV medicines can lead to both drug-food interactions and drug-condition interactions.

Food can affect the absorption of some HIV medicines and increase or reduce the concentration of the medicine in the blood. Depending on the HIV medicine, the change in concentration may be helpful or harmful. Directions on how to take HIV medicines specify whether to take the medicine with food or on an empty stomach. Some HIV medicines can be taken with or without food, because food does not affect their absorption.

Conditions, such as kidney disease, hepatitis, and pregnancy, can affect how the body processes HIV medicines. The dosing of some HIV medicines may need to be adjusted in people with certain medical conditions.

HOW CAN A PERSON AVOID DRUG INTERACTIONS?

You can take the following steps to avoid drug interactions:
- Tell your healthcare provider about all prescription and nonprescription medicines you are taking or plan

to take. Also tell your healthcare provider about any vitamins, nutritional supplements, and herbal products you take.

- Tell your healthcare provider about any other conditions you may have, such as high blood pressure or diabetes.
- Before taking a medicine, ask your healthcare provider or pharmacist the following questions:
  - What is the medicine used for?
  - How should I take the medicine?
  - While taking the medicine, should I avoid any other medicines or certain foods or beverages?
  - Can I take this medicine safely with the other medicines that I am taking?
  - Are there any possible drug interactions I should know about?
  - What are the signs of those drug interactions?
  - In the case of a drug interaction, what should I do?
- Take medicines according to your healthcare provider's instructions. Always read the information and directions that come with a medicine. Drug labels and package inserts include important information about possible drug interactions.

Section 30.2 | Risk of Muscle Injury

This section includes text excerpted from "FDA Drug Safety Communication: Interactions between Certain HIV or Hepatitis C Drugs and Cholesterol-Lowering Statin Drugs Can Increase the Risk of Muscle Injury," U.S. Food and Drug Administration (FDA), January 19, 2016. Reviewed February 2022.

FACTS ABOUT STATINS AND PROTEASE INHIBITORS

- Statins are a class of prescription drugs used together with diet and exercise to reduce blood levels of low-density lipoprotein (LDL) cholesterol ("bad cholesterol").

- HIV protease inhibitors are a class of prescription anti-viral drugs used to treat HIV.
- HCV protease inhibitors are a class of prescription anti-viral drugs used to treat hepatitis C infection.
- A side effect of taking HIV protease inhibitors is increased cholesterol and triglyceride (fat) levels. Therefore, some patients taking HIV protease inhibitors may need to take cholesterol-lowering medicines such as statins.

SAFETY ANNOUNCEMENT

The U.S. Food and Drug Administration (FDA) is issuing updated recommendations concerning drug-drug interactions between drugs for human immunodeficiency virus (HIV) or hepatitis C virus (HCV) known as "protease inhibitors" and certain cholesterol-lowering drugs known as "statins." Protease inhibitors and statins taken together may raise the blood levels of statins and increase the risk for muscle injury (myopathy). The most serious form of myopathy, called "rhabdomyolysis," can damage the kidneys and lead to kidney failure, which can be fatal.

The labels for both the HIV protease inhibitors and the affected statins have been updated to contain consistent information about the drug-drug interactions. These labels also have been updated to include dosing recommendations for those statins that may safely be co-administered with HIV or HCV protease inhibitors.

Healthcare professionals should refer to the current drug labels for protease inhibitors and statins for the latest recommendations on prescribing these drugs.

Patients should contact their healthcare professional if they have any questions or concerns about taking protease inhibitors and statins.

ADDITIONAL INFORMATION FOR PATIENTS

- Human immunodeficiency virus (HIV) and hepatitis C virus (HCV) protease inhibitors can interact with cholesterol-lowering statins to increase the risk of muscle injury.

- Patients should inform their healthcare professional about all medicines that they are taking or plan to take prior to starting an HIV or HCV protease inhibitor or statin.
- HIV and HCV protease inhibitors should never be taken (are contraindicated) with lovastatin (Mevacor) and simvastatin (Zocor).
- Patients should contact their healthcare professional if they have any questions or concerns about HIV or HCV protease inhibitors or statins.
- Patients should report side effects from the use of HIV or HCV protease inhibitors and/or statins to the FDA MedWatch program.

DATA SUMMARY
Table 30.1 shows the statin dose limitations.

Atorvastatin
The results from a drug-drug interaction study with atorvastatin and lopinavir/ritonavir that were previously in the atorvastatin label have not yet been validated. Therefore, these results have been removed from the label and the dose cap of atorvastatin 20 mg when co-administered with lopinavir/ritonavir has also been removed. Pending validation of the study, healthcare professionals should use caution when co-administering atorvastatin with lopinavir/ritonavir and use the lowest necessary dose of atorvastatin.

Lovastatin and Simvastatin
Lovastatin and simvastatin are sensitive in vivo cytochrome P450 3A4 (CYP3A4) substrates. Therefore, strong CYP3A4 inhibitors are predicted to significantly increase lovastatin and simvastatin exposures. A literature review indicates that itraconazole, a strong CYP3A4 inhibitor, increases lovastatin exposure up to 20-fold, and the drug interaction appears to result in rhabdomyolysis. Itraconazole increases simvastatin exposure up to 13-fold. Hence, other CYP3A4 inhibitors, including ketoconazole, posaconazole, erythromycin, clarithromycin, telithromycin, nefazodone, human

immunodeficiency virus (HIV) protease inhibitors, and the hepatitis C virus (HCV) protease inhibitors boceprevir and telaprevir, are also expected to significantly increase lovastatin and simvastatin exposures. Therefore, concomitant administration of lovastatin and simvastatin with HIV protease inhibitors or HCV protease inhibitors (boceprevir and telaprevir) is contraindicated.

Rosuvastatin

The HIV protease inhibitor combinations lopinavir/ritonavir and atazanavir/ritonavir increase rosuvastatin exposure up to 3-fold. For these combinations, the dose of rosuvastatin should be limited to 10 mg.

Table 30.1. Statin Dose Limitations

Statin	Interacting Protease Inhibitor(s)	Prescribing Recommendation
	Tipranavir + ritonavir Telaprevir	Avoid atorvastatin
	Lopinavir + ritonavir	Use with caution and use with the lowest atorvastatin dose necessary
	Darunavir + ritonavir Fosamprenavir Fosamprenavir + ritonavir Saquinavir + ritonavir	Do not exceed 20 mg atorvastatin daily
Atorvastatin	Nelfinavir	Do not exceed 40 mg atorvastatin daily
Fluvastatin		No data available
Lovastatin	HIV protease inhibitors Boceprevir Telaprevir	Contraindicated
Pitavastatin	Atazanavir ± ritonavir Darunavir + ritonavir Lopinavir + ritonavir	No dose limitations
Pravastatin	Darunavir + ritonavir Lopinavir + ritonavir	No dose limitations

Table 30.1. Continued

Statin	Interacting Protease Inhibitor(s)	Prescribing Recommendation
Rosuvastatin	Atazanavir ± ritonavir Lopinavir + ritonavir	Limit rosuvastatin dose to 10 mg once daily
Simvastatin	HIV protease inhibitors Boceprevir Telaprevir	Contraindicated

Chapter 31 | **Alternative (Complementary) Therapies for HIV/AIDS**

Many people use alternative (sometimes known as "complementary") health treatments in addition to the medical care they get from their provider. These therapies are sometimes called "alternative" because they do not fit into the more mainstream, western ways of looking at medicine and healthcare. They are called "complementary therapies" because usually they are used alongside the more standard medical care you receive. Some common complementary therapies include:

- Physical (body) therapies, such as yoga, massage, and acupuncture
- Relaxation techniques, such as meditation and visualization
- Herbal medicines (from plants)

With most complementary therapies, your health is looked at from a holistic (or "whole picture") point of view. Think of your body as working as one big system. From a holistic viewpoint, everything you do – from what you eat to what you drink to how stressed you are – affects your health and well-being.

This chapter includes text excerpted from "Alternative (Complementary) Therapies for HIV/AIDS," U.S. Department of Veterans Affairs (VA), April 30, 2019.

DO ALTERNATIVE THERAPIES WORK?

Healthy people use these kinds of therapies to try to make their immune systems stronger and to make themselves feel better in general. People who have diseases or illnesses, such as human immunodeficiency virus (HIV), use these therapies for the same reasons. They also can use these therapies to help deal with symptoms of the disease or side effects from the medicines that treat the disease. Many people report positive results from using complementary therapies. In many cases, however, there is not enough research to tell if these treatments really help people with HIV.

PHYSICAL THERAPIES

Physical, or body, therapies include such activities as yoga, massage, and aromatherapy. These types of therapies focus on using a person's body and senses to promote healing and well-being.

Yoga

Yoga is a set of exercises that people use to improve their fitness, reduce stress, and increase flexibility. Yoga can involve breathing exercises, stretching and strengthening poses, and meditation. Many people, including people with HIV, use yoga to reduce stress and to become more relaxed. There are many different types of yoga and various classes you can take. You can also try out yoga by following a video program. Before you begin any kind of exercise program, always talk with your healthcare provider.

Massage

Many people believe that massage therapy is an excellent way to deal with the stress and side effects that go along with having an illness, including HIV. During massage therapy, a trained therapist moves and rubs your body tissues (such as your muscles). There are many kinds of massage therapy. You can try massage therapy for reducing muscle and back pain, headaches, and soreness. Massages also can improve your blood flow (circulation) and reduce tension.

Acupuncture

Acupuncture is part of a whole healing system known as "traditional Chinese medicine." During an acupuncture treatment, tiny needles (about as wide as a hair) are inserted into certain areas of a person's body. Most people say that they do not feel any pain from the needles. Many people with HIV use acupuncture. Some people think that acupuncture can help treat symptoms of HIV and side effects from the medicine, like fatigue and nausea. Some people say that acupuncture can be used to help with neuropathy (body pain caused by nerve damage from HIV or the medicines used to treat HIV). Others report that acupuncture gives them more energy.

Aromatherapy

Aromatherapy is based on the idea that certain smells can change the way you feel. The smells used in aromatherapy come from plant oils, and they can be inhaled (breathed in) or used in baths or massages. People use aromatherapy to help them deal with stress or to help with fatigue. For example, some people report that lavender oil calms them down and helps them sleep better. Please remember! The oils used in aromatherapy can be very strong and even harmful. Always talk with an expert before using these oils yourself.

RELAXATION TECHNIQUES

Relaxation therapies, such as meditation and visualization, focus on how a person's mind and imagination can promote overall health and well-being.

Meditation

Meditation is a certain way of concentrating that may allow your mind and body to become very relaxed. Meditation helps people to focus and be quiet. There are many different forms of meditation. Most involve deep breathing and paying attention to your body and mind. Sometimes people sit still and close their eyes to meditate. Meditation also can be casual. For instance, you can meditate when you are taking a walk or watching a sunrise. People with HIV can use meditation to relax. It can help them deal with the stress that comes with any illness. Meditation can help you to calm down and focus if you are feeling overwhelmed. There may be meditation classes you can take.

Visualization

Visualization is another method people use to feel more relaxed and less anxious. People who use visualization imagine that they are in a safe, relaxing place (such as the beach). Most of us use visualization without realizing it – for example, when we daydream or remember a fun, happy time in our lives. Focusing on a safe, comfortable place can help you to feel less stress, and sometimes it can lessen the pain or side effects from HIV or the medicines you are taking. There are classes you can take, and there are self-help tapes that you can listen to that lead you through the process.

HERBAL MEDICINE

Herbal medicines are substances that come from plants, and they work like standard medicine. They can be taken from all parts of a plant, including the roots, leaves, berries, and flowers. People with HIV sometimes take these medicines to help deal with side effects from HIV medications or with symptoms from the disease.

An important note about St. John's wort. St. John's wort is an herbal medicine that is used by some people to treat depression. It interacts with the liver and can change how some drugs work in your body, including some HIV medications (e.g., protease inhibitors and nonnucleoside reverse transcriptase inhibitors (NNRTIs). If you are taking antiviral medications for your HIV, you should not take St. John's wort. Be sure you tell your provider if you are using St. John's wort. Also, do not take St. John's wort if you are taking other antidepressants.

POINTS TO REMEMBER

In addition to getting mainstream medical care, many people use complementary treatments to improve their overall health or to help with specific health problems.

Alternative (Complementary) Therapies for HIV/AIDS

Complementary therapies can include physical therapies (such as yoga and acupuncture), relaxation techniques (such as meditation), and herbal medicines. Many people report that these therapies make them feel better and help with symptoms and side effects.

It is important to remember that not all complementary therapies are safe for you. In fact, some therapies (including certain herbs) can be very dangerous because they can interact with your HIV medications or cause severe side effects.

Always be sure to let your provider know what medicines you are taking – whether they are prescription or not.

Chapter 32 | Medical Marijuana for HIV/AIDS

Marijuana is a green, brown, or gray mix of dried, crumbled parts from the marijuana plant. It can be rolled up and smoked like a cigarette or cigar or smoked in a pipe. Sometimes people mix it in food or inhale it using a vaporizer.

Marijuana can cause problems with memory, learning, and behavior. Smoking can cause some of the same coughing and breathing problems as smoking cigarettes. Some people get addicted to marijuana after using it for a while. It is more likely to happen if they use marijuana every day, or start using it when they were teenagers.

Some states have approved "medical marijuana" to ease symptoms of various health problems. The U.S. Food and Drug Administration (FDA) has not approved the marijuana plant as a medicine. However, there have been scientific studies of cannabinoids, the chemicals in marijuana. This has led to two FDA-approved medicines. They contain tetrahydrocannabinol (THC), the active ingredient in marijuana. They treat nausea caused by chemotherapy and increase appetite in patients who have severe weight loss from human immunodeficiency virus (HIV)/acquired immunodeficiency syndrome (AIDS). Scientists are doing more research on marijuana and its ingredients to treat many diseases and conditions.

This chapter contains text excerpted from the following sources: Text in this chapter begins with excerpts from "Marijuana," Effective Health Care Program, Agency for Healthcare Research and Quality (AHRQ), August 11, 2021; Text beginning with the heading "How Does Marijuana Produce Its Effects?" is excerpted from "How Does Marijuana Produce Its Effects?" National Institute on Drug Abuse (NIDA), July 2, 2020.

HOW DOES MARIJUANA PRODUCE ITS EFFECTS?

THC's chemical structure is similar to the brain chemical anandamide. The similarity in structure allows the body to recognize THC and to alter normal brain communication.

Endogenous cannabinoids such as anandamide function as neurotransmitters because they send chemical messages between nerve cells (neurons) throughout the nervous system. They affect brain areas that influence pleasure, memory, thinking, concentration, movement, coordination, and sensory and time perception. Because of this similarity, THC is able to attach to molecules called "cannabinoid receptors" on neurons in these brain areas and activate them, disrupting various mental and physical functions and causing the effects described earlier. The neural communication network that uses these cannabinoid neurotransmitters, known as the "endocannabinoid system," plays a critical role in the nervous system's normal functioning, so interfering with it can have profound effects.

For example, THC is able to alter the functioning of the hippocampus and orbitofrontal cortex, brain areas that enable a person to form new memories and shift his or her attentional focus. As a result, using marijuana causes impaired thinking and interferes with a person's ability to learn and perform complicated tasks. THC also disrupts the functioning of the cerebellum and basal ganglia, brain areas that regulate balance, posture, coordination, and reaction time. This is the reason people who have used marijuana may not be able to drive safely and may have problems playing sports or engaging in other physical activities.

THC, acting through cannabinoid receptors, also activates the brain's reward system, which includes regions that govern the response to healthy pleasurable behaviors such as sex and eating. Like most other drugs that people misuse, THC stimulates neurons in the reward system to release the signaling chemical dopamine at levels higher than typically observed in response to naturally rewarding stimuli. The surge of dopamine "teaches" the brain to repeat the rewarding behavior, helping account for marijuana's addictive properties.

IS MARIJUANA SAFE AND EFFECTIVE AS MEDICINE?

The potential medicinal properties of marijuana and its components have been the subject of research and heated debate for decades. THC itself has proven medical benefits in particular formulations. The FDA has approved THC-based medications, dronabinol (Marinol®) and nabilone (Cesamet®), prescribed in pill form for the treatment of nausea in patients undergoing cancer chemotherapy and to stimulate appetite in patients with wasting syndrome due to AIDS.

In addition, several other marijuana-based medications have been approved or are undergoing clinical trials. Nabiximols (Sativex®), a mouth spray that is currently available in the United Kingdom, Canada, and several European countries for treating the spasticity and neuropathic pain that may accompany multiple sclerosis, combines THC with another chemical found in marijuana called "cannabidiol" (CBD).

The FDA also approved a CBD-based liquid medication called "Epidiolex®" for the treatment of two forms of severe childhood epilepsy, Dravet syndrome and Lennox-Gastaut syndrome. It is being delivered to patients in a reliable dosage form and through a reproducible route of delivery to ensure that patients derive the anticipated benefits. CBD does not have the rewarding properties of THC.

Researchers generally consider medications like these, which use purified chemicals derived from or based on those in the marijuana plant, to be more promising therapeutically than use of the whole marijuana plant or its crude extracts. The development of drugs from botanicals such as the marijuana plant poses numerous challenges. Botanicals may contain hundreds of unknown, active chemicals, and it can be difficult to develop a product with accurate and consistent doses of these chemicals. Use of marijuana as medicine also poses other problems such as the adverse health effects of smoking and THC-induced cognitive impairment. Nevertheless, a growing number of states have legalized dispensing of marijuana or its extracts to people with a range of medical conditions.

An additional concern with "medical marijuana" is that little is known about the long-term impact of its use by people with health- and/or age-related vulnerabilities – such as older adults or people with cancer, AIDS, cardiovascular disease, multiple sclerosis, or other neurodegenerative diseases. Further research will be needed to determine whether people whose health has been compromised by disease or its treatment (e.g., chemotherapy) are at greater risk for adverse health outcomes from marijuana use.

Chapter 33 | **HIV/AIDS Treatments in Development**

Chapter Contents

Section 33.1 | Therapeutic HIV Vaccines

This section includes text excerpted from "What Is a Therapeutic HIV Vaccine?" HIVinfo, U.S. Department of Health and Human Services (HHS), August 4, 2021.

WHAT IS A THERAPEUTIC HIV VACCINE?

A therapeutic human immunodeficiency virus (HIV) vaccine is a vaccine that is designed to improve the body's immune response to HIV in a person who already has HIV. Researchers are developing and testing therapeutic HIV vaccines to slow down the progression of HIV to acquired immunodeficiency syndrome (AIDS). The hope is that treating people with these vaccines would ideally keep HIV at undetectable levels (known as "undetectable viral load") without the need for regular antiretroviral therapy (ART). ART is the recommended treatment for HIV infection and involves using a combination of different HIV medicines to prevent HIV from multiplying. Currently, a person with HIV must remain on ART to keep HIV at undetectable levels. A therapeutic HIV vaccine may also make it less likely that a person could transmit HIV to others.

In the future, therapeutic vaccines could:

- Prevent HIV from advancing to AIDS.
- Replace the use of daily HIV medicines.
- Helps in preventing HIV transmission.

ARE THERE ANY FDA-APPROVED THERAPEUTIC HIV VACCINES?

There are currently no U.S. Food and Drug Administration (FDA)-approved therapeutic HIV vaccines, but research is underway. You must be enrolled in a clinical trial to receive a therapeutic HIV vaccine.

HOW IS A THERAPEUTIC HIV VACCINE DIFFERENT FROM A PREVENTIVE HIV VACCINE?

A preventive HIV vaccine is given to people who do not have HIV, with the goal of preventing HIV infection in the future. The vaccine teaches the person's immune system to recognize and effectively fight HIV in case the virus ever enters the person's body.

A therapeutic HIV vaccine is given to people who already have HIV. The goal of a therapeutic HIV vaccine is to strengthen a person's immune response to the HIV that is already in the person's body.

Section 33.2 | Future Directions for HIV Treatment Research

This section includes text excerpted from "Future Directions for HIV Treatment Research," National Institute of Allergy and Infectious Diseases (NIAID), August 26, 2019.

A major goal of the National Institute of Allergy and Infectious Diseases (NIAID)-supported research on human immunodeficiency virus (HIV) treatment today is to develop long-acting therapies that – unlike current antiretrovirals, which require daily dosing – could be taken only once a week, once a month, or even less often. Such long-acting therapies might be easier for some people to stick to than daily pills, and might also be less toxic and more cost-effective. The three types of agents under study are long-acting drugs, broadly neutralizing antibodies, and therapeutic vaccines.

LONG-ACTING DRUGS

The NIAID-supported scientists aim to develop a new array of drugs for HIV treatment that include longer-acting pills as well as alternative formulations such as injections, patches, and implants. The complexity of developing such products has led NIAID to create a consortium of experts who can facilitate relationships among the many types of researchers needed to translate an idea for a long-acting HIV drug into a workable solution. Long-Acting/Extended Release Antiretroviral Resource Program (LEAP), the consortium includes scientists and clinicians from academia, industry, and government, as well as patient advocates.

NIAID also will investigate the effectiveness of two investigational long-acting HIV drugs, rilpivirine long-acting (LA) and cabotegravir LA, in people for whom adhering to conventional antiretroviral therapy has been a challenge. Another study is planned to test whether the combination of monthly injections of cabotegravir LA and monthly infusions of an NIAID-discovered broadly neutralizing antibody called "VRC01LS" can keep HIV suppressed in people whose infection was previously controlled by antiretroviral therapy.

BROADLY NEUTRALIZING ANTIBODIES

Scientists at the NIAID Vaccine Research Center (VRC) and NIAID-supported scientists at other institutions are developing and testing multiple antibodies for the treatment of HIV. Antibodies are good candidates for treatment because they have few side effects and can be modified to ensure they last a long time in the body, suggesting that dosing could be every other month or even less often. Importantly, the antibodies under investigation can powerfully stop a wide range of HIV strains from infecting human cells in the laboratory and thus are known as "broadly neutralizing antibodies," or "Broadly neutralizing HIV-1 antibodies (bNAbs)."

In the context of treatment, bNAbs can potentially thwart HIV in three ways:

- By binding directly to the virus, preventing it from entering a cell and accelerating its elimination
- By binding to an HIV-infected cell, recruiting immune-system components that facilitate cell killing
- By binding to a key fragment of HIV, forming a complex that may lead to the stimulation of immune cells in a manner similar to a vaccine, thereby preparing the immune system for future encounters with the virus.

Clinical studies have established that giving infusions of certain bNAbs to people living with HIV can suppress the virus, albeit to a limited degree. Further studies have shown that treating people living with HIV with just one bNAb fosters the emergence of HIV strains that are resistant to the antibody. Thus, just as antiretroviral therapy requires a combination of drugs to effectively suppress HIV, it appears that antibody-based therapy will require a combination of either multiple bNAbs or bNAbs and long-acting drugs to suppress the virus. Studies in monkeys infected with a simian version of HIV have already demonstrated that combinations of complementary bNAbs powerfully suppress the virus for an extended period. NIAID is now funding and conducting clinical trials of this strategy for treating HIV in people.

In addition, scientists are engineering changes to known bNAbs to optimize them for HIV treatment and prevention applications. These changes are designed to increase the number of HIV strains an antibody can block, how long the antibody lasts in the body, how powerfully the antibody attaches to the virus, and how efficiently the antibody triggers the immune system to attack both the virus and HIV-infected cells.

THERAPEUTIC HIV VACCINES

Perhaps the ideal treatment for HIV infection would be a therapeutic vaccine. Unlike a vaccine designed to prevent HIV infection, a therapeutic vaccine would be given to people already infected with the virus. Such a vaccine would stimulate the immune system to be ready to control any future emergence of HIV and thereby end the need for further therapy, perhaps save periodic booster shots. Such an approach could lead to sustained viral remission, meaning treatment or vaccination that would result in prolonged undetectable levels of HIV without regular antiretroviral therapy.

The presence of rare people living with HIV who can control the virus naturally either from the time of infection or after halting antiretroviral therapy is evidence that a therapeutic vaccine could theoretically alter the immune system to achieve long-term control of HIV. Nevertheless, attempts to create effective therapeutic HIV vaccines have so far been unsuccessful. To help improve results, NIAID is working to advance the underlying science – in particular, to improve understanding of immune responses that sustainably suppress HIV and to improve the potency of those responses.

Three of the NIAID-funded Martin Delaney Collaboratories are pursuing strategies that involve therapeutic vaccines to achieve long-term control of HIV or reduction of the reservoir of all virus-carrying cells.

FUTURE DIRECTIONS FOR DEVELOPING DAILY HIV DRUGS

At the same time, NIAID continues to support research to develop new drugs with unique mechanisms of action for daily antiretroviral therapy. Such drugs likely would be effective against HIV strains with resistance to other drug types.

For example, basic NIAID-supported research contributed to development of the experimental drug islatravir (also known as "EFdA" or "MK-8591"), which belongs to a class of drugs known as "nucleoside reverse transcriptase translocation inhibitors," or "NRTTIs." NIAID research also contributed to the development of maturation inhibitors, investigational drugs that target the same stage of the HIV lifecycle as protease inhibitors but act by a different mechanism.

Researchers also are attempting to target other parts of the HIV lifecycle. For example, the experimental inhibitor fostemsavir blocks HIV from infecting immune cells by attaching to the gp120 protein on the virus' surface. Another example is the development of capsid assembly inhibitors, which halt construction of the viral capsid, the protein shell that encloses HIV's genetic material.

Chapter 34 |
Investigational HIV Drug and Its Role in HIV Treatment

WHAT IS AN INVESTIGATIONAL HIV DRUG?

An investigational human immunodeficiency virus (HIV) drug is an experimental drug that is being studied to see whether it is safe and effective. Investigational HIV drugs are studied in medical research studies called "clinical trials." Once an investigational HIV drug has been proven safe and effective in a clinical trial, the U.S. Food and Drug Administration (FDA) may approve the drug for general use or sale in the United States.

WHAT TYPES OF INVESTIGATIONAL HIV DRUGS ARE BEING STUDIED?

Investigational HIV drugs being studied include drugs to treat HIV and prevent HIV. Some types of investigational HIV drugs being studied include microbicides, immune modulators, latency-reversing agents, gp120 attachment inhibitors, and rev inhibitors.

HIV researchers are also studying investigational vaccines to prevent HIV and treat HIV. The goal of a preventive HIV vaccine

This chapter includes text excerpted from "What Is an Investigational HIV Drug?" HIVinfo, U.S. Department of Health and Human Services (HHS), August 20, 2021.

is to prevent HIV in people who do not have HIV, but who may be exposed to the virus. A safe and effective HIV treatment vaccine (also called a "therapeutic HIV vaccine") could prevent HIV from advancing to acquired immunodeficiency syndrome (AIDS), replace the daily use of HIV medicines, and help prevent HIV transmission.

HOW ARE CLINICAL TRIALS OF INVESTIGATIONAL DRUGS CONDUCTED?

Clinical trials are conducted in phases. Each phase has a different purpose and helps researchers answer different questions about the investigational drug.

- **Phase 1 trial.** Initial testing in a small group of people (20–80) to evaluate the drug's safety and to identify side effects.
- **Phase 2 trial.** Testing in a larger group of people (100–300) to determine the drug's effectiveness and to further evaluate its safety.
- **Phase 3 trial.** Continued testing in large groups of people (1,000–3,000) to confirm the drug's effectiveness, monitor side effects, compare it with standard or equivalent treatments, and collect information to ensure that the investigational drug can be used safely. In most cases, an investigational drug must be proven effective and must show continued safety in a Phase 3 clinical trial to be considered for approval by the FDA for sale in the United States. (However, some drugs go through the FDA's accelerated approval process and are approved before a Phase 3 clinical trial is complete.)
- **Phase 4 trial.** Ongoing tracking that occurs after a drug is approved by the FDA for sale in the United States. The purpose of the tracking is to seek more information about the drug's risks, benefits, and optimal use.

HOW CAN A PERSON FIND A CLINICAL TRIAL THAT IS STUDYING AN INVESTIGATIONAL HIV DRUG?

To find an HIV and AIDS clinical trial that is studying an investigational HIV drug, use the find a study search feature on ClinicalTrials.gov.

For help with your search, call a Clinical Info health information specialist at 800-448-0440 or e-mail ContactUs@HIVinfo.NIH.gov.

You can also join ResearchMatch, which is a free, secure online tool that makes it easier for the public to become involved in clinical trials.

ARE INVESTIGATIONAL HIV DRUGS AVAILABLE FOR USE OUTSIDE OF A CLINICAL TRIAL?

In some cases, an investigational HIV drug may be available through an expanded access program. Expanded access allows for the use of an investigational drug outside of a clinical trial to treat a person who has a serious or immediate life-threatening disease and who has no FDA-approved treatment options. Drug companies must have permission from the FDA to make an investigational drug available for expanded access.

People seeking expanded access to an investigational HIV drug should talk to their healthcare provider to see if they may qualify to take part in an expanded access program.

IS IT SAFE TO USE AN INVESTIGATIONAL HIV DRUG?

One goal of HIV research is to identify safer, more effective HIV medicines. Researchers try to make clinical trials as safe as possible. However, taking an investigational HIV drug can involve both benefits and risks. Risks may include unexpected side effects from the drug, which can be unpleasant, serious, or even life-threatening.

The benefits and possible risks of participating in a clinical trial or an expanded access program are explained to people before they decide whether to participate.

Chapter 35 | HIV/AIDS Clinical Trials and Research

Section 35.1 | Basics of Clinical Trials

This section includes text excerpted from "HIV and AIDS Clinical Trials," HIVinfo, U.S. Department of Health and Human Services (HHS), August 13, 2021.

WHAT IS A CLINICAL TRIAL?

A clinical trial is a research study that evaluates new medical approaches in people. These approaches include:

- New medicines or new combinations of medicines
- New medical devices or surgical procedures
- New ways to use an existing medicine or device
- New ways to change behaviors to improve health

Clinical trials are conducted in several phases to determine whether new medical approaches are safe and effective in people. Results from a Phase 1 Trial, Phase 2 Trial, and Phase 3 Trial are used to determine whether a new drug should be approved for sale in the United States. Once a new drug is approved, researchers continue to track its safety in a Phase 4 Trial.

Interventional trial and observational trial are two main types of clinical trials.

WHAT IS AN HIV AND AIDS CLINICAL TRIAL?

Human immunodeficiency virus (HIV) and acquired immuno-deficiency syndrome (AIDS) clinical trials help researchers find better ways to prevent, detect, or treat HIV and AIDS. Every HIV medicine was first studied through clinical trials.

Examples of HIV and AIDS clinical trials include:

- Studies of new medicines to prevent or treat HIV and AIDS
- Studies of vaccines to prevent or treat HIV
- Studies of medicines to treat infections related to HIV and AIDS

CAN ANYONE PARTICIPATE IN AN HIV AND AIDS CLINICAL TRIAL?

It depends on the study. Some HIV and AIDS clinical trials enroll only people who have HIV. Other studies include people who do not have HIV.

Participation in an HIV and AIDS clinical trial may also depend on other factors, such as age, gender, HIV treatment history, or other medical conditions.

WHAT ARE THE BENEFITS OF PARTICIPATING IN AN HIV AND AIDS CLINICAL TRIAL?

Participating in an HIV and AIDS clinical trial can provide benefits. For example, many people participate in HIV and AIDS clinical trials, because they want to contribute to HIV and AIDS research. They may have HIV or know someone who has HIV.

People with HIV who participate in an HIV and AIDS clinical trial may benefit from new HIV medicines before they are widely available. HIV medicines being studied in clinical trials are called "investigational drugs."

Participants in clinical trials can receive regular and careful medical care from a research team that includes doctors and other health professionals. Often the medicines and medical care are free of charge.

Sometimes people get paid for participating in a clinical trial. For example, they may receive money or a gift card. They may be reimbursed for the cost of meals or transportation.

ARE HIV AND AIDS CLINICAL TRIALS SAFE?

Researchers try to make HIV and AIDS clinical trials as safe as possible. However, volunteering to participate in a study testing an experimental treatment for HIV can involve risks of varying degrees. Most volunteers do not experience serious side effects; however, potential side effects that may be serious or even life-threatening can occur from the treatment being studied.

Before enrolling in a clinical trial, potential volunteers learn about the study in a process called "informed consent." The process includes an explanation of the possible risks and benefits of participating in the study.

Once enrolled in a study, people continue to receive information about the study through the informed consent process.

IF A PERSON DECIDES TO PARTICIPATE IN AN HIV AND AIDS CLINICAL TRIAL, WILL THEIR PERSONAL INFORMATION BE SHARED?

The privacy of study volunteers is important to everyone involved in an HIV and AIDS clinical trial. The informed consent process includes an explanation of how a study volunteer's personal information is protected.

HOW CAN ONE FIND AN HIV AND AIDS CLINICAL TRIAL LOOKING FOR VOLUNTEER PARTICIPANTS?

There are several ways to find an HIV and AIDS clinical trial looking for volunteer participants.

- Use the find a study search feature on ClinicalTrials.gov to find HIV and AIDS studies looking for volunteer participants.
- Call a Clinical Info health information specialist at 800-448-0440 or e-mail ContactUs@HIVinfo.NIH.gov.
- Join ResearchMatch (www.researchmatch.org/about), which is a free, secure online tool that makes it easier for the public to become involved in clinical trials.

Section 35.2 | **Effectiveness of Prevention Strategies on HIV Prevention**

This section includes text excerpted from "HIV Risk Behaviors," Centers for Disease Control and Prevention (CDC), November 13, 2019.

HIV RISK BEHAVIORS

The risk of getting human immunodeficiency virus (HIV) varies widely depending on the type of exposure or behavior (such as sharing needles or having sex without a condom). Some exposures to HIV carry a much higher risk of transmission than other exposures. For some exposures, while transmission is biologically possible, the risk is so low that it is not possible to put a precise number on it. But risks do add up over time. Even relatively small risks can add up over time and lead to a high lifetime risk of getting HIV. In other words, there may be a relatively small chance of acquiring HIV when engaging in a risk behavior with an infected partner only once; but, if repeated many times, the overall likelihood of becoming infected after repeated exposures is actually much higher.

EVIDENCE SUPPORTING EFFECTIVENESS ESTIMATES OF ANTIRETROVIRAL THERAPY

- Effectiveness estimates based on suppressive ART ("Optimal Use" of ART) as indicated by achieving and maintaining viral suppression:
  - Optimal use of ART is defined as taking ART daily as prescribed and achieving and maintaining a suppressed viral load (or viral suppression).
  - Four key studies provide evidence for the effectiveness of ART, when used optimally, on preventing the sexual transmission of HIV. These studies – HPTN052, PARTNER, Opposites Attract, and PARTNER2 – observed zero linked sexual transmissions among HIV-discordant couples with viral suppression.
    - Each of these studies followed HIV-discordant couples while the HIV-positive partners were

treated with ART with the intent of suppressing HIV replication. The follow-up assessments, at frequencies typical of what experts recommend for clinical care, included regular measurement of plasma HIV RNA concentrations and HIV testing of the HIV-negative partner. In each study, new HIV infections in the uninfected partners were assessed phylogenetically to determine whether they were genetically linked to their HIV-positive partner in the study.

- The HPTN052 study followed 1,763 HIV-discordant couples (97 percent heterosexual; 3 percent MSM) for a median of 5.5 years. Zero genetically linked transmissions were observed while the HIV-positive partner was virally suppressed, defined as <400 copies/mL of plasma, resulting in a transmission rate estimate of 0.00 per 100 couple-years and an effectiveness estimate of 100 percent, if calculated (not reported in study). The confidence intervals for the effectiveness and transmission rate estimates were not reported and could not be calculated from data reported. The authors reported six partner infections that occurred during the study period where linkage could not be determined due to the inability to amplify HIV RNA; these infections were excluded from all analyses. Although linked infection could not be definitively ruled out, epidemiologic investigation strongly suggested most were not linked. Reported condom use was high (93 percent) among couples and likely contributed to the observed reduction in HIV transmission risk.

- The PARTNER study followed 1,166 HIV-discordant couples (62 percent heterosexual; 38 percent MSM) for a median of 1.3 years while the HIV-positive partner was treated with ART and virally suppressed at baseline. During the 1,238 couple-years of follow-up time included in the analysis, where nearly

900 couples engaged in over 58,000 condomless sex acts, the HIV-negative partner did not use PrEP or PEP, and the HIV-positive partner was virally suppressed, defined as VL <200 copies/mL of plasma, zero genetically linked transmissions were observed. The resulting transmission rate estimate per 100 couple-years was 0.00, with a 95 percent confidence interval (CI) = (0.00, 0.30). The upper 95 percent confidence limit varied by risk group and sexual behavior due to the range of couple-years observed across the subgroups. For example, the estimate for the sexual transmission rate of HIV among discordant couples while the HIV-positive partner was virally suppressed was:

- 0.00 (0.0 – 0.46) per 100 couple-years during any condomless sex among heterosexual women and men
- 0.00 (0.0 – 0.89) per 100 couple-years during condomless anal sex among MSM

- The Opposites Attract study followed 343 HIV-discordant male-male couples for a median of 1.7 years while the HIV-positive partner was treated with ART, with most taking ART at baseline (80 percent). During the 232 couple-years of follow-up time included in the analysis, where the HIV-positive partner was virally suppressed (defined as <200 copies/mLof plasma) and couples reported over 12,000 episodes of any condomless anal sex acts and no PrEP use, there were zero genetically linked transmissions observed. This translates to a transmission rate estimate of:
  - 0.00 (0.00 – 1.59) per 100 couple-years during condomless anal sex among MSM
- The PARTNER2 study was an extension of the PARTNER study that recruited more HIV-discordant male-male couples and extending the follow-up time for those enrolled in the PARTNER study, totaling

972 HIV-discordant male-male couples enrolled in PARTNER2. The final analysis included almost 800 couples followed for a median of 2.0 years. Over nearly 1,600 couple-years of follow-up while the HIV-positive partner was on ART and virally suppressed, defined as <200 copies/mL of plasma, and couples reported no PrEP use and over 76,000 episodes of condomless anal sex, zero genetically linked transmissions were observed. This translates to a transmission rate estimate of:

- 0.00 (0.00 – 0.23) per 100 couple-years during condomless anal sex among MSM

- Additional supporting evidence beyond the four individual studies includes:
  - Combining over 2,600 couple-years of follow-up and more than 125,000 episodes of sex without a condom or PrEP while the HIV-positive partner was virally suppressed, from the PARTNER, PARTNER2, and Opposites Attract studies, results in a combined HIV transmission risk estimate for condomless and PrEP-less sex among heterosexual or MSM couples of 0.00 (0.00 – 0.14) per 100 couple-years (www.cdc.gov/hiv/pdf/risk/art/cdc-hiv-art-viral-suppression.pdf).
  - A review at the 2019 CROI conference combined the four studies above along with several previous observational studies, accumulating over 4,000 couple-years of follow-up, and reported a combined HIV transmission risk estimate while the HIV-positive person was virally suppressed, excluding unconfirmed viral loads, of 0.00 (0.00 – 0.07) per 100 couple-years.
  - No cases of linked HIV transmission to sexual partners when the person with HIV was virally suppressed have been documented.
- **Earlier effectiveness estimates based on original RCT study:**

- Cohen was the first published RCT examining the protective benefits of ART for reducing HIV transmission. This paper reported the interim analysis of the HPTN 052 study, a randomized controlled trial (RCT) of providing early ART, compared with delayed ART, among 1,763 mostly heterosexual, serodiscordant couples followed for a median of 1.7 years. The effectiveness estimate for ART was 96 percent, based on the ITT results using verified linked cases of HIV.
  - Typically, findings from the primary analysis within an RCT include many participants assigned to the intervention strategy but, not necessarily using the strategy. In this study, however, most participants in the "early ART" arm were taking ART consistently as evidenced by a high level of adherence to ART (79 percent had at least 95 percent adherence via pill count) and a high rate of viral suppression (89 percent were virally suppressed by 3 months). Given that this ITT analysis included time periods where the HIV-positive person was not taking ART or not virally suppressed, this effectiveness estimate for consistent use of ART is not an accurate estimate for optimal use of ART, where the HIV-positive person would be taking ART as prescribed and would have achieved viral suppression.
  - The 96 percent effectiveness of taking early ART, as well as a significant reduction in morbidity and mortality among HIV-positive participants, led to ending the RCT and offering all couples ART. Cohen and colleagues have continued to follow participants from this original study and offer ART to participants in both arms (thereby turning the study from an RCT to an observational design, although they continue also to analyze participants per their original random assignment). By the end of the study, 96 percent of HIV-positive persons in the "delayed ART" arm

had started ART. The final HPTN 052 study ITT effectiveness estimate, including more than 5 years of follow-up, was 93 percent comparing "early ART" versus "delayed ART." Given that essentially all participants in both arms has started ART by the end of the study, this finding is not a better estimate of the effectiveness of taking ART (versus not taking ART) on reducing HIV transmission.

- Based on the HPTN 052 RCT, the best estimate for the overall effectiveness of taking ART consistently among heterosexuals is 96 percent. There are no comparable RCTs for MSM or PWID.

EVIDENCE SUPPORTING EFFECTIVENESS ESTIMATES OF ORAL DAILY PREPS

- **Effectiveness estimates based on "Optimal or Consistent Use" of oral daily PrEP**
  - The effectiveness of oral daily PrEP is highly dependent on PrEP adherence. The effectiveness estimate of PrEP, when taken daily or consistently, is presented here. The effectiveness estimates of PrEP as assigned within a trial or when used recently are presented below.
  - When taking oral PrEP daily or consistently, it is extremely effective in preventing HIV and HIV acquisition is extremely rare. Only three cases of seroconversion have been confirmed to date worldwide, while HIV-negative individuals were on PrEP with verified adherence (www.thebody.com/content/80972/has-anyone-gotten-hiv-when-they-were-on-prep.htmlexternal icon)
  - The United States Preventive Services Task Force (USPSTF) provides a Grade A recommendation for oral daily PrEP in preventing HIV acquisition in persons at high risk. The USPSTF also concludes with high certainty that the benefit of oral PrEP is substantial,

but that adherence to PrEP is central to maximizing its benefit.

- **MSM.** Several studies evaluated the effectiveness of PrEP use among MSM. These studies vary in study design methods (e.g., RCT, observational) as well as how PrEP adherence is measured; but, all provide evidence for the effectiveness of PrEP when taken daily or consistently.

  - **iPrEx OLE study.** This open-label extension (OLE) cohort study enrolled 1,603 MSM and transgender women previously enrolled in three PrEP trials (ATN 082; iPrEx; and United States Safety Study) and followed participants for 72 weeks. All were offered free daily oral PrEP (TDF/FTC or Truvada), and 1,225 elected to take PrEP. PrEP adherence was measured by drug concentration of TFV-DP in dried blood spots. No new HIV infections were observed among MSM taking PrEP where drug levels indicated they had taken 4 or more doses per week.

    - Among those with the highest drug concentrations indicating daily PrEP use, as verified by drug level of TFV-DP in dried blood spots of >1250 fmol/punch (equivalent to ~7 pills/week), there were no new HIV infections. This resulted in a risk reduction estimate of 100 percent when compared to the previous placebo group from the iPrEx trial or the concurrent group of participants not on PrEP.

    - In addition, among those with drug concentration levels indicating at least 4 pills/week (>700 fmol/punch), there were no new HIV infections, which resulted in a risk reduction estimate of 100 percent when compared to either comparison group.

  - **DEMO project.** This open-label observational study enrolled 557 MSM and transgender women in 2 STI clinics and a community health center in 3 U.S. cities and offered free daily oral PrEP (TDF/FTC) for 48 weeks. PrEP adherence was measured by drug concentration of TFV-DP in dried blood spots in a large sample of participants at all follow-up visits. At the end of follow-up, 527 had at least 1 follow-up visit, providing a total of 481 person-years of follow-up. Most of the participants (ranging from 80 percent to 86 percent of participants across the follow-up visits) of those assessed for PrEP adherence had drug levels considered protective (consistent with >4 pills/week). At the end of the study, 2 participants acquired HIV infection; however, both participants had drug levels indicative of < 2 doses/week or BLQ (below the limit of quantification) throughout the study. This means no new HIV infections were observed among those with protective levels of PrEP use.

- **PROUD study**. The PROUD study was a randomized-control trial (RCT) evaluating immediate daily oral PrEP (TDF/FTC) versus delayed PrEP among HIV-negative MSM patients in 13 clinics in England from 2012-2014. A total of 554 MSM were randomized, 275 to immediate PrEP and 269 to the delayed group. After an interim analysis, the trial stopped early and all deferred patients were offered PrEP. More than 90 percent of the patients in each group were retained at the end of the study, providing ~500 person-years of follow up. The mITT results from the trial are reported below. Although there were 3 new HIV infections among those assigned to the immediate PrEP group, there were no HIV infections observed among those actually taking PrEP. All 3 new HIV infections in the immediate PrEP group, based on clinical indications, attendance, and prescription info,were not taking PrEP near the time of seroconversion – 2 never started taking PrEP and 1 infection was identified over 40 weeks after last clinic visit (where 90 PrEP pills were provided).

- Kaiser Permanente observational study. This observational study followed 1,045 Kaiser Permanente (KP) patients, mostly MSM (98-99 percent), who were referred to a specialized PrEP program in KP San Francisco during 2012-2015, and then later extended through February 2017. PrEP use was measured based on pharmacy refill data. Among the 2,107 patients never starting PrEP, there were 22 new HIV infections. Among the 4,991 who started PrEP, although you do not know how many were always taking PrEP daily, there were no new HIV infections while PrEP prescriptions were filled (over 12.4 months; 5,104 person-years on PrEP). Of the 1,303 patients who stopped PrEP (prescription not re-filled), 11 new HIV infections were later observed after stopping PrEP, by the end of the follow-up.

- The effectiveness of PrEP among MSM when used daily or consistently is estimated to be 100 percent in studies. However, a few cases of new HIV infections have been reported with PrEP verified adherence, indicating that the risk has not been completely eliminated and that the effectiveness of PrEP cannot be exactly 100 percent. Given the number of persons on PrEP worldwide (prepwatch.org), the risk reduction (or effectiveness of PrEP) would likely need to be very high and close to 100 percent to observe only three confirmed cases of PrEP failure (new HIV infection despite taking PrEP daily or consistently) to date. To represent the protective value of PrEP while also acknowledging the small number of failures, it indicate the effectiveness of PrEP is about 99 percent.

- **Transgender women.** The iPrEx OLE cohort study enrolled mostly MSM, but included 175 transgender women previously enrolled in three PrEP trials (ATN 082; iPrEx; and United States Safety Study) and offered free daily oral PrEP (TDF/FTC or Truvada) for 72 weeks. PrEP adherence was measured by drug concentration of TFV-DP in dried blood spots. One transgender woman seroconverted while receiving PrEP and one seroconversion occurred in a woman who elected not to use PrEP. No new HIV infections were observed among transgender women who were taking PrEP where drug levels indicated they had taken 4 or more doses per week. However, the iPrEx trial results described below show no benefit of PrEP among transgender women, likely due to low PrEP adherence.

- **Heterosexual women and men.** There is no effectiveness estimate of PrEP when taken daily or consistently among heterosexuals. There is evidence for the effectiveness of PrEP, which is estimated to be 88–90 percent, as described below. These estimates come from subset analyses among heterosexual men or women with evidence of taking PrEP (based on detecting TFV in plasma). These subset analyses likely include people who vary in PrEP adherence, including those who used PrEP but not consistently, used PrEP consistently but not daily (e.g., ~4 times/week), or used PrEP daily. Given that the effectiveness of PrEP is highly dependent on PrEP adherence, the effectiveness of PrEP when taking PrEP daily or consistently is likely to be greater than when taking PrEP recently; therefore, likely to be greater than 90 percent and similar to what is observed for MSM. Data show that it takes longer (~13 days longer) to reach a maximum drug level of PrEP in vaginal tissue as compared to rectal tissue, but once maximum drug levels are reached, the effectiveness of PrEP in preventing acquisition during sex should be similar for vaginal or anal sex, and for men or women.

- **PWID**. The Bangkok Tenofovir Study (BTS) was an RCT evaluating oral daily PrEP use (TDF alone) against placebo among HIV-negative persons who inject drugs (PWID).
  - When taking PrEP (TDF) nearly daily, as verified by TFV detected in plasma and directly observed therapy (DOT) (with at least 70 percent of days were DOT, with no gaps of >2 days without DOT; equivalent to ~5 days/week), the risk of HIV acquisition was reduced by 74 percent among HIV-uninfected injecting drug users.
  - When taking PrEP (TDF) nearly daily, when defined as 97.5 percent adherence, based on daily diary (most often confirmed daily by DOT staff) and monthly pill count, the risk of HIV acquisition was reduced by about 84 percent. This study also showed a dose-response between adherence and protection from PrEP, with greater adherence resulting in a greater effectiveness estimate for PrEP.
  - This BTS study evaluated TDF (Tenofovir) rather than the combination drug TDF/FTC (Truvada). The effectiveness of two-drug oral therapy has not been assessed among PWID but may be higher than TDF alone. TDF alone had been shown to have a slightly lower efficacy than TDF/FTC, although not statistically different, among heterosexual HIV-discordant couples in the Partners PrEP study. In addition, since the measures used in the BTS study for assessing PrEP adherence included those taking PrEP nearly daily but not daily, the effectiveness of daily PrEP use may in fact be greater.
  - Note that TDF (Tenofovir) is recommended in the United States as an alternative to TDF/FTC (Truvada) among PWID (www.cdc.gov/hiv/pdf/risk/prep/cdc-hiv-prep-guidelines-2021.pdf).

- **Effectiveness estimates based on "Recent Use" of oral daily PrEP**
  - Recent use of oral PrEP is measured based on drug detected, typically detecting FTC or TFV, in plasma. All effectiveness estimates presented here come from subset analyses within larger RCTs restricting to participants with drug detected in plasma indicating recent use of PrEP. These estimates do not reflect optimal or consistent use of PrEP, which resulted in greater effectiveness estimates among MSM and PWID as described above.
  - MSM. The iPrEx Trial was an RCT evaluating oral daily PrEP use (TDF/FTC) against placebo among MSM. The findings from a case/control sub-analysis show that effectiveness of PrEP, when recently used, was estimated to be 92 percent. This measure of recent use of PrEP was based on detecting FTC or TFV in plasma or detecting FTC-TP or TFV-DP in PBMC.
  - Heterosexual women and men. The Partners PrEP Study was an RCT with three arms, evaluating oral daily PrEP use as TDF/FTC and as TDF alone against a placebo arm, among HIV-discordant heterosexual Women and Men.
    - The effectiveness of PrEP (TDF/FTC), when used recently, was estimated to be 88 percent – 90 percent, which comes from two separate sub-analyses from the Partners PrEP Study.
    - A case/control sub-analysis reported the effectiveness of PrEP, when used recently (based on detecting TFV in plasma), was estimated to be 90 percent among HIV-uninfected heterosexual Women and Men.
    - Another restricted analysis of the same study was based on TFV drug levels in plasma. When taking PrEP (TDF/FTC) recently, as defined by >40 ng/ml of TFV in plasma (unknown equivalent pills/week), the risk of HIV acquisition was reduced by 88

percent among HIV-uninfected heterosexual Women and Men. Given these levels of TFV in plasma do not translate to a known level of PrEP adherence or known number of pills/week, this finding more accurately corresponds to those taking PrEP recently rather than daily or consistently.

- **PWID**. The Bangkok Tenofovir Study (BTS) was an RCT evaluating oral daily PrEP use (TDF alone) against placebo among HIV-negative persons who inject drugs (PWID).
  - A case/control sub-analysis reported the effectiveness of PrEP (TDF), when used recently (based on detecting TFV in plasma), was estimated to be 70 percent among PWID.
  - This BTS study evaluated TDF (Tenofovir) rather than the combination drug TDF/FTC (Truvada). The effectiveness of two-drug oral therapy has not been assessed among PWID but may be higher than TDF alone. TDF alone has been shown to have a slightly lower efficacy than TDF/FTC when compared to placebo, although not statistically different, among heterosexual HIV-discordant couples in the Partners PrEP study.
  - Note that TDF (Tenofovir) is recommended in the United States as an alternative to TDF/FTC (Truvada) among PWID (www.cdc.gov/hiv/pdf/risk/prep/cdc-hiv-prep-guidelines-2021.pdf).
- **Effectiveness estimates based on modified intent-to-treat (mITT) analyses in trials, regardless of level of PrEP use**
  - **MSM**
    - The iPrEx Trial was an RCT designed to evaluate the efficacy of oral daily PrEP (TDF/FTC) versus placebo in preventing HIV acquisition among 2,499 HIV-uninfected MSM and transgender women. After a median of 1.2 years of follow-up, the risk of HIV acquisition was reduced by 44 percent among

HIV-uninfected MSM assigned to daily PrEP (TDF/FTC) (mITT analysis). This estimate includes all participants assigned to take daily PrEP, regardless of actual use.

- The PROUD Study was an RCT evaluating immediate daily oral PrEP (TDF/FTC) versus delayed PrEP among HIV-negative patients in 13 clinics in England from 2012-2014. A total of 554 MSM were randomized, 275 to immediate PrEP and 269 to the delayed group. After an interim analysis, the trial stopped early and all deferred patients were offered PrEP. More than 90 percent of the patients in each group were retained at the end of the study, providing ~500 person-years of follow-up.
  - RCT results (mITT analysis) – At the end of interim analysis, 3 new HIV infections were observed in the immediate PrEP group and 20 in delayed group, resulting in a risk reduction estimate of 86 percent.
  - There were no HIV infections observed among those taking PrEP. All 3 new HIV infections in immediate PrEP group, based on clinical indications, attendance, and prescription information, were not taking PrEP near the time of seroconversion – 2 never started taking PrEP and 1 infection was identified over 40 weeks after last clinic visit (where 90 PrEP pills were provided).
- The IPERGAY Trial was an RCT evaluating the efficacy of "on-demand" PrEP (TDF/FTC) regimen (defined as taking 2 pills 2-24 hours before sex, 1 pill 24 hours later, and a 4th pill 24 hours after the 3rd) versus placebo among 400 MSM. At the interim analysis of the trial, after 1 year of follow-up, the efficacy of "on-demand" PrEP was estimated to be 86 percent in the mITT analysis and 82 percent in the ITT analysis. By measured plasma drug levels in a

subset of those randomized to TDF/FTC, 86 percent had TDF levels consistent with having taken the drug during the previous week.

- **The IPERGAY OLE study.** Following the interim analysis where the efficacy of "on-demand" PrEP was determined, the placebo group was discontinued, all study participants were offered TDF/FTC in an OLE phase of the study, and 361 enrolled. Although not part of the trial, the IPERGAY OLE study reported the risk of HIV acquisition was reduced by 97 percent when comparing the MSM taking PrEP as part of the OLE cohort to the placebo arm of the IPERGAY trial. Seventy-one percent of those in the OLE cohort had TDF levels consistent with having taken the drug during the previous week.

- Two participants in the "on-demand" PrEP arm of the RCT seroconverted after enrollment and 1 participant in the OLE cohort seroconverted during follow-up. In all three cases, study records showed that the participants were not taking PrEP at the time of the diagnosis (no drug detected in plasma and all had returned all or most of their PrEP pills at the visit). No new HIV infections were observed among participants taking PrEP.

- A small sub-study of the IPERGAY trial reported high effectiveness of on-demand PrEP among those MSM participants with less frequent sexual intercourse. This subset analysis reported an estimated 100 percent reduction in HIV incidence among a subset of participants reporting less frequent sexual intercourse (median of 5 sex acts/month) when reportedly taking on-demand PrEP, about 9.5 pills/month (or ~2-3 pills/week), compared to placebo.

- Daily dosing is the only Food and Drug Administration (FDA)-approved schedule for taking PrEP to prevent HIV. However, the International Antiviral Society-USA supports the "off-label" but, evidence-based use of on-demand PrEP, as an alternative to daily PrEP, for gay, bisexual and other men who have sex with men with infrequent sexual exposures. Given limited data on the effectiveness of on-demand PrEP for heterosexual Women and Men, PWID, and transgender persons, IAS-USA does not recommend on-demand PrEP for these populations. Several health departments have developed guidance on off label use of on demand PrEP for MSM, including the New York City Department of Health (www1.nyc.gov/assets/doh/downloads/pdf/ah/prep-on-demand-dosing-guidance.pdf) and the San Francisco Department of Public Health (www.gettingtozerosf.org/wp-content/uploads/2018/11/HIVUpdate_02122019_v2.pdf)

- **Transgender women**. A follow-up sub-analysis of the iPrEx Trial evaluated the effectiveness of PrEP (TDF/FTC) versus placebo among 339 transgender women. No benefit of PrEP was identified (HR=1.1, 95 percent CI: 0.5–2.7); however, the transgender women appeared to have lower PrEP adherence than MSM within iPrEx.
- **Heterosexual women and men**
  - The Partners PrEP study was an RCT among 4747 HIV-discordant heterosexual couples assessing the efficacy of oral daily PrEP by comparing three treatment arms – TDF/FTC (Truvada), TDF alone, and placebo. The risk of HIV acquisition was reduced by 75 percent among HIV-uninfected heterosexual Women and Men assigned to TDF/FTC (Truvada) compared to placebo. This estimate included all participants assigned to take daily PrEP, regardless of actual use.

- The TDF2 study was an RCT among 1219 HIV-negative heterosexual Women and Men comparing TDF/FTC (Truvada) to placebo and found the risk of HIV acquisition was reduced by 62 percent. This estimate included all participants assigned to take daily PrEP, regardless of actual use. An as-treated analysis, restricting to those participants taking PrEP based on self-reported PrEP use in last 30 days, found the risk of HIV acquisition was reduced by 78 percent. This, however, was based on self-report and not an objective measure of use.
- There are additional PrEP trials among women reported in the literature not summarized here. Riddell and the USPSTF reviewed the trial findings for PrEP and described additional trials among women showing no significant effects of PrEP, primarily due to extremely low adherence among women in the studies.
- **PWIDs.** The Bangkok Tenofovir Study (BTS) was an RCT evaluating oral daily PrEP use (TDF alone) against placebo among HIV-negative persons who inject drugs. This trial showed the risk of HIV acquisition was reduced by 49 percent among HIV-uninfected injecting drug users assigned to oral daily PrEP (TDF). This estimate included all participants assigned to take daily PrEP, regardless of actual use.

EVIDENCE SUPPORTING EFFECTIVENESS ESTIMATES OF OPTIMAL CONDOM USE

- **Effectiveness estimates based on "optimal use" of condoms.**
  - Optimal use of condoms is defined here as both consistent and correct use during every sex act.
  - Laboratory studies show that (latex-based, polyurethane, or other synthetic material-based) condoms provide an impermeable barrier to passage of

HIV. Even during optimal use, however, condoms may not offer complete protection all the time due to the rare chance of product failure.

- Measures are in place to ensure high quality control on product development. Condoms are regulated as class II medical devices by the U.S. Food and Drug Administration (FDA). FDA requires every condom to be tested electronically for holes and weak spots before it is packaged and released for sale. In addition, samples of condoms undergo a series of additional laboratory tests for leakage, strength, and other factors. Condom samples must be at least 99.6 percent effective in laboratory "water leak" tests, which means that at least 996 out of every 1000 condoms sampled must pass the test.

- Other laboratory testing has estimated that the worst-case product failure would lead to less than 0.01 percent of volume leakage during sex. In other words, the worst-case scenario would still eliminate about 99.99 percent of volume exposure during sex, in the event of product failure.

- **Effectiveness estimates based on "consistent use" of condoms.**

  - Although rare, and not easily measured, condoms may break, slip, or leak during use, even if used correctly. In addition, not using condoms correctly (user failure) increases the risk of breakage, slippage, leakage, or incomplete coverage which can increase exposure to HIV and, thus, may decrease condom effectiveness. Because male condoms are applied by the user during sex, user error or failure is an ongoing risk during each sexual episode. User error is difficult to eliminate; however, over time, as the user becomes more experienced, it is minimized. In addition, not using condoms consistently, meaning during every sex act, may further increase potential exposure to HIV and decrease effectiveness even more. Below are effectiveness estimates for consistently using condoms in practice as measured in observational studies.

- **Heterosexual women and men.** The Weller Cochrane review of 13 longitudinal cohort studies among HIV discordant heterosexual couples reported results comparing those reporting "Always" versus "Never" using condoms during vaginal sex from 5 of the 13 studies with data available at the longest follow-up. Vaginal versus anal and insertive versus receptive sex were not distinguished in these analyses. Always using condoms, based on self-report, during sex with an HIV-positive partner reduces the risk of HIV acquisition per person-year of follow-up by an estimated 80 percent among heterosexual women and men. This measure does not account for the possibility of different numbers of sex acts over time between condom users and nonusers.
- **MSM.** Two studies have estimated the effectiveness of consistent condom use on HIV risk among HIV-negative MSM having sex with HIV-positive men.
  - The Smith study combined data from two longitudinal studies among MSM (EXPLORE and Vax004) and compared HIV-negative MSM who reported "Always" versus "Never" using condoms during receptive anal sex, during insertive anal sex, and during any anal sex, with HIV-positive partners.
    - **MSM, receptive anal sex.** Always using condoms, based on self-report, during receptive anal sex with HIV-positive partners reduced the risk of HIV acquisition per person-year by an estimated 72 percent among MSM.
    - **MSM, insertive anal sex.** Always using condoms, based on self-report, during insertive anal sex with HIV-positive partners reduced the risk of HIV acquisition per person-year by an estimated 63 percent among MSM. This analysis does not

take into account whether HIV-negative MSM also engaged in receptive anal sex, with or without condoms, which could affect this estimate.

- **MSM, any anal sex**. Always using condoms, based on self-report, during any (insertive or receptive) anal sex with HIV-positive partners reduced the risk of HIV acquisition per person-year by an estimated 70 percent among MSM.
- These measures do not account for the possibility of different numbers of sex acts over time between condom users and nonusers.
- The Johnson study examined condom effectiveness per partner in four cohorts of MSM (EXPLORE, Vaxx004, JumpStart, and Vaccine Preparedness Study) by comparing those "Always" using condoms versus "Not always" using condoms, based on self-report, throughout the sexual partnerships. Among HIV-uninfected MSM engaging in receptive anal sex with their HIV-positive partner, always using condoms during receptive anal sex throughout the partnership reduced the risk of HIV acquisition per partner by an estimated 91 percent. This measure does not account for the possibility of different numbers of sex acts per partner between condom users and nonusers.
- The estimates provided here likely underestimate the effectiveness of condoms when used consistently and correctly in practice due to measurement error regarding both aspects of condom use – consistent use and correct use.
  - These estimates for "consistent use" are based on observational cohort studies because no RCTs exist, due to ethical and feasibility concerns with assigning a no condom use arm. In addition, only subjective measures of condom use (self-report) are available in studies with HIV as an outcome, which may overestimate actual condom use, resulting in

underestimating condom effectiveness. Therefore, the effectiveness of consistent condom use is likely greater.

- These studies also did not measure whether condoms were used correctly. If used incorrectly, condoms may break, slip, leak, or not provide complete coverage, which may increase exposure to HIV. The studies among MSM, however, did ask MSM to count "breakage" and "slippage" as "not using a condom" in an attempt to account for user failure – but, this relies on knowledge of failure and self-report and likely underestimates true failure. If these analyses included any data where condoms were used incorrectly but misclassified as consistent and correct use, then these estimates are likely underestimating condom effectiveness when used correctly, and the effectiveness of correct condom use is likely greater.

STRENGTHS AND LIMITATIONS OF EFFECTIVENESS ESTIMATES OF CIRCUMCISION STATUS

- Most of the evidence is based on observational studies and circumcision status is primarily based on self-report; only some studies are based on medical exam (objective measure of exposure).
- **MSM insertive anal sex**. A Cochrane review of 7 observational studies among MSM reporting mainly or only "insertive" sex reports a significant protective effect of circumcision on acquiring HIV through insertive anal sex, 73 percent risk reduction. Exposure (circumcision) was primarily measured via self-report (subjective measure), although genital exams occurred in some studies. Two more published observational studies show nonsignificant effects of circumcision on HIV acquisition during insertive anal sex. With conflicting results, the evidence is inconclusive and an updated meta-analysis is needed.

- **MSM receptive anal sex.** A Cochrane review of 3 observational studies among MSM reporting primarily "receptive" sex reports a nonsignificant effect estimate for circumcision (of the insertive partner) on HIV acquisition during receptive anal sex, with exposure measured by self-report. The published observational study reports a significant effect of circumcision (based on self-report) on HIV acquisition during receptive anal sex among MSM. With conflicting results, the evidence is inconclusive, and an updated meta-analysis is needed.
- **Heterosexual men.** A Cochrane review of 3 RCTs synthesizes ITT results on the effects of circumcision on risk of HIV acquisition during sex among HIV-negative heterosexual men.
- **Heterosexual women.** A meta-analysis (including one RCT and several observational studies) reports that there is insufficient evidence to conclude that male circumcision reduces the risk of HIV acquisition during sex among HIV-negative heterosexual women. Two more reports, 1 RCT and 1 observational study, also show nonsignificant effects of male circumcision (confirmed by medical exam) on HIV acquisition in women among HIV-discordant heterosexual couples. The evidence is inconclusive, and an updated meta-analysis is needed.

Section 35.3 | **HIV Research Activities**

This section contains text excerpted from the following sources: Text under the heading "Supporting Research to Effectively Prevent, Diagnose, and Treat HIV" is excerpted from "HIV Research Activities," HIV.gov, U.S. Department of Health and Human Services (HHS), September 19, 2018. Reviewed February 2022; Text under the heading "National Leadership for HIV Prevention Research" is excerpted from "HIV – Research," Centers for Disease Control and Prevention (CDC), March 12, 2020.

SUPPORTING RESEARCH TO EFFECTIVELY PREVENT, DIAGNOSE, AND TREAT HIV

In the three decades since the first cases of acquired immunodeficiency syndrome (AIDS) were reported, federal investments in basic, biomedical, behavioral, and social science research have led to numerous HIV prevention interventions and life-saving treatments. Several federal agencies conduct or support HIV research activities.

Leading the Way in HIV Research

The National Institutes of Health (NIH), a part of the U.S. Department of Health and Human Services (HHS), is the Nation's primary medical research agency, making important discoveries that improve health and save lives. NIH conducts and supports a comprehensive program of basic, behavioral, clinical, and translational research on HIV/AIDS and its associated coinfections, comorbidities, and other complications. Since HIV crosses nearly every area of medicine and scientific investigation, the response to the HIV pandemic requires a multi-Institute, multidisciplinary, global research program. At NIH, this research is coordinated by the Office of AIDS Research (OAR) and carried out by nearly all the NIH Institutes and Centers, in both at NIH and at NIH-funded institutions worldwide. The NIH HIV/AIDS Research Program represents the world's largest public investment in AIDS research.

Within NIH, the National Institute of Allergy and Infectious Diseases (NIAID) manages the largest portfolio of HIV/AIDS research activities. NIAID-supported investigators have made groundbreaking scientific discoveries that have led to significant progress in the fight against HIV/AIDS. Among these discoveries,

NIAID-supported research has demonstrated that people living with HIV who take antiretroviral medications daily as prescribed and who achieve and maintain an undetectable viral load have effectively no risk of sexually transmitting the virus to an HIV-negative partner.

The NIAID-supported HPTN 052 study, which involved more than 1,600 heterosexual couples over 10 years, found that starting and sustaining treatment for HIV infection early, when the immune system is relatively healthy, essentially eliminated the transmission of HIV. No HIV transmission was observed when antiretroviral therapy consistently, durably suppressed the virus in the partner living with HIV. While some transmission events did occur in the study, new infections resulted when the partner living with HIV was not fully virally suppressed due to either having just started antiretroviral therapy, or for whom treatment no longer was working and the virus was replicating. The study also showed that early treatment initiation improved health outcomes for people living with HIV.

The HPTN 052 results, along with those of another NIAID-funded trial (the START study), which showed that those living with HIV who received early treatment significantly reduced their risk of illness and death, helped influence the World Health Organization (WHO) in 2015 to recommend that everyone living with HIV should begin treatment upon diagnosis.

Seeking a Cure for HIV

The NIAID also invests in basic and clinical research with the goal of developing a safe, affordable and scalable cure for HIV and AIDS. NIAID's research efforts include studies to identify the precise locations where HIV hides in the body (known as "viral reservoirs"), determine how those reservoirs are established and maintained, and develop strategies to minimize or deplete them. An HIV cure in the classic sense, meaning it removes all HIV from the body, would require eradication of viral reservoirs. Treatment-free remission, also known as a "functional cure," would not eradicate reservoirs but would allow a person living with HIV to control the virus without daily medication.

Making Progress toward an HIV Vaccine

Historically, vaccination has been the best method for protecting people from infectious diseases. While many HIV prevention techniques are available, the development of a safe and effective HIV vaccine remains key to realizing a durable end to the HIV/AIDS pandemic. NIAID and its global partners are pursuing numerous research strategies to develop next-generation vaccine candidates.

Developing Safe and Effective HIV Treatments

One of NIAID's greatest success stories is that its research led to the development of numerous antiretroviral drugs to treat HIV/AIDS, turning what was once a uniformly fatal disease into a manageable chronic condition for many. The NIAID is working to find new and more effective therapeutic products, drug classes, and combinations as well as safe and effective treatments for related co-infections and complications.

Research to Prevent HIV Infection and Transmission

The NIAID also conducts and supports research to develop and improve cutting-edge tools and techniques that can work to prevent HIV in diverse populations around the world.

The Centers for Disease Control and Prevention (CDC) also provides national leadership for HIV prevention research, including the development of biomedical and behavioral interventions to prevent HIV transmission and reduce disease progression in the United States and internationally. CDC's research efforts include identifying scientifically proven, cost-effective, and scalable interventions and prevention strategies to be implemented as part of a high-impact prevention approach for maximal impact on the HIV epidemic.

Advancing the National HIV Priorities through Research

The National HIV/AIDS Strategy: Updated to 2020 calls for numerous ongoing research efforts, including the prioritization and promotion of research to fill in gaps in prevention science among the highest risk populations and communities; the promotion and prioritization of research to fill in gaps in knowledge along the HIV care continuum; the scaling up of effective, evidence-based programs that address social determinants of health; support for research to better understand the scope of the intersection of HIV and violence against women and girls, as well as the development of effective interventions; and the strengthening of the timely availability and use of data. Across the federal government, agencies and programs are engaged in these efforts.

NATIONAL LEADERSHIP FOR HIV PREVENTION RESEARCH

The CDC provides national leadership for HIV prevention research, including the development and evaluation of HIV biomedical and behavioral interventions to prevent HIV transmission and reduce HIV disease progression in the United States and internationally. The CDC's research efforts also include identifying those scientifically proven, cost-effective, and scalable interventions and prevention strategies to be implemented as part of a high-impact prevention approach for maximal impact on the HIV epidemic.

Serostatus Approach

The AIDS epidemic, although first recognized only 20 years ago, has had a profound impact in communities throughout the United States. The serostatus approach to fighting the HIV epidemic (SAFE): Prevention Strategies for Infected Individuals.

Intervention Research

The CDC has provided funding to HIV partners to help implement programs that will help curb the increase of HIV infections. These programs facilitated with the partners and grantees are critical in the goal of eliminating HIV infection in the United States.

Biomedical Research

The CDC has researched several HIV prevention interventions that have proven effective in helping to prevent HIV infection in certain populations and communities.

Demonstration Projects

The CDC has worked with key cities to create effective policies and programs to curb the tide of HIV infections in those cities. These cities have higher rates of HIV due to a number of factors therefore making them key locations for studies.

Medical Monitoring Project

The Medical Monitoring Project (MMP) is a surveillance system designed to learn more about the experiences and needs of people who are living with HIV. It is supported by several government agencies and conducted by state and local health departments along with the CDC.

Section 35.4 | Drug Combination Reduces Risk of HIV Infection among Teen Males

This section includes text excerpted from "Drug Combination Reduces Risk of HIV Infection among Teen Males," National Institutes of Health (NIH), September 5, 2017. Reviewed February 2022.

A National Institutes of Health (NIH) network study has confirmed that a combination of two drugs taken daily to reduce the chances of HIV infection among high-risk adults also works well and appears safe in males ages 15 to 17 years.

Truvada, a single pill containing the drugs tenofovir and emtricitabine (TDF/FTC), is approved for daily use in adults. The drug is the cornerstone of pre-exposure prophylaxis (PrEP), a strategy in which healthy people at risk for HIV infection take one or more anti-HIV drugs to reduce this risk.

The study published in JAMA Pediatrics was funded by NIH's *Eunice Kennedy Shriver* National Institute of Child Health and Human Development (NICHD), National Institute on Drug Abuse (NIDA), and National Institute of Mental Health (NIMH).

"Several studies have shown that daily oral PrEP is effective in preventing HIV among people at high risk of becoming

390

infected, but none of them included adolescents under age 18," said study author Bill Kapogiannis, M.D., of NICHD's Maternal and Pediatric Infectious Diseases Branch (MPIDB). "The study suggests that this therapy can safely reduce HIV risk for those under 18."

The study was conducted by researchers in the NICHD-funded Adolescent Medicine Trials Network for HIV/AIDS Interventions. When the study began, participants ranging in age from 15 to 17 years old were not infected with HIV, and were considered at-risk for HIV because of factors such as having unprotected sex with a male partner who had HIV or whose HIV status was unknown, having at least three male partners, or having a sexually transmitted infection other than HIV. Youth with poor kidney function and a history of bone fractures were excluded from the study because the drug combination may sometimes stress the kidneys and cause bone loss.

Study participants received periodic tests for HIV and other sexually transmitted diseases, counseling, and other interventions to help them avoid risky behaviors. The 72 youth who took part in the study also received daily oral TDF/FTC for 48 weeks.

As the study progressed, many participants skipped doses of their medication. Levels of the drug sufficient to prevent HIV infection were found in 54 percent of participants by week four, 49 percent by week 12, 28 percent by week 24, and 22 percent by week 48. The principal reason that the participants gave for skipping the medications was worry that others would see them taking pills and think that they are HIV-positive. Other reasons for missing doses included being away from home (32 percent), being too busy (28 percent), forgetting (26 percent), and experiencing changes in routine (19 percent).

In general, study participants tolerated the drug well, and there were no reports of effects on the kidneys or bones. Three participants were diagnosed with HIV during the study: one at weeks 32, 36, and 48. All three had no detectable blood levels of TDF/FTC at the visit before their HIV infection was first diagnosed, indicating that they likely were missing doses or not taking the medicine at all.

The authors concluded that the lack of significant adverse health events during the study indicates that the drug is safe for males under age 18. Similarly, the lack of HIV infection among participants who had sufficiently high blood levels of medication is consistent with studies in adults and suggests that the drug can be effective in this population when taken appropriately. The researchers added that the tendency of youth to skip medications demonstrates the need for more contact with clinical staff during therapy, and for the development of strategies to ensure that at-risk youth take the drug as prescribed.

The NIH also is funding studies of PrEP therapy for girls and young women. In an upcoming NIH-funded study in several African countries, adolescent females ages 16-21 will use a vaginal ring for six months, oral PrEP for six months, then choose which method they want to use for the final six months of the study.

Section 35.5 | Potential Source of HIV Persistence Confirmed

This section includes text excerpted from "Potential Source of HIV Persistence Confirmed," National Institute of Mental Health (NIMH), April 18, 2017. Reviewed February 2022.

Research with a unique animal model provides new evidence that a class of immune cells not thought to be a primary reservoir for HIV can harbor the virus even following antiretroviral treatment (ART). While earlier work has reported persistence of HIV in these cells – macrophages – investigators in this work developed a mouse model with an immune system generated from human cells but lacking T cells, which are a primary target of and reservoir for HIV. The absence of T cells enabled the team to establish definitively the persistence of HIV in macrophages.

Jenna Honeycutt, Ph.D., and J. Victor Garcia, Ph.D., at the University of North Carolina at Chapel Hill, along with scientists at several collaborating centers, conducted this work. The persistence of HIV in this type of cell – macrophages – means that treatment to eradicate HIV will have to target these cells in addition to those already demonstrated to have a role in the rebounding of HIV if ART is stopped.

The study is reported in the journal Nature Medicine, online April 17; it was funded by the National Institute of Mental Health (NIMH) and the National Institute of Allergy and Infectious Diseases. NIMH's Division of AIDS Research supports a broad range of studies on HIV/AIDS, including research aimed at understanding and alleviating the consequences of HIV infection of the central nervous system.

Section 35.6 | Biomarker Tracks Accelerated HIV-Associated Aging

This section includes text excerpted from "Biomarker Tracks Accelerated HIV-Associated Aging," National Institute of Mental Health (NIMH), April 21, 2016. Reviewed February 2022.

By measuring a molecular signature of aging, researchers have found that HIV infection accelerates aging, adding an average of five years to someone's biological age. The more rapid aging is occurring in people receiving antiretroviral treatment, so that even though treatment enables them to live for many decades, they remain at higher risk of aging-related chronic disease.

Studies of people with HIV infection have noted a higher risk of diseases associated with aging, such as liver and kidney failure, cancer, and heart disease. While the observations have suggested that HIV infection causes accelerated aging, there has not been a biologically based marker of aging with which scientists could clarify and quantify the impact of HIV on aging.

In search of such a marker, scientists at the University of Nebraska Medical Center, led by Howard Fox, M.D., Ph.D., in collaboration with scientists at the University of California, San Diego School of Medicine, led by Trey Ideker, Ph.D., turned to epigenetics, a term for changes to DNA that affect its function without altering the sequence of bases that make up DNA. Through epigenetic processes, experience can alter the genome, silencing or activating genes.

Previous research by Ideker's group had found that aging is associated with an epigenetic change called "methylation," the addition of a chemical (methyl) group to specific sites on the DNA chain. In this new work, analysis of the "methylomes" in the blood cells of 137 HIV-positive individuals found marked differences in methylation in comparison with 44 matched but HIV-negative individuals. The investigators controlled for factors besides HIV infection that might alter methylation, such as other health conditions and differences in the methylation levels of different types of cells, given that HIV can alter cell populations. Building on information from previous research on methylation and aging, the team found that methylation tracked well with chronological age in those without HIV. In HIV-positive individuals, however, the changes in methylation were accelerated, adding an average of five years to "epigenetic" age. This fast forward occurred even in those who had had HIV for short duration, less than five years. Previous models found that aging-related changes in methylation parallel increases in mortality; the changes found here in HIV positive patients suggest a 19 percent increase in mortality.

"The medical issues in treating people with HIV have changed," says Fox. "You are no longer as worried about infections that come from being immunocompromised. Now you worry about diseases related to aging, such as cardiovascular disease, neurocognitive impairment, and liver problems."

The team also found that one region of the genome was particularly rich in HIV-associated changes in methylation: this region, the human leukocyte antigen locus, encompasses genes that encode molecules that are central to immune responses. The authors suggest that epigenetic processes may contribute to the changes in regulation of this region of the genome and thus the progression, or control, of HIV.

The work provides an objective method of assessing the impact in individuals of HIV on biological age. It provides insight into the mechanisms behind the accelerated aging, and may offer a means of identifying individuals vulnerable to aging-related chronic disease, and who may benefit from more careful attention to monitoring and preventive treatments. Given epigenetic changes observed in the HLA region, it may provide clues to future approaches to controlling infection.

"Among the areas that NIH has identified as high priority for HIV research in the next three to five years are studies on the impact of HIV-associated comorbidities such as premature aging associated with long-term HIV disease and antiretroviral therapy," said NIMH's Division of AIDS Research Director Dianne M. Rausch, Ph.D. "This work is important for the insight it provides into the mechanism of HIV-associated accelerated aging and the potential it offers in terms of a biomarker for identifying individuals with HIV infection who are at greatest risk of aging-related disease as well as the development of targeted interventions."

Section 35.7 | Experimental Combination Surprises with Anti-HIV Effectiveness

This section includes text excerpted from "Experimental Combination Surprises with Anti-HIV Effectiveness," National Institute of Mental Health (NIMH), January 20, 2016. Reviewed February 2022.

A compound developed to protect the nervous system from HIV surprised researchers by augmenting the effectiveness of an investigational antiretroviral drug beyond anything expected. The potency of the combination treatment, tested so far in mice, suggests that it would be possible to rid the body of HIV for months, reducing the frequency with which patients must take these medications from daily to several times a year.

Even when people with HIV infection take antiretroviral drugs, more than 50 percent have HIV-associated neurocognitive disorders (HAND), which can result in any of a variety of symptoms, including confusion and problems with memory. NIH-supported scientists led by Harris A. Gelbard, M.D., Ph.D., at the University of Rochester School of Medicine and Dentistry developed the compound URMC-099 to protect against HIV-associated neurologic damage. This and similar compounds would always be administered with an antiretroviral medication; the objective of this research was to test URMC-099 as such an adjunct.

The antiretroviral medication used is in a class of antiretroviral drugs (protease inhibitors) commonly used to treat HIV, but in this case, NIH-supported researchers at the University of Nebraska Medical Center, led by Howard E. Gendelman, M.D., used nanotechnology to reconstitute the compound in an effort to enhance its ability to reach and remain in target tissues. (Nanotechnology involves use or creation of materials in very small dimensions – billionths of a meter.) The process renders the drug into crystal form and adds a protective coat. The small scale formulation of nano-antiretroviral therapy (nanoART) enables it to penetrate and endure in immune cells, forming reservoirs of antiretroviral activity.

Previous work had shown that URMC-099 was anti-inflammatory and protected neuronal tissue. Used alone it is not antiviral, but it was possible, the researchers reasoned, that its anti-inflammatory effects could enhance the beneficial effects of an antiviral. They tested the combination therapy in HIV-infected mice that have what is essentially a human immune system; human immune stem cells are introduced in mice that are born lacking components of a normal immune system. On a number of measures, URMC-099 enhanced the effects of nanoART beyond expectations. It reduced HIV levels beyond what nanoART could achieve alone and below what is detectable. It increased the ability of nanoART to form persistent antiretroviral "depots" in immune cells which are thought to be central to these drugs' ability to inhibit HIV replication.

"Our ultimate hope is that you are able to create a therapy that could be given less frequently than the daily therapy that is required," said Gelbard. "If a drug could be given once every six months or longer, that would greatly increase compliance, reduce side effects, and help people manage the disease, because they will not have to think about taking medication every day."

"The NIH Office of AIDS Research has identified the development of long acting HIV therapies and research towards a cure as high priority topics for research support," said Dianne M. Rausch, Ph.D., director of NIMH's Division of AIDS Research. "The nanoformulation strategies reported here could facilitate targeting HIV anatomic reservoirs such as lymph nodes and brain which are difficult to reach because of limited penetration of antiretroviral drugs into tissue compartments."

This work was supported by the National Institute of Mental Health along with the National Institute of Allergy and Infectious Diseases, the National Institute on Drug Abuse, the National Institute of Neurological Disorders and Stroke, and the National Institute on Aging.

Section 35.8 | HIV Can Spread Early, Evolve in Patients' Brains

This section includes text excerpted from "HIV Can Spread Early, Evolve in Patient's Brains," National Institutes of Health (NIH), March 26, 2015. Reviewed February 2022.

The acquired immunodeficiency virus (AIDS) virus can genetically evolve and independently replicate in patient's brains early in the illness process, researchers funded by the National Institutes of Health have discovered. An analysis of cerebral spinal fluid (CSF), a window into brain chemical activity, revealed that for a subset of patients human immunodeficiency virus (HIV) had started replicating within the brain within the first four months of infection. CSF in 30 percent of HIV-infected patients tracked showed at least transient signs of inflammation – suggesting an active infectious process – or viral replication within the first two years of infection. There was also evidence that the mutating virus can evolve a genome in the central nervous system that is distinct from that in the periphery.

"These results underscore the importance of early diagnosis and treatment with antiretroviral therapy," said Dianne Rausch, Ph.D., director of the Division of AIDS Research (DAR) of the NIH's National Institute of Mental Health (NIMH). "Any delay runs the risk that the virus could find refuge and cause damage in the brain, where some medications are less effective – potentially enabling it to re-emerge, even after it is suppressed in the periphery."

Prior to the study, it was known that HIV readily penetrates the brain and can trigger neurological problems and eventually cause dementia over the course of the infection. Yet there was little evidence about how quickly it can take hold and thrive there. Nor was it clear to what extent the brain serves as a hard-to-reach hideout from which the virus might re-infect the body – even if it is eliminated from peripheral blood and lymph node tissue by treatment.

The researchers compared evidence of HIV activity in CSF versus blood from 72 untreated HIV-infected patients over the first two years of their infection. Overall, 10-22 percent of the patients showed evidence of HIV replication or inflammation in the brain at the different time points analyzed within the first two years – and the signs persisted over time in about 16 percent of the participants.

The evidence suggests that in most patients peripheral forms of the virus infect immune cells that spread to the brain via blood. Yet in some patients, genetic versions of the virus not found in blood evolve in the brain environment. So it could become an independent, compartmentalized viral reservoir, capable of generating treatment-resistant mutant forms that could break out and re-infect the rest of the body after seemingly successful treatment, explained Rausch.

Whether the potential brain damage caused by early HIV replication and inflammation might be reversible with antiviral therapy awaits further research, said Swanstrom.

Section 35.9 | Starting Antiretroviral Treatment Early Improves Outcomes for HIV-Infected Individuals

This section includes text excerpted from "Starting Antiretroviral Treatment Early Improves Outcomes for HIV-Infected Individuals," HIV.gov, U.S. Department of Health and Human Services (HHS), May 27, 2015. Reviewed February 2022.

A major international randomized clinical trial has found that human immunodeficiency virus (HIV)-infected individuals have a considerably lower risk of developing AIDS or other serious illnesses if they start taking antiretroviral drugs sooner, when their cluster of differentiation 4 (CD4+) T-cell count – a key measure of immune system health – is higher, instead of waiting until the CD4+ cell count drops to lower levels. Together with data from previous studies showing that antiretroviral treatment reduced the risk of HIV transmission to uninfected sexual partners, these findings support offering treatment to everyone with HIV.

The finding is from the Strategic Timing of AntiRetroviral Treatment (START) study, the first large-scale randomized clinical trial to establish that earlier antiretroviral treatment benefits all HIV-infected individuals. The National Institute of Allergy and Infectious Diseases (NIAID), part of the National Institutes of Health, provided primary funding for the START trial. Though the study was expected to conclude at the end of 2016, an interim review of the study data by an independent data and safety monitoring board (DSMB) recommended that results be released early.

"We now have clear-cut proof that it is of significantly greater health benefit to an HIV-infected person to start antiretroviral therapy sooner rather than later," said NIAID Director Anthony S. Fauci, M.D. "Moreover, early therapy conveys a double benefit, not only improving the health of individuals but at the same time, by lowering their viral load, reducing the risk they will transmit HIV to others. These findings have global implications for the treatment of HIV."

"This is an important milestone in HIV research," said Jens Lundgren, M.D., of the University of Copenhagen and one of the cochairs of the START study. "We now have strong evidence that early treatment is beneficial to the HIV-positive person. These results support treating everyone irrespective of CD4+ T-cell count."

The START study, which opened widely in March 2011, was conducted by the International Network for Strategic Initiatives in Global HIV Trials (INSIGHT) at 215 sites in 35 countries. The trial enrolled 4,685 HIV-infected men and women ages 18 and older, with a median age of 36. Participants had never taken antiretroviral therapy and were enrolled with CD4+ cell counts in the normal range – above 500 cells per cubic millimeter (cells/mm3).

Approximately half of the study participants were randomized to initiate antiretroviral treatment immediately (early treatment), and the other half were randomized to defer treatment until their CD4+ cell count declined to 350 cells/mm3. On average, participants in the study were followed for three years.

The study measured a combination of outcomes that included serious AIDS events (such as AIDS-related cancer), serious non-AIDS events (major cardiovascular, renal and liver disease and cancer), and death. Based on data from March 2015, the DSMB found 41 instances of AIDS, serious non-AIDS events or death among those enrolled in the study's early treatment group compared to 86 events in the deferred treatment group. The DSMB's interim analysis found risk of developing serious illness or death was reduced by 53 percent among those in the early treatment group, compared to those in the deferred group.

Rates of serious AIDS-related events and serious non-AIDS-related events were both lower in the early treatment group than the deferred treatment group. The risk reduction was more pronounced for the AIDS-related events. Findings were consistent across geographic regions, and the benefits of early treatment were similar for participants from low- and middle-income countries and participants from high-income countries.

"The study was rigorous and the results are clear," said INSIGHT principal investigator James D. Neaton, Ph.D., a professor of biostatistics at the University of Minnesota, Minneapolis. "The definitive findings from a randomized trial like START are likely to influence how care is delivered to millions of HIV-positive individuals around the world." The University of Minnesota served as the trial's regulatory sponsor and statistical and data management center.

Prior to the START trial, there was no randomized controlled trial evidence to guide initiating treatment for individuals with higher CD4+ cell counts. Previous evidence to support early treatment among HIV-positive people with CD4+ cell counts above 350 was limited to data from nonrandomized trials or observational cohort studies, and on expert opinion.

START is the first large-scale randomized clinical trial to offer concrete scientific evidence to support the U.S. HIV treatment guidelines, which recommend that all asymptomatic HIV-infected individuals take antiretrovirals, regardless of CD4+ cell count. The World Health Organization HIV treatment guidelines recommend that HIV-infected individuals begin antiretroviral therapy when CD4+ cell counts fall to 500 cells/mm3 or less.

In light of the DSMB findings, study investigators are informing all participants of the interim results. Participants will be offered treatment if they are not already on antiretroviral therapy, and they will continue to be followed through 2016.

The HIV medicines used in the trial are approved medications donated by AbbVie, Inc., Bristol-Myers Squibb, Gilead Sciences, GlaxoSmithKline/ViiV Healthcare, Janssen Scientific Affairs, LLC, and Merck Sharp and Dohme Corp.

In addition to NIAID, funding for the START trial came from other NIH entities, including the National Cancer Institute (NCI), the National Heart, Lung and Blood Institute (NHLBI); the National Institute of Mental Health (NIMH); the National Institute of Neurological Disorders and Stroke (NINDS); the *Eunice Kennedy Shriver* National Institute of Child Health and Human Development (NICHHD); the NIH Clinical Center; and the National Institute of Arthritis and Musculoskeletal and Skin Diseases (NIAMS). Funding was also provided by the National Agency for Research on AIDS and Viral Hepatitis (ANRS) in France, the Federal Ministry of Education and Research in Germany, the European acquired immunodeficiency syndrome (AIDS) Treatment Network and government organizations based in Australia, Denmark, and the United Kingdom.

Chapter 36 | **Paying for HIV Care and Treatment**

PAYING FOR HIV CARE

Human immunodeficiency virus (HIV) care and treatment involves taking antiretroviral therapy (ART) and having regular check-ups with your healthcare provider who will monitor your health status on an ongoing basis.

These things are important because with the proper care and treatment, you can reduce your viral load, protect your health, enjoy a long and healthy life, and reduce the potential of transmitting the virus to others.

But, you might have concerns about how to pay for this. There are resources that can help you pay for the care you need.

PRIVATE INSURANCE

- **Job-based and individual insurance**. Many people have private health insurance through their employer (or a family member's employer), or they have individual insurance they have purchased. Under the Affordable Care Act (ACA), most job-based and individual plans are required to offer new benefits and protections. For example, plans cannot drop you or deny you coverage just because you have a preexisting health condition, like HIV. And insurers cannot impose lifetime caps on your insurance benefits. However, you will still need to pay any deductibles, copayments, and coinsurance your plan

This chapter includes text excerpted from "Paying for HIV Care and Treatment," HIV.gov, U.S. Department of Health and Human Services (HHS), January 17, 2022.

requires. Make sure you read your plan carefully so that you know what your plan will (and will not) cover. When you leave a job, you may be able to keep your job-based health insurance for a period, usually up to 18 months. This is called "Continuation of Health Coverage (COBRA) continuation coverage." With COBRA coverage, you usually have to pay the entire monthly premium yourself, plus a small administrative fee. Your former employer no longer pays any of your insurance costs.

- **The health insurance marketplace**. Established under the ACA, the Health Insurance Marketplace, available at Healthcare.gov, helps uninsured people find and apply for quality, affordable health coverage. Private plans in the Marketplace are required to cover a set of essential health benefits, including HIV screening, sexually transmitted infections (STIs) prevention counseling, and pre-exposure prophylaxis (PrEP). And, low and middle-income people may qualify for lower costs, based on their household size and income. To see if you can enroll in a health insurance plan or change plans, visit HealthCare.gov or find local help (localhelp.healthcare.gov). Some states run their health insurance exchanges. You can still get connected to them through HealthCare.gov.

FEDERAL RESOURCES

If you do not have private health insurance – or you need help because your insurance does not pay for the HIV care and treatment you need – there are federal resources that may help you.

- **Getting help**. Figuring out which programs and services you qualify for can be confusing. But, do not worry! There are case managers and benefits counselors who can help you. They know what services are available and can help you get care. Their services are free. Someone may provide this service at your healthcare provider's office or clinic. You also can find one near you by contacting a local human immunodeficiency virus (HIV)/Acquired immunodeficiency syndrome (AIDS) service organization. Toll-free state HIV/AIDS Hotlines will help put you in touch with agencies that can determine what programs and services you may be eligible for and help you access them.

Here are federal resources that are available:

- **Medicaid.** A state and federal partnership, Medicaid provides coverage for people with lower incomes, older people, people with disabilities, and some families and children. It is a critical source of coverage for many people living with HIV. States establish and administer their own Medicaid programs and determine they type, amount, duration, and scope of services within broad federal guidelines. States are required to cover certain mandatory benefits and can choose to provide other optional benefits, including prescription drugs. The eligibility rules for Medicaid are different in each state, but most states offer coverage for adults with children at some income level. And, under the ACA, states have the option, with significant federal matching funds, to expand Medicaid eligibility to generally include people below certain income levels, including low-income childless adults who were previously not generally eligible for Medicaid. As a result, in states that opt for Medicaid expansion, people with HIV who meet the income threshold no longer have to wait for an AIDS diagnosis in order to become eligible for Medicaid. You can apply for and enroll in Medicaid at any time. There is no limited enrollment period. If you qualify, your coverage can begin immediately. As of October 2021, 39 states (including the District of Columbia (DC)) have adopted the Medicaid expansion and 12 states have not adopted the expansion. Even if your state has not expanded Medicaid, you should still apply for coverage to see if you qualify under your state's existing rules.

- **The Ryan White HIV/AIDS program**. The Ryan White HIV/AIDS program works with cities, states, and local community-based organizations to provide HIV-related services to more than half a million people living with HIV each year. The program is for those who do not have sufficient healthcare coverage or financial resources to cope with HIV disease. Ryan White fills gaps in care not covered by these other sources. The program is divided into several "parts" to meet the needs of different communities and populations and includes support for an AIDS Drug Assistance Program (ADAP). To find a Ryan White clinic near you, use the HIV Testing and Care Services Locator.

- **The health center program**. Health centers provide high-quality preventive and primary healthcare services, including HIV testing and medical care, to patients regardless of their ability to pay. Some patients receive services directly at the health center itself, while others are referred to an HIV specialist in the community. Major investments in the network of community health centers over the past several years have created more opportunities for HIV care delivery. You can find a health center near you by going to the HIV Testing and Care Services Locator.

- **Medicare**. Medicare is health insurance for people age 65 or older, people under 65 with certain disabilities, and people of all ages with End-Stage Renal Disease. Medicare coverage for eligible individuals includes outpatient care, prescription drugs, and inpatient hospital care. It covers all medically necessary treatments for a person with HIV. To learn more about Medicare coverage and choices, visit Medicare.gov.

- **Federal programs for women and children**. There are several federal programs to help low-income women and children access healthcare. The Children's Health Insurance Program (CHIP) provides free or low-cost health insurance coverage for children up to age 19.

Each state has its own rules about who qualifies for CHIP. You can apply for and enroll a child in CHIP at any time. There is no limited enrollment period. If the child qualifies, her/his coverage can begin immediately. Visit www.insurekidsnow.gov to learn more and see if you are eligible for coverage or call 877-543-7669. In addition, programs supported by the Maternal and Child Health Services Block Grant, authorized by Title V of the Social Security Act (SSA), serve low-income women, children, and youth with limited access to healthcare, including children with special needs. Specifically, the Title V Maternal and Child Health program seek to assure access to quality care, especially for those with low incomes or limited availability of care.

- **American Indian and Alaska Native programs**. The Indian Health Service (IHS) provides healthcare services – including HIV services – for members and descendants of federally-recognized American Indian and Alaska Native Tribes.

- **Veterans programs**. The U.S. Department of Veterans Affairs (VA) is the largest single provider of medical care to people with HIV in the United States, supporting over 31,000 Veterans with HIV. If you are eligible, you may be able to receive HIV care through the Veterans Health Administration. VA offers an online benefits website (www.ebenefits.va.gov/ebenefits/homepage) with detailed information about healthcare benefits.

NON-FEDERAL RESOURCES

Patient Assistance Programs (PAPs) are programs administered by pharmaceutical companies to offer free or reduced-cost antiretroviral (ARV) medicines to low-income people living with HIV who are uninsured or underinsured, and who do not qualify for federal assistance programs such as Medicaid, Medicare, or AIDS Drug Assistance Programs. Each pharmaceutical company has different eligibility criteria for qualifying for its PAP.

The U.S. Department of Health and Human Services, seven pharmaceutical companies, the National Alliance of State and Territorial AIDS Directors (NASTAD), and community stakeholders worked together to develop a common patient assistance program application (CPAPA) and companion document that can be used by patients and providers to access these programs.

Part 5 | Common Co-occurring Infections and Complications of HIV/AIDS

Chapter 37 | Opportunistic Infections and Their Relationship to HIV/AIDS

WHAT ARE OPPORTUNISTIC INFECTIONS?

- Opportunistic infections (OIs) are illnesses that occur more frequently and are more severe in people with human immunodeficiency virus (HIV). This is because they have damaged immune systems.
- Nowadays, OIs are less common in people with HIV because of effective HIV treatment.
- But, some people with HIV still develop OIs because,
  - They may not know they have HIV
  - They may not be on HIV treatment or
  - Their HIV treatment may not be working properly

HOW CAN YOU PREVENT OPPORTUNISTIC INFECTIONS?

Taking HIV medicine is the best way to prevent getting OIs. HIV medicine can keep your immune system strong and healthy. If you develop an OI, talk to your healthcare provider about how to treat it.

There are also steps you can take to prevent getting OIs:

- Talk to your healthcare provider about medicines and vaccines that prevent certain OIs.

This chapter contains text excerpted from the following sources: Text beginning with the heading "What Are Opportunistic Infections?" is excerpted from "AIDS and Opportunistic Infections," Centers for Disease Control and Prevention (CDC), May 20, 2021; Text beginning with the heading "What Causes Opportunistic Infections" is excerpted from "Opportunistic Infections," HIV.gov, U.S. Department of Health and Human Services (HHS), January 14, 2022.

- Prevent exposure to other sexually transmitted diseases.
- Do not share needles, syringes, or other drug-injection equipment (e.g., cookers).
- Limit your exposure to germs that could make you very sick. This includes tuberculosis or germs found in the stools, saliva, or on the skin of animals.
- Do not consume certain foods, including undercooked eggs, raw milk and cheeses, unpasteurized fruit juices, or raw seed sprouts.
- Do not drink untreated water, such as water directly from lakes or rivers. Avoid drinking tap water in foreign countries. Use bottled water or water filters.
- Talk to your healthcare provider about things that could expose you to OIs at work, at home, and on vacation.

Few common opportunistic infections:
- Candidiasis
- Invasive cervical cancer
- Coccidioidomycosis
- Cryptococcosis
- Cryptosporidiosis (Crypto)
- Cystoisosporiasis
- Cytomegalovirus (CMV)
- Encephalopathy, HIV-related
- Herpes simplex virus (HSV)
- Histoplasmosis
- Kaposi sarcoma (KS)
- Lymphoma
- Tuberculosis (TB)
- *Mycobacterium avium* complex (MAC)
- *Pneumocystis* pneumonia (PCP)
- Pneumonia
- Progressive multifocal leukoencephalopathy
- *Salmonella* septicemia
- Toxoplasmosis

WHAT CAUSES OPPORTUNISTIC INFECTIONS

OIs are caused by a variety of germs (viruses, bacteria, fungi, and parasites). These germs spread in different ways, such as in the air, in body fluids, or in contaminated food or water. They can cause health problems when a person's immune system is weakened by HIV disease.

CAN OPPORTUNISTIC INFECTIONS BE TREATED?

If you develop OIs, there are treatments available such as antiviral, antibiotic, and antifungal drugs. The type of medicine your health-care provider prescribes will depend on the OI.

Once an OI is successfully treated, a person may continue to use the same medicine or an additional medicine to prevent the OI from coming back. Having an OI may be a very serious medical situation and its treatment can be challenging.

Chapter 38 | **Preventing Opportunistic Infections**

Opportunistic infections (OIs) can be caused by viruses, bacteria, fungus, even parasites. One way to avoid these infections is to reduce your risk of exposure to these germs. Here are some practical suggestions.

SEXUAL EXPOSURES
- Use condoms every time you have sex.
- Avoid oral-anal sex.
- Use waterproof gloves if you are going to insert your finger into your partner's anus.
- Frequently wash hands and genitals with warm soapy water after any sex play that brings them in contact with feces.

INJECTION DRUG USE
- Do not inject drugs.
- If you cannot stop using, avoid sharing needles and other equipment.
- Get vaccinated against hepatitis A and hepatitis B.

JOB EXPOSURE
Certain types of jobs or facilities can put a person with human immunodeficiency virus (HIV) at risk of OIs.

This chapter includes text excerpted from "Preventing Opportunistic Infections (OIs)," U.S. Department of Veterans Affairs (VA), December 27, 2019.

These include work in:
- Healthcare facilities
- Homeless shelters
- Day-care centers
- Prisons
- Places that involved work with animals (such as farms, veterinary clinics, pet stores)

PET EXPOSURE
Pets can carry diseases that do not affect a healthy person but can pose a serious risk to someone with HIV. For that reason, if you have a pet, follow these suggestions.

General
- Wash your hands after handling your pet (especially before eating).
- Avoid contact with your pet's feces. If your pet has diarrhea, ask a friend or family member to take care of it.
- If you are getting a new pet, try not to get one that is younger than a year old, especially if it has diarrhea. (Young animals are more likely to carry certain germs such as Salmonella.) Avoid stray animals.

Cats
- Keep your cat indoors. They should not be allowed to hunt and should not be fed raw or undercooked meat.
- Clean the litter box daily. If you do it yourself, wear gloves and wash your hands thoroughly afterward.
- Control fleas (ask your vet how to do this).
- Avoid playing with your cat in ways that may result in scratches or bites. If you do get scratched or bitten, wash the area right away. Do not let your cat lick your cuts or wounds.

Birds
- Avoid areas where there are any bird droppings. Do not disturb soil underneath bird-roosting sites.

Others

- Avoid touching reptiles, such as snakes, lizards, iguanas, and turtles.
- Wear gloves if you are cleaning an aquarium.
- Avoid areas where there are any bird droppings. Do not disturb soil underneath bird-roosting sites.

CAUTIONS ABOUT FOOD AND WATER

- Avoid raw or undercooked eggs (including hollandaise sauce, Caesar salad dressing, some mayonnaise, eggnog, cake, and cookie batter).
- Avoid raw or undercooked poultry, meat, and seafood (especially raw seafood). Use a meat thermometer. Cook poultry to 180 °F, and other meats to 165 °F. If you do not have a meat thermometer, cook meat until no traces of pink remain.
- Avoid unpasteurized dairy products and fruit juice.
- Avoid raw seed sprouts (such as alfalfa, mung beans).
- Thoroughly wash fruits and vegetables before eating.
- Do not let uncooked meats come into contact with other uncooked foods. (Wash thoroughly hands, cutting boards, counters, knives, and other utensils after contact with uncooked meats.)
- Do not drink water directly from lakes or rivers. Filtered water is preferable, particularly if your immune system is weak.

People with HIV whose immune systems are severely weakened may want to:

- Avoid soft cheeses (feta, brie, camembert, blue-veined, and Mexican-style cheeses, such as queso fresco).
- Cook leftover foods or ready-to-eat foods, such as hot dogs, until they are steaming hot.
- Avoid food from delicatessens, such as prepared meats, salads, and cheeses – or heat these foods until steaming before eating.

CAUTIONS ABOUT TRAVEL

Before you travel to other countries, particularly developing countries, talk to your provider about ways you can avoid getting sick on your trip. People with weakened immune systems are at risk and should discuss travel plans well in advance. Be sure to check with your provider regarding recommended or required immunizations, as well as indications and precautions of travel vaccines, before traveling out of the country.

When traveling in developing countries, people who have HIV should be especially cautious of food and water that may be contaminated. It is best to avoid:

- Raw fruits and vegetables (unless you peel them first)
- Raw or undercooked seafood or meat
- Tap water or ice made with tap water (drink bottled water instead)
- Unpasteurized milk or dairy products
- Swallowing water when swimming

Talk to your healthcare provider about whether you need to get vaccinated before your trip and whether you need to take drugs to prevent diseases that are common in the country you are going to visit.

Chapter 39 | **HIV/AIDS and Co-occurring Bacterial Infections**

Chapter Contents

Section 39.1 | *Mycobacterium avium* Complex

This section includes text excerpted from "Mycobacterium avium Complex Infections," Genetic and Rare Diseases Information Center (GARD), National Center for Advancing Translational Sciences (NCATS), November 8, 2018. Reviewed February 2022.

Mycobacterium avium complex (MAC) refers to infections caused by two types of bacteria: *Mycobacterium avium* and *Mycobacterium intracellulare.* MAC bacteria do not make most people sick. However, people with immune systems that do not work well (from human immunodeficiency virus (HIV)/acquired immunodeficiency syndrome (AIDS) or certain cancers for example) or people with lung disease (such as chronic obstructive pulmonary disease (COPD) or cystic fibrosis) are at the greatest risk for getting sick from MAC Infections. Elderly women are also at higher risk to get sick from MAC infections.

There are 3 types of MAC infections:

- Pulmonary MAC infections. Affect the lungs and are the most common type. These mainly affect elderly women and people who already have lung disease.
- Disseminated MAC infections. Have spread throughout the body. This type is usually seen in people with advanced AIDS.
- MAC-associated lymphadenitis. Causes swelling of the lymph nodes (especially in the neck) and are the most common in young children who have normal immune systems.

While the symptoms are different for each type of infection, general symptoms include fever, night sweats, weight loss, and fatigue. MAC bacteria are found in water, soil, and dust. They infect people when the bacteria are inhaled or swallowed. MAC bacteria are not usually spread from person to person. MAC infections are diagnosed by a combination of imaging scans and identifying the bacteria in cultures of cells from the infected area. Treatment for MAC infection depends on the type and may include antibiotics, antiviral medications, or surgery.

SYMPTOMS OF *MYCOBACTERIUM AVIUM* COMPLEX

MAC infections can cause various symptoms depending on the site of the infection. For example, pulmonary MAC mainly affects the lungs; disseminated MAC affects the whole body, and MAC lymphadenitis causes swollen lymph nodes. The symptoms of pulmonary MAC infection start slowly, get worse over time, and may last for weeks to months. People with pulmonary MAC infections may experience cough, weight loss, fever, fatigue, and night sweats. Symptoms of disseminated MAC infection include:

- Fever
- Sweating
- Weight loss
- Fatigue
- Diarrhea
- Shortness of breath
- Abdominal pain
- Anemia

People with disseminated MAC infection may also have symptoms associated with an infection of the breast tissue (mastitis); an infection of the skeletal muscle (pyomyositis), abscesses of the skin or brain, and gastrointestinal problems. MAC lymphadenitis generally affects children with normal immune systems. Symptoms of MAC lymphadenitis usually only include swollen lymph nodes mainly on one side of the neck

CAUSES OF *MYCOBACTERIUM AVIUM* COMPLEX

MAC infections are caused by two types of bacteria: *Mycobacterium avium* and *Mycobacterium intracellulare*. These bacteria are found in many places including water (fresh or salt), household dust, and soil. MAC bacteria get into the body when the bacteria are inhaled into the lungs or swallowed. Most people have MAC bacteria in their bodies and never get sick. MAC bacteria primarily cause illness in people who have poorly working immune systems or lung disease. Touching the same objects or having a close relationship with people who are sick from a MAC infection does not seem to increase the chance of getting sick. MAC infections are not thought to be contagious from one person to another.

INHERITANCE OF *MYCOBACTERIUM AVIUM* COMPLEX

MAC infection is caused by bacteria and is not an inherited condition. To become infected with MAC bacteria and get sick, a person must first be exposed to one of the associated types of bacteria.

There have been a few reports of families with more than one family member with a MAC infection. In these families, it is thought that there is a variation in a gene or genes involved with the body's immune response. A genetic variant in an immune system gene may make some people more likely to get sick from infection than others. There are many genes involved in the human immune response, and there is no single gene known to be responsible for MAC infections.

DIAGNOSIS OF *MYCOBACTERIUM AVIUM* COMPLEX

Diagnosis of a pulmonary MAC infection is based on a combination of physical exam findings, laboratory test results, and lung x-rays or computerized tomography (CT) scan results. The laboratory tests include cultures of mucus spit up from the lungs (sputum) and special staining (acid-fast bacillus test). A laboratory culture involves placing cells from a sputum sample in an environment that encourages the bacteria to grow. Results identifying the bacteria may take several days or longer. Because the symptoms of MAC infections are similar to those of other types of infections, other types of infections and diseases must also be ruled out.

Diagnosis of disseminated MAC infection is suspected based on symptoms and is confirmed in cultures of blood and often lymph node cells. Cultures of cells from urine, stool, liver, or bone marrow may also be helpful. CT scans may be used to try to determine the different sites of infection in the body. If pulmonary or disseminated MAC infection is suspected, an HIV test may be done, as well as other tests, to rule out other associated medical conditions.

A diagnosis of MAC lymphadenitis is confirmed by finding the bacteria in the culture of lymph node cells. These cells are collected by a biopsy of a swollen lymph node.

TREATMENT OF *MYCOBACTERIUM AVIUM* COMPLEX

MAC infection is classified into several different types including:
- Pulmonary MAC infection, which affects the lungs
- Disseminated MAC infection, which affects many different parts of the body
- MAC lymphadenitis, which causes swollen lymph nodes

Treatment options for MAC infections vary by type of infection and by the presence of other medical conditions such as AIDS, cystic fibrosis, COPD, or cancer.

Pulmonary MAC infections and disseminated MAC infections are usually treated with a combination of antibiotic medications. There are many types of antibiotics approved for treating MAC infections. A combination of medicines is used because some of the disease-causing bacteria can be resistant to certain types of antibiotics. Using more than one antibiotic reduces the chance for the MAC bacteria to come back after treatment is over.

For people who have both HIV/AIDS and a MAC infection, treatment usually involves a combination of different antibiotics for the MAC infection and antiretroviral therapy (ART) to treat the HIV infection.

In special circumstances, there is some evidence to suggest that surgery to remove a single spot of infection in one lung can be helpful in people who have had a poor response to drug therapy. Surgery is usually only done when the infection is found in only one lung and the surgery will not cause any long-term harm.

Treatment of MAC lymphadenitis usually involves surgical removal of affected lymph nodes. Antibiotics may also be prescribed depending on the severity of infection and the response to surgery.

FDA-Approved Treatments

The medication(s) listed below have been approved by the U.S. Food and Drug Administration (FDA) as orphan products for the treatment of this condition.

- **Liposomal amikacin (brand name: Arikayce).** Manufactured by Insmed Incorporated FDA-approved indication: September 2018, liposomal amikacin (Arikayce) was approved for the treatment of MAC lung disease as part of a combination antibacterial drug regimen in patients who do not achieve negative sputum cultures after a minimum of six consecutive months of a multidrug background regimen therapy.

PROGNOSIS OF *MYCOBACTERIUM AVIUM* COMPLEX

The long-term outlook (prognosis) for people who are sick from MAC infections depends on the type of infection and whether or not the person has other medical conditions or health problems. One published study reviewed the long-term outlook of people with MAC infections with and without other diseases, and found a 75 percent chance for survival five years after their first diagnosis.

People who are HIV-positive with MAC infections may have a shortened lifespan depending on their immune systems and their response to HIV medications. For people who have had successful treatment, there is still a chance that the infection will come back, so people who have been sick from a MAC infection need to be monitored over time.

In HIV-negative people with lung disease from a MAC infection, the treatment success rates range from 20–90 percent in different studies. People with certain types of lung disease, people who are underweight, and people with anemia are more likely to have a poor outcome than other HIV-negative people affected by a MAC infection.

MAC lymphadenitis in children generally does not impact their health. In some cases, the condition may go away even without treatment.

Section 39.2 | Tuberculosis

This section includes text excerpted from "Basic TB Facts," Centers for Disease Control and Prevention (CDC), March 20, 2016. Reviewed February 2022.

Tuberculosis (TB) is caused by a bacterium called "*Mycobacterium tuberculosis.*" The bacteria usually attack the lungs, but TB bacteria can attack any part of the body such as the kidney, spine, and brain. Not everyone infected with TB bacteria becomes sick. As a result, two TB-related conditions exist latent TB infection (LTBI) and TB disease. If not treated properly, TB disease can be fatal.

HOW TUBERCULOSIS SPREADS

TB bacteria are spread through the air from one person to another. The TB bacteria are put into the air when a person with TB disease of the lungs or throat coughs, speaks or sings. People nearby may breathe in these bacteria and become infected. TB is not spread by:

- Shaking someone's hand
- Sharing food or drink
- Touching bed linens or toilet seats
- Sharing toothbrushes
- Kissing

When a person breathes in TB bacteria, the bacteria can settle in the lungs and begin to grow. From there, they can move through the blood to other parts of the body, such as the kidney, spine, and brain.

TB disease in the lungs or throat can be infectious. This means that the bacteria can be spread to other people. TB in other parts of the body, such as the kidney or spine, is usually not infectious.

People with TB disease are most likely to spread it to people they spend time with every day. This includes family members, friends, and coworkers or schoolmates.

TUBERCULOSIS AND HIV COINFECTION

TB is a serious health threat, especially for people living with the human immunodeficiency virus (HIV). People living with HIV are more likely than others to become sick with TB. Worldwide, TB is one of the leading causes of death among people living with HIV.

Without treatment, as with other opportunistic infections, HIV and TB can work together to shorten their lifespan.

- Someone with untreated LTBI and HIV infection is much more likely to develop TB disease during his or her lifetime than someone without HIV infection.
- Among people with LTBI, HIV infection is the strongest known risk factor for progressing to TB disease.
- A person who has both HIV infection and TB disease has an acquired immunodeficiency syndrome (AIDS)-defining condition.

People infected with HIV who also have either LTBI or TB disease can be effectively treated. The first step is to ensure that people living with HIV are tested for TB infection. If found to have TB infection, further tests are needed to rule out TB disease. The next step is to start treatment for LTBI or TB disease based on test results.

TREATMENT

Untreated LTBI infection can quickly progress to TB disease in people living with HIV since the immune system is already weakened. And without treatment, TB disease can progress from sickness to death. Fortunately, there are a number of treatment options for people living with HIV who also have either LTBI or TB disease.

Chapter 40 | **HIV/AIDS and Co-occurring Fungal Infections**

Chapter Contents

Section 40.1 | Risk of Fungal Infections among People with HIV/AIDS

This section includes text excerpted from "People Living with HIV/AIDS," Centers for Disease Control and Prevention (CDC), December 17, 2020.

As a person living with human immunodeficiency virus (HIV)/ acquired immunodeficiency syndrome (AIDS), you have many opportunities for a healthy and full life. You may also have some health challenges. One of those challenges is avoiding infections.

Many fungal infections are called "opportunistic infections," which means that they usually affect people with weak immune systems. Because HIV weakens the immune system, you have a greater chance of getting some types of fungal infections such as cryptococcosis, coccidioidomycosis, histoplasmosis, and pneumocystis pneumonia (PCP).

WHAT YOU NEED TO KNOW ABOUT FUNGAL INFECTIONS

- **Your CD4 count is important**. You are at the greatest risk for fungal infection when your CD4 count is less than 200. Keeping your CD4 count above 200 may help you avoid serious illness.
- **Antiretroviral therapy (ART) is important**. Starting ART helps slow the progress of HIV and can reduce your chances of getting a fungal infection.
- **Fungal infections can range from mild to life-threatening**. Some fungal infections are mild skin rashes, but others can be deadly, such as fungal meningitis. Because of this, it is important to seek treatment as soon as possible to try to avoid serious infection.
- **Fungal infections can look like bacterial or viral infections**. If you are taking medicine to fight infection and you are not getting better, ask your doctor about testing you for a fungal infection.
- **Where you live (geography) matters**. Some disease-causing fungi are more common in certain parts of the

world. If you have HIV/AIDS and live in or visit these areas, you are more likely to get these infections than the general population.

- **Your activities matter**. Disease-causing fungi can be found in air, dust, and soil, especially soil that contains bird or bat droppings. Doing activities that disturb the soil, such as gardening, cleaning chicken coops, construction, demolition, and visiting caves can cause you to inhale more fungi and increase your chance of infection.
- **Some fungal infections can interfere with taking your medications**. Thrush, an infection in the mouth and throat, is sometimes seen among people living with HIV/AIDS. This infection is not usually life-threatening but can be painful, make it difficult to eat, or interfere with taking your medications. Your nutrition is an important part of staying healthy, so it is important to seek care for this infection.

PREVENTING FUNGAL INFECTIONS IN PEOPLE LIVING WITH HIV/AIDS

Fungi are difficult to avoid because they are a natural part of the environment. Fungi live outdoors in soil, on plants, trees, and other vegetation. They are also on many indoor surfaces and on your skin. However, there may be some ways for you to lower your chances of getting a serious fungal infection.

- **Learn about fungal infections**. There are different types of fungal infections. Learning about them can help you and your healthcare provider recognize the symptoms early, which may prevent serious illness.
- **Find out about your risk**. The danger of getting a fungal infection can change depending on your location and your CD4 count. Learning what things can put you at risk may prevent serious illness.
- **Get additional medical care if necessary**. Fungal infections often resemble other illnesses. Visiting your healthcare provider may help with faster diagnosis and may prevent serious illness.

- **Antifungal medication**. Your healthcare provider may prescribe medication to prevent fungal infections. For example, they may recommend medication (TMP-SMX, also called "Bactrim," "Septra," or "Cotrim") to prevent a type of fungal pneumonia called "*Pneumocystis jirovecii* pneumonia" (PCP).
- **Protect yourself from the environment**. There may be some ways to lower your chances of getting a serious fungal infection by trying to avoid disease-causing fungi in the environment. It is important to note that although these actions are recommended, they have not been proven to prevent fungal infections.
  - Try to avoid areas with a lot of dust such as construction or excavation sites.
  - Stay inside during dust storms.
  - Stay away from areas with bird and bat droppings. This includes places such as chicken coops and caves.
  - Wear gloves when handling materials such as soil, moss, or manure.
  - Wear shoes, long pants, and a long-sleeved shirt when doing outdoor activities such as gardening, yard work, or visiting wooded areas.

HIV/AIDS AND FUNGAL INFECTIONS
The United States
One of the first signs that the HIV/AIDS epidemic was beginning in the United States was a cluster of five cases of a type of fungal pneumonia called "*Pneumocystis jirovecii* pneumonia" (PCP) in California in 1981. Before antiretroviral therapy was discovered, fungal and other opportunistic infections were a major problem for people with HIV/AIDS. Since then, the numbers of fungal infections and deaths due to fungal infections in people living with HIV/AIDS have decreased substantially. For example, one study showed that the incidence of cryptococcosis in AIDS patients decreased by approximately 90 percent in the 1990s. The decrease in opportunistic infections is primarily because ART helps keep people with

HIV from reaching the stage where their immune systems are most vulnerable to fungal infections and other infections. However, fungal diseases are still a concern for people living with HIV/AIDS in the United States. Awareness is your best protection, and learning about the different fungal diseases will help you safeguard your health.

Global

Even with the growing availability of HIV care and treatment in less developed countries, fungal infections, particularly cryptococcosis and histoplasmosis, are still a problem for people living with HIV/AIDS in many resource-limited settings. For example, worldwide, approximately 220,000 new cases of cryptococcal meningitis occur each year, resulting in 181,000 deaths, the majority of which occur in sub-Saharan Africa. In Latin America, histoplasmosis is one of the most common opportunistic infections among people living with HIV/AIDS, and approximately 30 percent of HIV/AIDS patients diagnosed with histoplasmosis die from this infection. Some of the reasons that explain the public health burden of fungal diseases in these areas of the world are that there is a lack of laboratory infrastructure needed to diagnose fungal infections, or because the antifungal medications needed to treat these infections are expensive or unavailable.

Section 40.2 | Candidiasis

This section includes text excerpted from "Candidiasis," Centers for Disease Control and Prevention (CDC), October 30, 2020.

Candidiasis is a fungal infection caused by a yeast (a type of fungus) called "*Candida*." Some species of *Candida* can cause infection in people; the most common is *Candida albicans*. *Candida* normally lives on the skin and inside the body, in places such as the mouth, throat, gut, and vagina, without causing any problems. *Candida* can cause infections if it grows out of control or if it enters deep into the body (e.g., the bloodstream or internal organs such as the kidney, heart, or brain).

CANDIDA INFECTIONS OF THE MOUTH, THROAT, AND ESOPHAGUS

Candida can multiply and cause an infection if the environment inside the mouth, throat, or esophagus changes in a way that encourages fungal growth. Candidiasis in the mouth and throat is also called "thrush" or "oropharyngeal candidiasis." Candidiasis in the esophagus (the tube that connects the throat to the stomach) is called "esophageal candidiasis" or "*Candida* esophagitis." Esophageal candidiasis is one of the most common infections in people living with HIV/AIDS.

Symptoms of *Candida* Infections of the Mouth, Throat, and Esophagus

Candidiasis in the mouth and throat can have many different symptoms, including:

- White patches on the inner cheeks, tongue, roof of the mouth, and throat
- Redness or soreness
- Cotton-like feeling in the mouth
- Loss of taste
- Pain while eating or swallowing
- Cracking and redness at the corners of the mouth

Symptoms of candidiasis in the esophagus usually include pain when swallowing and difficulty swallowing.

Contact your healthcare provider if you have symptoms that you think are related to candidiasis in the mouth, throat, or esophagus.

Risk of *Candida* Infections of the Mouth, Throat, and Esophagus

Candidiasis in the mouth, throat, or esophagus is uncommon in healthy adults. People who are at higher risk for getting candidiasis in the mouth and throat include babies, especially those younger than 1 month of age, and people with at least one of these factors:

- Wear dentures
- Have diabetes
- Have cancer
- Have HIV/AIDS
- Take antibiotics or corticosteroids, including inhaled corticosteroids for conditions such as asthma
- Take medications that cause dry mouth or have medical conditions that cause dry mouth
- Smoke

Most people who get candidiasis in the esophagus have weakened immune systems, meaning that their bodies do not fight infections well. This includes people living with HIV/AIDS and people who have blood cancers such as leukemia and lymphoma. People who get candidiasis in the esophagus often also have candidiasis in the mouth and throat.

Prevention of *Candida* Infections of the Mouth, Throat, and Esophagus

Ways to help prevent candidiasis in the mouth and throat include:
- Maintain good oral health
- Rinse your mouth or brush your teeth after using inhaled corticosteroids

Sources

Candida normally lives in the mouth, throat, and the rest of the digestive tract without causing any problems. Sometimes, *Candida* can multiply and cause an infection if the environment inside the mouth, throat, or esophagus changes in a way that encourages its growth.

This can happen when:
- A person's immune system becomes weakened,
- If antibiotics affect the natural balance of microbes in the body,
- Or for a variety of other reasons in other groups of people.

Diagnosis and Testing of *Candida* Infections of the Mouth, Throat, and Esophagus

Healthcare providers can usually diagnose candidiasis in the mouth or throat simply by looking inside. Sometimes a healthcare provider will take a small sample from the mouth or throat. The sample is sent to a laboratory for testing, usually to be examined under a microscope.

Healthcare providers usually diagnose candidiasis in the esophagus by doing an endoscopy. An endoscopy is a procedure to examine the digestive tract using a tube with a light and a camera. A healthcare provider might prescribe antifungal medicine without doing an endoscopy to see if the patient's symptoms get better.

Treatment of *Candida* Infections of the Mouth, Throat, and Esophagus

Candidiasis in the mouth, throat, or esophagus is usually treated with antifungal medicine. The treatment for mild to moderate infections in the mouth or throat is usually an antifungal medicine applied to the inside of the mouth for 7 to 14 days. These medications include clotrimazole, miconazole, or nystatin. For severe infections, the most common treatment is fluconazole (an antifungal medication) taken by mouth or through a vein. If the patient does not get better after taking fluconazole, healthcare providers may prescribe a different antifungal. The treatment for candidiasis in the esophagus is usually fluconazole. Other types of prescription antifungal medicines can also be used for people who cannot take fluconazole or who do not get better after taking fluconazole.

Statistics of *Candida* Infections of the Mouth, Throat, and Esophagus

The exact number of cases of candidiasis in the mouth, throat, and esophagus in the United States is difficult to determine. This is because there is no national surveillance for these infections. In one study, about one-third of patients with advanced HIV infection had candidiasis in the mouth and throat.

VAGINAL CANDIDIASIS

Candida can multiply and cause an infection if the environment inside the vagina changes in a way that encourages its growth. Candidiasis in the vagina is commonly called a "vaginal yeast infection." Other names for this infection are "vaginal candidiasis," "vulvovaginal candidiasis," or "candidal vaginitis."

Symptoms of Vaginal Candidiasis

The symptoms of vaginal candidiasis include:

- Vaginal itching or soreness
- Pain during sexual intercourse
- Pain or discomfort when urinating
- Abnormal vaginal discharge

Although most vaginal candidiasis is mild, some women can develop severe infections involving redness, swelling, and cracks in the wall of the vagina.

Contact your healthcare provider if you have any of these symptoms. These symptoms are similar to those of other types of vaginal infections, which are treated with different types of medicines. A healthcare provider can tell you if you have vaginal candidiasis and how to treat it.

Risk of Vaginal Candidiasis

Vaginal candidiasis is common, though more research is needed to understand how many women are affected. Women who are more likely to get vaginal candidiasis include those who:

- Are pregnant
- Use hormonal contraceptives (e.g., birth control pills)
- Have diabetes
- Have a weakened immune system (e.g., due to HIV infection or medicines that weaken the immune system, such as steroids and chemotherapy)
- Are taking or have recently taken antibiotics

Prevention of Vaginal Candidiasis

Wearing cotton underwear might help reduce the chances of getting a yeast infection. Because taking antibiotics can lead to vaginal candidiasis, take these medicines only when prescribed and exactly as your healthcare provider tells you.

Sources

Scientists estimate that about 20 percent of women normally have *Candida* in the vagina without having any symptoms. Sometimes, *Candida* can multiply and cause an infection if the environment inside the vagina changes in a way that encourages its growth. This can happen because of hormones, medicines, or changes in the immune system.

Diagnosis and Testing of Vaginal Candidiasis

Healthcare providers usually diagnose vaginal candidiasis by taking a small sample of vaginal discharge to be examined under a microscope in the medical office or sent to a laboratory for a fungal culture. However, a positive fungal culture does not always mean that *Candida* is causing symptoms because some women can have *Candida* in the vagina without having any symptoms.

Treatment of Vaginal Candidiasis

Vaginal candidiasis is usually treated with antifungal medicine. For most infections, the treatment is an antifungal medicine applied inside the vagina or a single dose of fluconazole taken by mouth. Other treatments may be needed for infections that are more severe, that do not get better, or that keep coming back after getting better. These treatments include more doses of fluconazole taken by mouth or other medicines applied inside the vagina, such as boric acid, nystatin, or flucytosine.

Statistics of Vaginal Candidiasis

Vaginal candidiasis is common. In the United States, it is the second most common type of vaginal infection after bacterial vaginal infections. An estimated 1.4 million outpatient visits for vaginal candidiasis occur annually in the United States. The number of vaginal candidiasis cases in the United States is unknown.

INVASIVE CANDIDIASIS
What Is Invasive Candidiasis?

Invasive candidiasis is an infection caused by a yeast (a type of fungus) called "*Candida*." Unlike *Candida* infections in the mouth and throat (also called "thrush") or vaginal "yeast infections," which are localized to one part of the body, invasive candidiasis is a serious infection that can affect the blood, heart, brain, eyes, bones, or other parts of the body.

Candida normally lives inside the body (in places such as the mouth, throat, gut, and vagina) and on the skin without causing any problems. However, in certain patients who are at risk, *Candida* can enter the bloodstream or internal organs and cause an infection. A *Candida* bloodstream infection, also called "candidemia," is the most common form of invasive candidiasis. In the United States, candidemia is one of the most common causes of bloodstream infections in hospitalized patients, and it often results in long hospital stays and death. It is also responsible for high medical costs.

Antifungal medication can treat invasive candidiasis. Certain patients such as those with cancer or bone marrow or organ transplants might receive antifungal medication to prevent invasive candidiasis.

ANTIFUNGAL RESISTANCE IN *CANDIDA*

Antifungal resistance is an increasing problem with the fungus *Candida*, a yeast. *Candida* infections may resist antifungal drugs, making them difficult to treat.

About 7 percent of all *Candida* blood samples tested at Centers for Disease Control and Prevention (CDC) are resistant to the antifungal drug fluconazole. Although one *Candida* species, *Candida albicans*, is the most common cause of severe *Candida* infections, resistance is most common in other species, particularly *Candida auris*, *Candida glabrata*, and *Candida parapsilosis*.

Resistance to another class of antifungal drugs, echinocandins, is particularly concerning. Echinocandin resistance appears to be increasing, especially in the species *Candida glabrata*. *C. glabrata* already has high levels of resistance to the antifungal fluconazole, and this resistance has remained fairly constant over the past 20 years, according to CDC surveillance data. Echinocandins are the preferred treatment for *C. glabrata*, and echinocandin resistance could severely limit treatment options for patients with candidiasis caused by *C. glabrata*.

Patients with *Candida* infections that are resistant to both fluconazole and echinocandin drugs have very few treatment options. The primary treatment option is amphotericin B, a drug that can be toxic for patients who are already very sick. Growing evidence suggests that patients who have drug-resistant *Candida* bloodstream infections (also known as "candidemia") are less likely to survive than patients who have candidemia that can be treated by antifungal drugs.

Concern is rising over the emerging fungus *Candida auris*, which is rare in most areas of the United States but is a growing threat. Resistance rates for *C. auris* are much higher than for other *Candida* species, with:

- About 90 percent of U.S. *C. auris* samples being resistant to fluconazole, and
- Up to one-third are resistant to the antifungal drug amphotericin B.

Although most *C. auris* samples are being susceptible to echinocandins, resistance to echinocandin drugs can also develop while the patient is being treated with these types of drugs. Moreover, *C. auris* is a concerning public health issue especially because it can be difficult to identify with standard laboratory methods and spreads easily in healthcare settings, such as hospitals and long-term care facilities with patients who have high care needs.

Section 40.3 | *Cryptococcus neoformans*

This section includes text excerpted from "*C. neoformans* Infection," Centers for Disease Control and Prevention (CDC), December 29, 2020.

Cryptococcus neoformans (abbreviated *C. neoformans*) is a fungus that lives in the environment throughout the world. People can become infected with *C. neoformans* after breathing in the microscopic fungus, although most people who are exposed to the fungus never get sick from it.

Infection with the fungus *Cryptococcus* (either *C. neoformans* or *C. gattii*) is called "cryptococcosis." Cryptococcosis usually affects the lungs or the central nervous system (the brain and spinal cord), but it can also affect other parts of the body. Brain infections due to the fungus *Cryptococcus* are called "cryptococcal meningitis."

C. neoformans infections are rare in people who are otherwise healthy. Most cases of *C. neoformans* infection occur in people who have weakened immune systems, particularly those who have advanced HIV/AIDS.

SYMPTOMS OF *C. NEOFORMANS* INFECTION

C. neoformans usually infects the lungs or the central nervous system (the brain and spinal cord), but it can also affect other parts of the body. The symptoms of the infection depend on the parts of the body that are affected.

In the Lungs

A *C. neoformans* infection in the lungs can cause a pneumonia-like illness. The symptoms are often similar to those of many other illnesses, and can include:

- Cough
- Shortness of breath
- Chest pain
- Fever

In the Brain (Cryptococcal Meningitis)

Cryptococcal meningitis is an infection caused by the fungus *Cryptococcus* after it spreads from the lungs to the brain. The symptoms of cryptococcal meningitis include:

- Headache
- Fever
- Neck pain
- Nausea and vomiting
- Sensitivity to light
- Confusion or changes in behavior

If you have symptoms that you think may be due to a *C. neoformans* infection, please contact your healthcare provider.

C. NEOFORMANS INFECTION RISK AND PREVENTION
Who Gets *C. neoformans* Infections

C. neoformans infections are rare among people who are otherwise healthy. Most cases of *C. neoformans* infection occur in people who have weakened immune systems, such as people who:

- Have advanced HIV/AIDS
- Have had an organ transplant or
- Are taking corticosteroids, medications to treat rheumatoid arthritis or other medications that weaken the immune system.

Is *C. neoformans* Infection Contagious?

No. The infection cannot spread between people or between people and animals.

Can Pets Get *C. neoformans* Infections?

Yes. Pets can get *C. neoformans* infections, but it is very rare, and the infection cannot spread between animals and people. If you are concerned about your pet's risk of getting a *C. neoformans* infection, or if you think that your pet has the infection, please talk to a veterinarian.

How Can You Prevent a *C. neoformans* Infection?

It is difficult to avoid breathing in *C. neoformans* because it is thought to be common in the environment. Most people who breathe in *C. neoformans* never get sick from it. However, in people who have weakened immune systems, *C. neoformans* can stay hidden in the body and cause infection later when the immune system becomes too weak to fight it off. This leaves a window of time when the silent infection can be detected and treated early, before symptoms develop.

Detecting Silent Cryptococcal Infections in People Who Have HIV/AIDS

One approach to prevent cryptococcal meningitis is called "targeted screening." Research suggests that *C. neoformans* is able to live in the body undetected, especially when a person's immune system is weaker than normal. In a targeted screening program, a simple blood test is used to detect cryptococcal antigen (an indicator of cryptococcal infection) in HIV-infected patients before they begin taking antiretroviral treatment (ART). A patient who tests positive for cryptococcal antigen can take fluconazole, an antifungal medication, to fight off the silent fungal infection and prevent it from developing into life-threatening meningitis.

What Is CDC Doing about *C. neoformans*?

The Centers for Disease Control and Prevention (CDC) is assisting areas of the world where the prevalence of cryptococcal infections is high, such as sub-Saharan Africa and Southeast Asia, to prevent deaths from cryptococcal infections by helping implement targeted screening programs to detect early cryptococcal disease in HIV-infected persons. Because many of the countries in these areas of the world often do not have the resources needed to detect *Cryptococcus* as the underlying cause of meningitis, the CDC is also helping these countries build their laboratory capacity. Early identification of cryptococcal-infected patients in resource-limited settings may lead to more timely treatment, reduced mortality due to cryptococcal meningitis, and overall improved quality of life.

WHERE *C. NEOFORMANS* INFECTION COMES FROM
Where Does *C. neoformans* Live?

C. neoformans lives in the environment throughout the world. The fungus is typically found in soil, on decaying wood, in tree hollows, or in bird droppings.

How Does Someone Get a *C. neoformans* Infection?

C. neoformans infections are not contagious. Humans and animals can get the infection after inhaling the microscopic fungus from the environment. Some research suggests that people may be exposed to *C. neoformans* in the environment when they are children. Most people who breathe in *C. neoformans* never get sick from it. However, in people who have weakened immune systems, *C. neoformans* can stay hidden in the body and cause infection later when the immune system becomes too weak to fight it off.

DIAGNOSIS AND TESTING FOR *C. NEOFORMANS* INFECTION

Healthcare providers rely on your medical history, symptoms, physical examinations, and laboratory tests to diagnose a *C. neoformans* infection.

Your healthcare provider will take a sample of tissue or body fluid (such as blood, cerebrospinal fluid, or sputum) and send the sample to a laboratory to be examined under a microscope, tested with an antigen test, or cultured. Your healthcare provider may also perform tests such as a chest x-ray or computed tomography (CT) scan of your lungs, brain, or other parts of the body.

TREATMENT OF *C. NEOFORMANS* INFECTION

People who have *C. neoformans* infection need to take prescription antifungal medication for at least 6 months, often longer. The type of treatment usually depends on the severity of the infection and the parts of the body that are affected.

- For people who have asymptomatic infections (e.g., diagnosed via targeted screening) or mild-to-moderate pulmonary infections, the treatment is usually fluconazole.

- For people who have severe lung infections or infections in the central nervous system (brain and spinal cord), the recommended initial treatment is amphotericin B in combination with flucytosine. After that, patients usually need to take fluconazole for an extended time to clear the infection.

The type, dose, and duration of antifungal treatment may differ for certain groups of people, such as pregnant women, children, and people in resource-limited settings. Some people may also need surgery to remove fungal growths (cryptococcomas).

Section 40.4 | Valley Fever (Coccidioidomycosis)

This section includes text excerpted from "Valley Fever (Coccidioidomycosis)," Centers for Disease Control and Prevention (CDC), December 29, 2020.

Valley fever is an infection caused by the fungus *Coccidioides*. The scientific name for Valley fever is "*coccidioidomycosis*," and it is also sometimes called "San Joaquin Valley fever" or "desert rheumatism." The term "Valley fever" usually refers to *Coccidioides* infection in the lungs, but the infection can spread to other parts of the body in severe cases (this is called "disseminated *coccidioidomycosis*").

The fungus is known to live in the soil in the southwestern United States and parts of Mexico and Central and South America. The fungus was also recently found in south-central Washington. People can get Valley fever by breathing in the microscopic fungal spores from the air in these areas.

Most people who breathe in the spores do not get sick, but some people do. Usually, people who get sick with Valley fever will get better on their own within weeks to months, but some people will need antifungal medication. Certain groups of people are at higher risk for developing severe forms of the infection, and these people typically need antifungal treatment. It is difficult to prevent exposure to *Coccidioides* in areas where it is common in the environment, but people who are at higher risk for severe Valley fever should try to avoid breathing in large amounts of dust if they are in these areas.

SYMPTOMS OF VALLEY FEVER (COCCIDIOIDOMYCOSIS)

Many people who are exposed to the fungus *Coccidioides* never have symptoms. Other people may have symptoms that go away on their own after weeks to months. If your symptoms last for more than a week, contact your healthcare provider.

Symptoms of Valley fever include:
- Fatigue (tiredness)
- Cough
- Fever
- Shortness of breath
- Headache
- Night sweats
- Muscle aches or joint pain
- Rash on upper body or legs

In extremely rare cases, the fungal spores can enter the skin through a cut, wound, or splinter and cause a skin infection.

How Soon Do the Symptoms Appear?

Symptoms of Valley fever may appear between 1 and 3 weeks after a person breathes in the fungal spores.

How Long Do the Symptoms Last?

The symptoms of Valley fever usually last for a few weeks to a few months. However, some patients have symptoms that last longer than this, especially if the infection becomes severe.

Severe Valley Fever

Approximately 5 to 10 percent of people who get Valley fever will develop serious or long-term problems in their lungs. an even smaller percent of people (about 1 percent), the infection spreads from the lungs to other parts of the body, such as the central nervous system (brain and spinal cord), skin, or bones and joints.

RISK AND PREVENTION
Who Gets Valley Fever

Anyone who lives in or travels to the southwestern United States (Arizona, California, Nevada, New Mexico, Texas, or Utah), or parts of Mexico or Central or South America can get Valley fever. Valley fever can affect people of any age, but it is most common in adults aged 60 and older. Certain groups of people may be at higher risk for developing the severe forms of Valley fever, such as:

- People who have weakened immune systems, for example, people who:
  - Have HIV/AIDS
  - Have had an organ transplant
  - Are taking medications such as corticosteroids or TNF-inhibitors
- Pregnant women
- People who have diabetes
- People who are Black or Filipino

Is Valley Fever Contagious?

No. The fungus that causes Valley fever, *Coccidioides*, cannot spread from the lungs between people or between people and animals. However, in extremely rare instances, a wound infection with *Coccidioides* can spread Valley fever to someone else, or the infection can be spread through an organ transplant with an infected organ.

Traveling to an Endemic Area
SHOULD YOU WORRY ABOUT VALLEY FEVER IF YOU ARE TRAVELING TO AN AREA WHERE THE FUNGUS IS COMMON?

The risk of getting Valley fever is low when traveling to an area where *Coccidioides* lives in the environment, such as the southwestern

United States, Mexico, or Central or South America. Your risk for infection could increase if you will be in a very dusty setting, but even then the risk is still low. If you have questions about your risk of getting Valley fever while traveling, talk to your healthcare provider.

Could You Get It Again If You Have Had It Before?

Usually not. If you have already had Valley fever, your immune system will most likely protect you from getting it again. Some people can have the infection come back again (a relapse) after getting better the first time, but this is very rare.

Can Pets Get Valley Fever?

Yes. Pets, particularly dogs, can get valley fever, but it is not contagious between animals and people. Valley fever in dogs is similar to valley fever in humans. Like humans, many dogs that are exposed to *Coccidioides* never get sick. Dogs that do develop symptoms often have symptoms that include coughing, lack of energy, and weight loss. If you are concerned about your pet's risk of getting Valley fever or if you think that your pet has Valley fever, please talk to a veterinarian.

Coccidioides at Your Workplace
WHAT SHOULD YOU DO IF YOU THINK YOU HAVE BEEN EXPOSED TO *COCCIDIOIDES* AT YOUR WORKPLACE OR IN A LABORATORY?

If you think you have been exposed to *Coccidioides* at work or in a laboratory, you should contact your Occupational Health, Infection Control, Risk Management, or Safety/Security Department. If your workplace or laboratory does not have these services, you should contact your local city, county, or state health department. There is no evidence showing that antifungal medication (i.e., prophylaxis) prevents people from getting sick with Valley fever after a workplace exposure to *Coccidioides*. If you develop symptoms of Valley fever, contact your healthcare provider.

How Can You Prevent Valley Fever?

It is very difficult to avoid breathing in the fungus *Coccidioides* in areas where it is common in the environment. People who live in these areas can try to avoid spending time in dusty places as much as possible. People who are at risk for severe Valley fever (such as people who have weakened immune systems, pregnant women, people who have diabetes, or people who are Black or Filipino) may be able to lower their chances of developing the infection by trying to avoid breathing in the fungal spores.

The following are some common-sense methods that may be helpful to avoid getting Valley fever. It is important to know that although these steps are recommended, they have not been proven to prevent Valley fever.

- Try to avoid areas with a lot of dust such as construction or excavation sites. If you cannot avoid these areas, wear an N95 respirator (a type of face mask) while you are there.
- Stay inside during dust storms and close your windows.
- Avoid activities that involve close contact to dirt or dust, including yard work, gardening, and digging.
- Use air filtration measures indoors.
- Clean skin injuries well with soap and water to reduce the chances of developing a skin infection, especially if the wound was exposed to dirt or dust.
- Take preventive antifungal medication if your healthcare provider says you need it.

Is There a Vaccine for Valley Fever?

No. Currently, there is no vaccine to prevent Valley fever.

WHERE VALLEY FEVER (COCCIDIOIDOMYCOSIS) COMES FROM
Where Does *Coccidioides* Live?

Coccidioides live in dust and soil in some areas in the southwestern United States, Mexico, and South America. In the United States, *Coccidioides* lives in Arizona, California, Nevada, New Mexico, Texas, and Utah. The fungus was also found in south-central Washington.

Life Cycle of *Coccidioides*

Coccidioides spores circulate in the air after contaminated soil and dust are disturbed by humans, animals, or the weather. The spores are too small to see without a microscope. When people breathe in the spores, they are at risk for developing Valley fever. After the spores enter the lungs, the person's body temperature allows the spores to change shape and grow into spherules. When the spherules get large enough, they break open and release smaller pieces (called "endospores") which can then potentially spread within the lungs or to other organs and grow into new spherules.

Uncommon Sources of Valley Fever

The most common way for someone to get Valley fever is by inhaling *Coccidioides* spores that are in the air. In extremely rare cases, people can get the infection from other sources, such as:

- From an organ transplant if the organ donor had Valley fever
- From inhaling spores from a wound infected with *Coccidioides*
- From contact with objects (such as rocks or shoes) that have been contaminated with *Coccidioides*

Testing Soil

ARE YOU WORRIED THAT COCCIDIOIDES IS IN THE SOIL NEAR YOUR HOME AND LOOKING FOR SOMEONE TEST THE SOIL TO FIND OUT IF THE FUNGUS IS THERE?

In this situation, testing soil for *Coccidioides* is not likely to be useful because the fungus is thought to be common in the soil in certain areas. A soil sample that tests positive for *Coccidioides* does not necessarily mean that the soil will release the fungus into the air and cause infection. Also, there are no commercially-available tests to detect *Coccidioides* in soil. Testing soil for *Coccidioides* is currently only done for scientific research.

TESTING SOIL FOR RESEARCH

Scientists sometimes test soil or other environmental samples for *Coccidioides* to understand more about its habitat and how weather or climate patterns may affect its growth. The available methods to detect *Coccidioides* in the soil do not always detect *Coccidioides* spores even if they are present. However, new tests are being developed so that researchers can better detect *Coccidioides* in the environment.

Valley Fever and the Weather

Scientists continue to study how weather and climate patterns affect the habitat of the fungus that causes Valley fever. *Coccidioides* is thought to grow best in soil after heavy rainfall and then disperse into the air most effectively during hot, dry conditions. For example, hot and dry weather conditions have been shown to correlate with an increase in the number of Valley fever cases in Arizona and in California (but to a lesser extent). The ways in which climate change may be affecting the number of Valley fever infections, as well as the geographic range of *Coccidioides*, is not known yet, but is a subject for further research.

Geographic Range of Valley Fever Expands to Washington State

Scientists believed that *Coccidioides* only lived in the Southwestern United States and parts of Latin America until discovering it in south-central Washington in 2013 after several residents developed Valley fever without recent travel to areas where the fungus is known to live. Samples from one patient and soil from the suspected exposure site were analyzed using a laboratory technique called "whole genome sequencing" and were found to be identical, proving that the infection was acquired in Washington.

After this discovery, many unanswered questions remain: How widespread is *Coccidioides* in Washington? How did it get there? How long has it been living there? Information about where a person was most likely infected with Valley fever, how strains are related, and which areas could pose a risk is essential for raising awareness about the disease among public health officials, healthcare providers, and the public. The CDC is working with state and local public health officials and other agencies to better understand where the fungus lives so that healthcare providers and the public can be aware of the risk for Valley fever.

DIAGNOSIS AND TESTING FOR VALLEY FEVER (COCCIDIOIDOMYCOSIS)

How Is Valley Fever Diagnosed?

Healthcare providers rely on your medical and travel history, symptoms, physical examinations, and laboratory tests to diagnose Valley fever. The most common way that healthcare providers test for Valley fever is by taking a blood sample and sending it to a laboratory to look for *Coccidioides* antibodies or antigens.

Healthcare providers may do imaging tests such as chest x-rays or CT scans of your lungs to look for Valley fever pneumonia. They may also perform a tissue biopsy, in which a small sample of tissue is taken from the body and examined under a microscope. Laboratories may also see if *Coccidioides* will grow from body fluids or tissues (this is called a "culture").

Where Can You Get Tested for Valley Fever?

Any healthcare provider can order a test for Valley fever.

How Long Will It Take to Get the Test Results?

It depends on the type of test. Results from a blood test will usually be available in a few days. If your healthcare provider sends a sample to a laboratory to be cultured, the results could take a few days to a couple of weeks.

Skin Testing

A skin test can detect whether you have developed an immune response to the fungus *Coccidioides*, the cause of Valley fever. This test became available again in the United States in 2014 for the first time since the late 1990s. Your healthcare provider might do this test if you have a history of Valley fever.

The test involves getting a small injection on the inside of your forearm, similar to a skin test for tuberculosis. If the test is positive, a bump will appear at the injection site. A healthcare provider must examine the injection site two days (48 hours) after the test was given to measure the size of the bump.

A positive test result means that you have an immune response to *Coccidioides* because of a past or current *Coccidioides* infection. Some people with a positive test result have been sick with Valley fever, but many people with a positive test have not had symptoms from the infection. A positive skin test generally means that you are immune to *Coccidioides* and will not get Valley fever in the future.

A negative skin test can mean that you have not been exposed to *Coccidioides* and have not had Valley fever. However, some people may not react to the skin test even though they have had a *Coccidioides* infection. This is called a "false-negative result." False-negative results occur more commonly in people who:

- Have had a *Coccidioides* infection that is recent or severe
- Have a condition or illness that interferes with the skin test results
- Are taking a medication that interferes with the skin test results

TREATMENT FOR VALLEY FEVER (COCCIDIOIDOMYCOSIS)
How Is Valley Fever Treated?

For many people, the symptoms of Valley fever will go away within a few months without any treatment. Healthcare providers choose to prescribe antifungal medication for some people to try to reduce the severity of symptoms or prevent the infection from getting worse. Antifungal medication is typically given to people who are at higher risk for developing severe Valley fever. The treatment is usually 3 to 6 months of fluconazole or another type of antifungal medication. There are no over-the-counter medications to treat Valley fever. If you have Valley fever, you should talk to your healthcare provider about whether you need treatment. The healthcare provider who diagnoses you with Valley fever may suggest that you see other healthcare providers who specialize in treating Valley fever.

People who have severe lung infections or infections that have spread to other parts of the body always need antifungal treatment and may need to stay in the hospital. For these types of infections, the course of treatment is usually longer than 6 months. Valley fever that develops into meningitis is fatal if it is not treated, so lifelong antifungal treatment is necessary for those cases.

Does Valley Fever Have Any Long-Term Effects?

Most people who have Valley fever will make a full recovery. A small percentage of people develop long-term lung infections that can take several years to get better. In very severe cases of Valley fever, the nervous system can be affected and there may be long-term damage, but this is very rare.

Section 40.5 | Histoplasmosis

This section includes text excerpted from "Histoplasmosis," Centers for Disease Control and Prevention (CDC), December 29, 2020.

Histoplasmosis is an infection caused by the fungus *Histoplasma*. The fungus lives in the environment, particularly in soil that contains large amounts of bird or bat droppings. In the United States, *Histoplasma* mainly lives in soil in the central and eastern states, especially areas around the Ohio and Mississippi River valleys. The fungus also lives in parts of Central and South America, Africa, Asia, and Australia.

People can get histoplasmosis after breathing in the microscopic fungal spores from the air, often after participating in activities that disturb the soil. Although most people who breathe in the spores do not get sick, those who do may have a fever, cough, and fatigue. Many people who get sick will get better on their own without medication. In some people, such as those who have weakened immune systems, the infection can become severe, especially if it spreads from the lungs to other organs.

SYMPTOMS OF HISTOPLASMOSIS

Most people who are exposed to the fungus Histoplasma never have symptoms. Other people may have symptoms that go away on their own.

Symptoms of histoplasmosis include:

- Fever
- Cough
- Fatigue (extreme tiredness)
- Chills
- Headache
- Chest pain
- Body aches

How Soon Do the Symptoms of Histoplasmosis Appear?

Symptoms of histoplasmosis may appear between 3 and 17 days after a person breathes in the fungal spores.

How Long Do the Symptoms of Histoplasmosis Last?

For most people, the symptoms of histoplasmosis will go away within a few weeks to a month. However, some people have symptoms that last longer than this, especially if the infection becomes severe.

Severe Histoplasmosis

In some people, usually, those who have weakened immune systems, histoplasmosis can develop into a long-term lung infection, or it can spread from the lungs to other parts of the body, such as the central nervous system (the brain and spinal cord).

HISTOPLASMOSIS RISK AND PREVENTION
Who Gets Histoplasmosis

Anyone can get histoplasmosis if they have been in an area where Histoplasma lives in the environment. Histoplasmosis is often associated with activities that disturb the soil, particularly soil that contains bird or bat droppings. Certain groups of people are at higher risk for developing the severe forms of histoplasmosis:

People who have weakened immune systems, for example, people who:

- Have HIV/AIDS
- Have had an organ transplant
- Are taking medications such as corticosteroids or TNF-inhibitors
- Infants
- Adults aged 55 and older

Is Histoplasmosis Contagious?

No. Histoplasmosis cannot spread from the lungs between people or between people and animals. However, in extremely rare cases, the infection can be passed through an organ transplant with an infected organ.

If You Have Already Had Histoplasmosis, Could You Get It Again?

It is possible for someone who has already had histoplasmosis to get it again, but the body's immune system usually provides some partial protection so that the infection is less severe the second time. In people who have weakened immune systems, histoplasmosis can remain hidden in the body for months or years and then cause symptoms later (also called a "relapse of infection").

Can Your Pets Get Histoplasmosis?

Yes. Pets, particularly cats, can get histoplasmosis, but it is not contagious between animals and people. Histoplasmosis in cats and dogs is similar to histoplasmosis in humans. Like humans, many cats and dogs that are exposed to Histoplasma never get sick. Cats and dogs that do develop symptoms often have symptoms that include coughing, lack of energy, and weight loss. The fungus that causes histoplasmosis grows well in soil that contains bird droppings, but birds do not appear to be able to get histoplasmosis. If you are concerned about your pet's risk of getting histoplasmosis or if you think that your pet has histoplasmosis, please talk to a veterinarian.

How Can You Prevent Histoplasmosis?

It can be difficult to avoid breathing in Histoplasma in areas where it is common in the environment. In areas where Histoplasma is known to live, people who have weakened immune systems (e.g., by HIV/AIDS, an organ transplant, or medications such as corticosteroids or TNF-inhibitors) should avoid doing activities that are known to be associated with getting histoplasmosis, including:

- Disturbing material (e.g., digging in soil or chopping wood) where there are bird or bat droppings
- Cleaning chicken coops
- Exploring caves
- Cleaning, remodeling, or tearing down old buildings

Large amounts of bird or bat droppings should be cleaned up by professional companies that specialize in the removal of hazardous waste. Before starting a job or activity where there is a possibility of being exposed to Histoplasma, consult the document Occupational Histoplasmosis: Epidemiology and Prevention Measures.

What Are Public Health Agencies Doing about Histoplasmosis?

- **Surveillance.** In some states, healthcare providers and laboratories are required to report histoplasmosis cases to public health authorities. Disease reporting helps government officials and healthcare providers understand how and why outbreaks occur and allows them to monitor trends in the number of histoplasmosis cases.
- **Developing better diagnostic tools**. The symptoms of histoplasmosis can be similar to those of other respiratory diseases. Faster, more reliable methods to diagnosis histoplasmosis are in development, which could help minimize delays in treatment, save money and resources looking for other diagnoses, and reduce unnecessary treatment for other suspected illnesses.
- **Building laboratory capacity**. Equipping laboratories in Latin America to be able to diagnose histoplasmosis and

perform laboratory-based surveillance will help reduce the burden of HIV-associated histoplasmosis in these areas.

WHERE HISTOPLASMOSIS COMES FROM
Where Does Histoplasma Live?

Histoplasma, the fungus that causes histoplasmosis, lives throughout the world, but it is most common in North America and Central America. In the United States, Histoplasma mainly lives in soil in the central and eastern states, particularly areas around the Ohio and Mississippi River Valleys, but it can likely live in other parts of the country as well. The fungus also lives in parts of Central and South America, Africa, Asia, and Australia. Figure 40.1 shows estimated areas with histoplasmosis and the biology of histoplasmosis.

The Life Cycle of Histoplasma

Histoplasma spores circulate in the air after contaminated soil is disturbed. The spores are too small to see without a microscope. When people breathe in the spores, they are at risk for developing histoplasmosis. After the spores enter the lungs, the person's body temperature allows the spores to transform into yeast. The yeast can then travel to lymph nodes and can spread to other parts of the body through the bloodstream.

DIAGNOSIS AND TESTING FOR HISTOPLASMOSIS
How Is Histoplasmosis Diagnosed?

Healthcare providers rely on your medical and travel history, symptoms, physical examinations, and laboratory tests to diagnose histoplasmosis. The most common way that healthcare providers test for histoplasmosis is by taking a blood sample or a urine sample and sending it to a laboratory.

Healthcare providers may do imaging tests such as chest x-rays or CT scans of your lungs. They may also collect a sample of fluid from your respiratory tract or perform a tissue biopsy, in which a small sample of affected tissue is taken from the body and examined

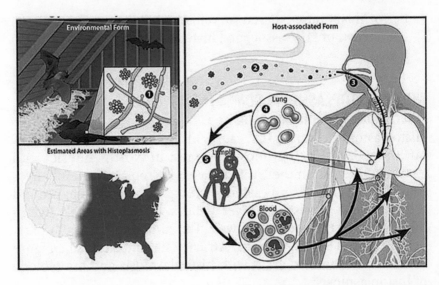

Figure 40.1. Biology of Histoplasmosis

Note: In the environment, Histoplasma capsulatum exists as a mold (1) with aerial hyphae. The hyphae produce macroconidia and microconidia (2) spores that are aerosolized and dispersed. Microconidia are inhaled into the lungs by a susceptible host (3). The warmer temperature inside the host signals a transformation to an oval, budding yeast (4). The yeast are phagocytized by immune cells and transported to regional lymph nodes (5). From there they travel in the blood to other parts of the body (6).

under a microscope. Laboratories may also see if Histoplasma will grow from body fluids or tissues (this is called a "culture").

Where Can You Get Tested for Histoplasmosis?

Most healthcare providers can order a test for histoplasmosis.

How Long Will It Take to Get Your Test Results?

It depends on the type of test. Results from a blood test or a urine test will usually be available in a few days. If your healthcare provider sends a sample to a laboratory to be cultured, the results could take a couple of weeks.

TREATMENT OF HISTOPLASMOSIS
How Is Histoplasmosis Treated?

For some people, the symptoms of histoplasmosis will go away without treatment. However, prescription antifungal medication is needed to treat severe histoplasmosis in the lungs, chronic histoplasmosis, and infections that have spread from the lungs to other parts of the body (disseminated histoplasmosis). Itraconazole is one type of antifungal medication that is commonly used to treat histoplasmosis. Depending on the severity of the infection and the person's immune status, the course of treatment can range from 3 months to 1 year.

Section 40.6 | *Pneumocystis* Pneumonia

This section includes text excerpted from "*Pneumocystis* Pneumonia," Centers for Disease Control and Prevention (CDC), October 13, 2021.

Pneumocystis pneumonia (PCP) is a serious infection caused by the fungus *Pneumocystis* jirovecii.

Most people who get PCP have a medical condition that weakens their immune system, such as human immunodeficiency virus (HIV)/acquired immunodeficiency syndrome (AIDS) or take medicines (such as corticosteroids) that lower the body's ability to fight germs and sickness. In the United States, people with HIV/AIDS are less likely to get PCP today than before the availability of antiretroviral therapy (ART). However, PCP is still a substantial public health problem. Much of the information we have about PCP and its treatment comes from caring for patients with HIV/AIDS.

Scientists have changed both the classification and the name of this organism since it first appeared in patients with HIV in the 1980s. *Pneumocystis* jirovecii used to be classified as a protozoan, but is now considered a fungus. *Pneumocystis* jirovecii used to be called "*Pneumocystis* carinii." When scientists renamed P. carinii to P. jirovecii, some people considered using the abbreviation "PJP," but to avoid confusion, *Pneumocystis* jirovecii pneumonia is still abbreviated "PCP."

SYMPTOMS OF *PNEUMOCYSTIS* PNEUMONIA

The symptoms of PCP can develop over several days or weeks and include:

- Fever
- Cough
- Difficulty breathing
- Chest pain
- Chills
- Fatigue (tiredness)

Contact your healthcare provider if you have symptoms that you think are related to PCP.

RISK OF *PNEUMOCYSTIS* PNEUMONIA

Pneumocystis pneumonia (PCP) is extremely rare in healthy people, but the fungus that causes this disease can live in their lungs without causing symptoms. In fact, up to 20 percent of adults might carry this fungus at any given time, and the immune system removes the fungus after several months.

Most people who get PCP have weakened immune systems, meaning that their bodies do not fight infections well. About 30–40 percent of people who get PCP have HIV/AIDS. The other people who get PCP are usually taking medicine (such as corticosteroids) that lowers the body's ability to fight germs or sickness or have other medical conditions, such as:

- Chronic lung diseases
- Cancer
- Inflammatory diseases or autoimmune diseases (e.g., lupus or rheumatoid arthritis)
- Solid-organ or stem cell transplant

PREVENTION OF *PNEUMOCYSTIS* PNEUMONIA

There is no vaccine to prevent PCP. A healthcare provider might prescribe medicine to prevent PCP for people who are more likely to develop the disease. The medicine most commonly used to prevent PCP is called "trimethoprim/sulfamethoxazole" (TMP/

SMX), which is also known as "co-trimoxazole" and by several different brand names, including Bactrim, Septra, and Cotrim. Other medicines are available for people who cannot take TMP/SMX.

Medicine to prevent PCP is recommended for some people infected with HIV, stem cell transplant patients, and some solid organ transplant patients. Healthcare providers might also prescribe medicine to prevent PCP in other patients, such as people who are taking long-term, high-dose corticosteroids.

HOW *PNEUMOCYSTIS* PNEUMONIA SPREADS

PCP spreads from person to person through the air. Some healthy adults can carry the *Pneumocystis* fungus in their lungs without having symptoms, and it can spread to other people, including those with weakened immune systems.

Many people are exposed to *Pneumocystis* as children, but they likely do not get sick because their immune systems prevent the fungus from causing an infection. 18 In the past, scientists believed that people who had been exposed to *Pneumocystis* as children could later develop PCP from that childhood infection if their immune systems become weakened. However, it is more likely that people get PCP after being exposed to someone else who has PCP or who is carrying the fungus in their lungs without having symptoms.

DIAGNOSIS AND TESTING OF *PNEUMOCYSTIS* PNEUMONIA

PCP is diagnosed using a sample from a patient's lungs. The sample is usually mucus that is either coughed up by the patient (called "sputum") or collected by a procedure called "bronchoalveolar lavage." Sometimes, a small sample of lung tissue (a biopsy) is used to diagnose PCP. The patient's sample is sent to a laboratory, usually to be examined under a microscope. Polymerase chain reaction (PCR) can also be used to detect *Pneumocystis* DNA in different types of samples. A blood test to detect β-D-glucan (a part of the cell wall of many different types of fungi) can also help diagnose PCP.

TREATMENT AND OUTCOMES OF *PNEUMOCYSTIS* PNEUMONIA

PCP must be treated with prescription medicine. Without treatment, PCP can cause death. The most common form of treatment is trimethoprim/sulfamethoxazole (TMP/SMX), which is also known as "co-trimoxazole" and by several different brand names, including Bactrim, Septra, and Cotrim. This medicine is given by mouth or through a vein for 3 weeks.

TMP/SMX can cause side effects such as rash and fever. Other medicines are available for patients who cannot take TMP/SMX.

STATISTICS

The exact number of cases of PCP in the United States is difficult to determine because there is no national surveillance for the disease.

Before the beginning of the HIV/AIDS epidemic in the 1980s, PCP was uncommon. In fact, clusters of PCP were one of the first signs that the HIV/AIDS epidemic was beginning in the United States. PCP soon became one of the main AIDS-defining illnesses in the United States. In the late 1980s, an estimated 75 percent of people living with AIDS developed PCP. Since then, PCP in people living with HIV/AIDS has decreased substantially due to antiretroviral therapy (ART) and preventive treatment with TMP/SMX.

Now, PCP is still a serious health concern for people living with HIV/AIDS or other conditions that weaken the immune system. In a study of HIV-infected patients in the United States and Canada, PCP was the most common opportunistic infection during 2008–2010. There were 10,590 estimated U.S. hospitalizations due to *Pneumocystis* pneumonia in 2017.

PCP is also a common opportunistic infection among people living with HIV/AIDS in developing countries.

Chapter 41 | **HIV/AIDS and Co-occurring Parasitic Infections**

Section 41.1 | **Cryptosporidiosis**

This section includes text excerpted from "Cryptosporidiosis," Centers for Disease Control and Prevention (CDC), May 20, 2019.

CAUSAL AGENTS

Many species and genotypes of the apicomplexan protozoan *Cryptosporidium* can infect humans and have a wide range of host animals. Zoonotic species and genotypes of *Cryptosporidium* are those transmitted from animal hosts to humans, and non zoonotic species and genotypes are host-adapted without evidence of transmission from animals to humans. *Cryptosporidium parvum* (formerly known as "*C. parvum* genotype II") and *C. hominis* (formerly known as "*C. parvum* genotype I") are the leading causes of human cryptosporidiosis. *C. meleagridis, C. felis, C. canis, C. ubiquitum, C. cuniculus, C. viatorum*, Chipmunk genotype I, *Cryptosporidium* mink genotype, and *C. muris* can also infect humans.

LIFE CYCLE

Sporulated oocysts, containing four sporozoites, are excreted by the infected host through feces (1) (and possibly other routes such as respiratory secretions). Transmission of *Cryptosporidium* spp. occurs mainly through ingestion of fecally contaminated water (e.g., drinking or recreational water) or food (e.g., raw milk) or following direct contact with infected animals or people (2). Following ingestion (and possibly inhalation) by a suitable host, excystation (a) occurs. The sporozoites are released and parasitize the epithelial cells (b,c) of the gastrointestinal tract (and possibly the respiratory tract). In these cells, usually within the brush border, the parasites undergo asexual multiplication (schizogony or merogony) (d,e,f) and then sexual multiplication (gametogony) producing microgamonts (male) (g) and macrogamonts (female) (h). Upon fertilization of the macrogamonts by the microgametes (i) that rupture from the microgamont, oocysts develop and sporulate in the infected host. Zygotes give rise to two different types

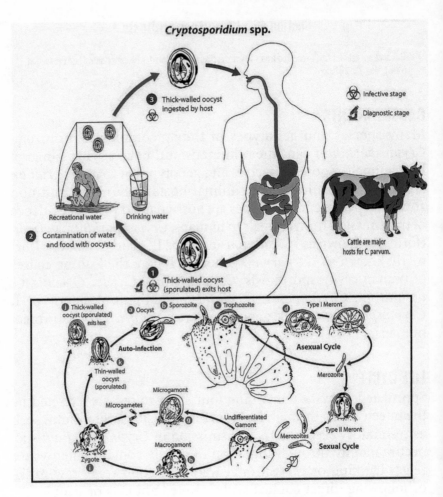

Figure 41.1. Cryptosporidium Life Cycle

of oocysts (thick-walled and thin-walled). Thick-walled oocysts are excreted from the host into the environment (j), whereas thin-walled oocysts are involved in the internal autoinfective cycle and are not recovered from stools (k). Oocysts are infectious upon excretion, thus enabling direct and immediate fecal-oral transmission. Extracellular stages have been reported, but their relevance in the overall life cycle is unclear.

HOSTS

Cryptosporidium can infect a wide range of vertebrate hosts, including birds, reptiles, and mammals. Many species and genotypes are host-adapted, but human cases caused by species and genotypes that are pathogens in other mammals or animals have been reported (e.g., *C. meleagridis*). predominantly infects humans and is generally considered anthroponotic, though sporadic reports in animal hosts exist. Zoonotic subtype families of *C. parvum* implicated in human infections are commonly associated with cattle, particularly calves. Figure 41.1 shows cryptosporidium lifecycle.

GEOGRAPHIC RANGE

Zoonotic and nonzoonotic *Cryptosporidium* spp. and genotypes are ubiquitous worldwide. Outbreaks of cryptosporidiosis have been and continue to be reported in several countries. Cryptosporidiosis outbreaks in the United States have been linked to swimming pools, water playgrounds, and other swimming venues; unpasteurized cider, juice, and milk; contact with animals; childcare settings; camps; and ill food handlers

CLINICAL PRESENTATION

Infection with *Cryptosporidium* spp. and genotypes results in a wide range of signs and symptoms. The incubation period is an average of 7 days (range: 2–10 days). Immunocompetent patients may present with a diarrheal illness that is self-limiting, typically resolving within 2–3 weeks. Immunocompromised patients may have more severe complications, such as life-threatening malabsorption and wasting. Diarrheal illness may be accompanied by fever or fatigue). While the small intestine is primarily affected, extraintestinal cryptosporidiosis (e.g., in the pulmonary or biliary tract, rarely in the pancreas) has been reported.

Section 41.2 | **Toxoplasmosis**

This section includes text excerpted from "Parasites - Toxoplasmosis (Toxoplasma Infection)," Centers for Disease Control and Prevention (CDC), August 29, 2018. Reviewed February 2022.

ABOUT TOXOPLASMOSIS

Toxoplasmosis is considered to be a leading cause of death attributed to foodborne illness in the United States. More than 40 million men, women, and children in the United States carry the *Toxoplasma* parasite, but very few have symptoms because the immune system usually keeps the parasite from causing illness. However, women newly infected with *Toxoplasma* during or shortly before pregnancy and anyone with a compromised immune system should be aware that toxoplasmosis can have severe consequences. Toxoplasmosis is considered one of the neglected parasitic infections of the United States, a group of five parasitic diseases that have been targeted by the Centers for Disease Control and Prevention (CDC) for public health action.

EPIDEMIOLOGY AND RISK FACTORS OF TOXOPLASMOSIS

Toxoplasmosis is caused by the protozoan parasite *Toxoplasma gondii*. In the United States it is estimated that 11 percent of the population 6 years and older have been infected with *Toxoplasma*. In various places throughout the world, it has been shown that more than 60 percent of some populations have been infected with *Toxoplasma*. Infection is often highest in areas of the world that have hot, humid climates and lower altitudes, because the oocysts survive better in these types of environments. Toxoplasmosis is not passed from person-to-person, except in instances of mother-to-child (congenital) transmission and blood transfusion or organ transplantation. People typically become infected by three principal routes of transmission.

Foodborne Transmission

The tissue form of the parasite (a microscopic cyst consisting of bradyzoites) can be transmitted to humans by food.

People become infected by:

- Eating undercooked, contaminated meat (especially pork, lamb, and venison) or shellfish (like oysters, clams, and mussels)
- Accidentally ingesting undercooked, contaminated meat or shellfish after handling it and not washing hands thoroughly (*Toxoplasma* cannot be absorbed through intact skin)
- Eating food that was contaminated by knives, utensils, cutting boards or other foods that had contact with raw, contaminated meat or shellfish.
- Drinking unpasteurized goat's milk (tachyzoites).

Animal-to-Human (Zoonotic) Transmission

Cats play an important role in the spread of toxoplasmosis. They become infected by eating infected rodents, birds, or other small animals. The parasite is then passed in the cat's feces in an oocyst form, which is microscopic. Kittens and cats can shed millions of oocysts in their feces for as long as 3 weeks after infection. Mature cats are less likely to shed *Toxoplasma* if they have been previously infected. A *Toxoplasma*-infected cat that is shedding the parasite in its feces contaminates the litter box. If the cat is allowed outside, it can contaminate the soil or water in the environment as well. People can be infected by:

- Accidental ingestion of oocysts after cleaning a cat's litter box when the cat has shed *Toxoplasma* in its feces
- Accidental ingestion of oocysts after touching or ingesting anything that has come into contact with a cat's feces that contain *Toxoplasma*
- Accidental ingestion of oocysts in contaminated soil (e.g., not washing hands after gardening or eating unwashed fruits or vegetables from a garden)
- Drinking water contaminated with the *Toxoplasma* parasite

Mother-to-Child (Congenital) Transmission

A woman who is newly infected with *Toxoplasma* during or just before pregnancy can pass the infection to her unborn child (congenital infection). The woman may not have symptoms, but there can be severe consequences for the unborn child, such as diseases of the nervous system and eyes.

Rare Instances of Transmission

Organ transplant recipients can become infected by receiving an organ from a *Toxoplasma*-positive donor. Rarely, people can also become infected by receiving infected blood via transfusion. Laboratory workers who handle infected blood can also acquire infection through accidental inoculation.

SIGNS AND SYMPTOMS OF TOXOPLASMOSIS
Healthy People (Nonpregnant)

Healthy people who become infected with *Toxoplasma gondii* often do not have symptoms because their immune system usually keeps the parasite from causing illness. When illness occurs, it is usually mild with "flu-like" symptoms (e.g., tender lymph nodes, muscle aches, etc.,) that last for weeks to months and then go away. However, the parasite remains in the person's body in an inactive state. It can become reactivated if the person becomes immunosuppressed.

Mother-to-Child (Congenital)

Generally, if a woman has been infected before becoming pregnant, the unborn child will be protected because the mother has developed immunity. If a woman becomes newly infected with *Toxoplasma* during or just before pregnancy, she can pass the infection to her unborn baby (congenital transmission). The damage to the unborn child is often more severe the earlier in pregnancy the transmission occurs. Potential results can be:

- A miscarriage
- A stillborn child

- A child born with signs of congenital toxoplasmosis (e.g., abnormal enlargement or smallness of the head)

Infants infected before birth often show no symptoms at birth but may develop them later in life with potential vision loss, mental disability, and seizures.

Persons with Ocular Disease

Eye disease (most frequently retinochoroiditis) from *Toxoplasma* infection can result from congenital infection or infection after birth by any of the modes of transmission. Eye lesions from congenital infection are often not identified at birth but occur in 20–80 percent of congenitally-infected persons by adulthood. However, in the United States <2 percent of persons infected after birth develop eye lesions. Eye infection leads to an acute inflammatory lesion of the retina, which resolves leaving retinochoroidal scarring. Symptoms of ocular disease include:

- Eye pain
- Sensitivity to light (photophobia)
- Tearing of the eyes
- Blurred vision

The eye disease can reactivate months or years later, each time causing more damage to the retina. If the central structures of the retina are involved there will be a progressive loss of vision that can lead to blindness.

Persons with Compromised Immune Systems

Persons with compromised immune systems may experience severe symptoms if they are infected with *Toxoplasma* while immune suppressed. Persons who acquire human immunodeficiency virus (HIV) infection and were not infected previously with *Toxoplasma* are more likely to develop a severe primary infection. Immunocompromised persons who were infected with *Toxoplasma* at some point before they become immunosuppressed are at risk for developing a relapse (reactivation) of toxoplasmosis. For example, a person who is HIV-infected and who has reactivated *Toxoplasma* infection can have symptoms that include fever, confusion, headache, seizures, nausea, and poor coordination.

Toxoplasma infection can reactivate in immunocompromised pregnant women who were infected with *Toxoplasma* before their pregnancy, and this can lead to congenital infection.

DIAGNOSIS OF TOXOPLASMOSIS

The diagnosis of *toxoplasmosis* is typically made by serologic testing. A test that measures immunoglobulin G (IgG) is used to determine if a person has been infected. If it is necessary to try to estimate the time of infection, which is of particular importance for pregnant women, a test that measures immunoglobulin M (IgM) is also used along with other tests such as an avidity test.

Diagnosis can also be made by direct observation of the parasite in stained tissue sections, cerebrospinal fluid (CSF), or other biopsy material. These techniques are used less frequently because of the difficulty of obtaining these specimens.

Parasites can also be isolated from blood or other body fluids (e.g., CSF), but this process can be difficult and requires considerable time. Molecular techniques that can detect the parasite's deoxyribonucleic acid (DNA) in the amniotic fluid can be useful in cases of possible mother-to-child (congenital) transmission.

Ocular disease is diagnosed based on the appearance of the lesions in the eye, symptoms, course of disease, and often serologic testing.

TREATMENT OF TAXOPLASMOSIS
Healthy People (Nonpregnant)

Most healthy people recover from toxoplasmosis without treatment. Persons who are ill can be treated with a combination of drugs such as pyrimethamine and sulfadiazine, plus folinic acid.

Pregnant Women, Newborns, and Infants

Pregnant women, newborns, and infants can be treated, although the parasite is not eliminated completely. The parasites can remain within tissue cells in a less active phase; their location makes it difficult for the medication to completely eliminate them.

Persons with Ocular Disease

Persons with ocular toxoplasmosis are sometimes prescribed medicine to treat active disease by their ophthalmologist. Whether or not medication is recommended depends on the size of the eye lesion, the location, and the characteristics of the lesion (acute active, versus chronic not progressing).

Persons with Compromised Immune Systems

Persons with compromised immune systems need to be treated until they have improvement in their condition. For acquired immunodeficiency syndrome (AIDS) patients, it may be necessary to continue medication for the rest of their lives, or for as long as they are immunosuppressed.

PREVENTION AND CONTROL

People who are healthy should follow some steps to reduce risk of toxoplasmosis.

Reduce Risk from Food

To prevent the risk of toxoplasmosis and other infections from food:

- Cook food to safe temperatures. A food thermometer should be used to measure the internal temperature of cooked meat. Color is not a reliable indicator that meat has been cooked to a temperature high enough to kill harmful pathogens such as *Toxoplasma*. Do not sample meat until it is cooked. The U.S. Department of Agriculture (USDA) recommends the following for meat preparation:
  - **For Whole Cuts of Meat (Excluding Poultry).** Cook to at least 145 °F (63 °C) as measured with a food thermometer placed in the thickest part of the

meat, then allow the meat to rest for three minutes before carving or consuming. According to USDA, "A 'rest time' is the amount of time the product remains at the final temperature, after it has been removed from a grill, oven, or other heat source. During the three minutes after meat is removed from the heat source, its temperature remains constant or continues to rise, which destroys pathogens."

- **For Ground Meat (Excluding Poultry).** Cook to at least 160 °F (71 °C); ground meats do not require a rest time.
- **For All Poultry (Whole Cuts and Ground).** Cook to at least 165 °F (74 °C). The internal temperature should be checked in the innermost part of the thigh, innermost part of the wing, and the thickest part of the breast. Poultry do not require a rest time.
- Freeze meat for several days at sub-zero (0 °F) temperatures before cooking to greatly reduce chance of infection. Freezing does not reliably kill other parasites that may be found in meat (like certain species of Trichinella) or harmful bacteria. Cooking meat to USDA recommended internal temperatures is the safest method to destroy all parasites and other pathogens.
- Peel or wash fruits and vegetables thoroughly before eating.
- Wash cutting boards, dishes, counters, utensils, and hands with soapy water after contact with raw meat, poultry, seafood, or unwashed fruits or vegetables.
- Do not drink unpasteurized goat's milk.
- Do not eat raw or undercooked oysters, mussels, or clams (these may be contaminated with *Toxoplasma* that has washed into seawater).

The U.S. Government and the meat industry continue their efforts to reduce *T. gondii* in meat.

Reduce Risk from the Environment

- Avoid drinking untreated water.
- Wear gloves when gardening and during any contact with soil or sand because it might be contaminated with cat feces that contain *Toxoplasma*.
- Wash hands with soap and water after gardening or contact with soil or sand.
- Teach children the importance of washing hands to prevent infection.
- Keep outdoor sandboxes covered.
- Feed cats only canned or dried commercial food or well-cooked table food, not raw or undercooked meats.
- Ensure that the cat litter box is changed daily. The *Toxoplasma* parasite does not become infectious until 1 to 5 days after it is shed in a cat's feces.
- If you are pregnant or immunocompromised:
  - Avoid changing cat litter if possible. If no one else can perform the task, wear disposable gloves and wash your hands with soap and water afterwards.
  - Keep cats indoors to prevent them from hunting and reduce the chances they will become infected with *Toxoplasma*.
  - Do not adopt or handle stray cats, especially kittens. Do not get a new cat while you are pregnant or immunocompromised.

Chapter 42 | **HIV/AIDS and Co-occurring Viral Infections**

Chapter Contents

Section 42.1 | Cytomegalovirus

This section includes text excerpted from "Cytomegalovirus (CMV) and Congenital CMV Infection," Centers for Disease Control and Prevention (CDC), August 18, 2020.

WHAT IS CYTOMEGALOVIRUS?

Cytomegalovirus (CMV) is a common virus for people of all ages; however, a healthy person's immune system usually keeps the virus from causing illness.

The COVID-19 pandemic is changing rapidly and continues to affect communities across the United States differently.

In the United States, nearly one in three children are already infected with cytomegalovirus by age five. Over half of adults have been infected with CMV by age 40. Once CMV is in a person's body, it stays there for life and can reactivate. A person can also be re-infected with a different strain (variety) of the virus. Most people with CMV infection have no symptoms and aren't aware that they have been infected.

SIGNS AND SYMPTOMS OF CYTOMEGALOVIRUS

In some cases, infection in healthy people can cause mild illness that may include:

- Fever
- Sore throat
- Fatigue
- Swollen glands

Occasionally, CMV can cause mononucleosis or hepatitis (liver problem).

People with weakened immune systems who get CMV can have more serious symptoms affecting the eyes, lungs, liver, esophagus, stomach, and intestines.

Babies born with CMV can have brain, liver, spleen, lung, and growth problems. The most common long-term health problem in babies born with congenital CMV infection is hearing loss, which may be detected soon after birth or may develop later in childhood.

TRANSMISSION FOR CYTOMEGALOVIRUS

People with CMV may pass the virus in body fluids, such as saliva, urine, blood, tears, semen, and breast milk. CMV is spread from an infected person in the following ways:

- From direct contact with saliva or urine, especially from babies and young children
- Through sexual contact
- From breast milk to nursing infants
- Through transplanted organs and blood transfusions

DIAGNOSIS AND TREATMENT FOR CYTOMEGALOVIRUS

Blood tests can be used to diagnose CMV infection in adults who have symptoms. However, blood is not the best fluid to test newborns with suspected CMV infection. Tests of saliva or urine are preferred for newborns.

Healthy people who are infected with CMV usually do not require medical treatment. Medications are available to treat CMV infection in people who have weakened immune systems and babies with signs of congenital CMV. For babies with signs of congenital CMV infection at birth, antiviral medications, primarily valganciclovir, may improve hearing and developmental outcomes. Valganciclovir can have serious side effects and has only been studied in babies with signs of congenital CMV infection. There is limited information on the effectiveness of valganciclovir to treat infants with hearing loss alone.

BABIES BORN WITH CONGENITAL CYTOMEGALOVIRUS

When a baby is born with cytomegalovirus infection, it is called "congenital CMV." Most babies with congenital CMV never show signs or have health problems. However, some babies have health problems at birth or that develop later.

SIGNS AND SYMPTOMS OF BABIES BORN WITH CONGENITAL CYTOMEGALOVIRUS

Some babies with congenital CMV infection have health problems that are apparent at birth or that develop later during infancy or childhood. In the most severe cases, CMV can cause the death of an unborn baby (pregnancy loss).

Some babies with congenital CMV infection have signs at birth. These signs include:

- Rash
- Jaundice (yellowing of the skin or whites of the eyes)
- Microcephaly (small head)
- Low birth weight
- Hepatosplenomegaly (enlarged liver and spleen)
- Seizures
- Retinitis (damaged eye retina)

Some babies with signs of congenital CMV infection at birth may have long-term health problems, such as:

- Hearing loss
- Developmental and motor delay
- Vision loss
- Microcephaly (small head)
- Seizures

Some babies without signs of congenital CMV infection at birth may have hearing loss. Hearing loss may be present at birth or may develop later, even in babies who passed the newborn hearing test.

TRANSMISSION FOR BABIES BORN WITH CONGENITAL CYTOMEGALOVIRUS

A pregnant woman can pass CMV to her unborn baby. The virus in the woman's blood can cross through the placenta and infect the baby. This can happen when a pregnant woman is infected with CMV for the first time or is infected with CMV again during pregnancy.

Childcare Providers and Parents of Young Children

People who have frequent contact with young children may be at greater risk of CMV infection because young children are a common source of CMV. By the age of five years, one in three children has been infected with CMV, but usually does not have symptoms.

CMV can be present in a child's body fluids for months after they become infected.

Most people with CMV infection have no symptoms and are not aware that they have been infected. A woman who is infected with CMV can pass the virus to her developing baby during pregnancy.

As a parent of a young child or a childcare provider, you may be able to lessen your risk of getting CMV by reducing contact with saliva and urine from babies and young children. The saliva and urine of children with CMV have high amounts of the virus. You can avoid getting a child's saliva in your mouth by, for example, not sharing food, utensils, or cups with a child. Also, you should wash your hands after changing diapers. These cannot eliminate your risk of getting CMV but may lessen the chances of getting it.

DIAGNOSIS FOR BABIES BORN WITH CONGENITAL CYTOMEGALOVIRUS

Congenital CMV infection can be diagnosed by testing a newborn baby's saliva, urine (preferred specimens), or blood. These specimens must be collected for testing within two to three weeks after the baby is born in order to confirm a diagnosis of congenital CMV infection.

TREATMENT BABIES BORN WITH CONGENITAL CYTOMEGALOVIRUS

For babies with signs of congenital CMV infection at birth, antiviral medications, primarily valganciclovir, may improve hearing and developmental outcomes. Valganciclovir can have serious side effects and has only been studied in babies with signs of congenital CMV infection. There is limited information on the effectiveness of valganciclovir to treat infants with hearing loss alone.

Section 42.2 | Genital Herpes

This section includes text excerpted from "Genital Herpes – CDC Fact Sheet," Centers for Disease Control and Prevention (CDC), January 3, 2022.

People who are sexually active can get genital herpes, a common sexually transmitted disease (STD).

WHAT IS GENITAL HERPES?

Genital herpes is a STD caused by two types of viruses – herpes simplex virus type 1 (HSV-1) and herpes simplex virus type 2 (HSV-2).

WHAT IS ORAL HERPES?

HSV-1 often causes oral herpes, which can result in cold sores or fever blisters on or around the mouth. However, most people with oral herpes do not have any symptoms. Most people with oral herpes get it during childhood or young adulthood from nonsexual contact with saliva.

IS THERE A LINK BETWEEN GENITAL HERPES AND ORAL HERPES?

Yes. Oral herpes caused by HSV-1 can spread from the mouth to the genitals through oral sex. This is why some cases of genital herpes are due to HSV-1.

HOW COMMON IS GENITAL HERPES?

Genital herpes is common in the United States. In 2018, The Centers for Disease Control and Prevention (CDC) estimates show there were 572,000 new genital herpes infections in the United States among people aged 14 to 49.

HOW IS GENITAL HERPES SPREAD?

You can get genital herpes by having vaginal, anal, or oral sex with someone who has the infection. You can get herpes if you have contact with:

- A herpes sore
- Saliva from a partner with an oral herpes infection
- Genital fluids from a partner with a genital herpes infection
- Skin in the oral area of a partner with oral herpes or
- Skin in the genital area of a partner with genital herpes.

You also can get genital herpes from a sex partner who does not have a visible sore or is unaware of their infection. It is also possible to get genital herpes if you receive oral sex from a partner with oral herpes.

You will not get herpes from toilet seats, bedding, or swimming pools. You also will not get it from touching objects, such as silverware, soap, or towels.

If you have more questions about herpes, consider discussing your concerns with a healthcare provider.

HOW CAN YOU KNOW IF YOU HAVE GENITAL HERPES?

Most people with genital herpes have no symptoms or have very mild symptoms. Mild symptoms may go unnoticed or be mistaken for other skin conditions such as a pimple or ingrown hair. Because of this, most people do not know they have a herpes infection.

Herpes sores usually appear as one or more blisters on or around the genitals, rectum or mouth. This is known as "having an outbreak." The blisters break and leave painful sores that may take a week or more to heal. Flu-like symptoms (e.g., fever, body aches, or swollen glands) also may occur during the first outbreak.

People who experience an initial outbreak of herpes can have repeated outbreaks, especially if they have HSV-2. However, repeat outbreaks are usually shorter and less severe than the first outbreak. Although genital herpes is a lifelong infection, the number of outbreaks may decrease over time.

Ask a healthcare provider to examine you if:
- Do you notice any symptoms; or
- Your partner has an STD or symptoms of an STD.

STD symptoms can include an unusual sore, a smelly genital discharge, burning when peeing, or bleeding between periods (if you have a menstrual cycle).

HOW WILL YOUR HEALTHCARE PROVIDER KNOW IF YOU HAVE GENITAL HERPES?

Your healthcare provider may diagnose genital herpes by simply looking at any sores that are present. Providers can also take a sample from the sore(s) and test it. If sores are not present, a blood test may be used to look for HSV antibodies.

Have an honest and open talk with your healthcare provider about herpes testing and other STDs.

Please note: A herpes blood test can help determine if you have herpes infection. It cannot tell you who gave you the infection or when you got the infection.

HOW CAN YOU PREVENT GENITAL HERPES?

The only way to completely avoid STDs is to not have vaginal, anal, or oral sex.

If you are sexually active, you can do the following things to lower your chances of getting genital herpes:
- Being in a long-term mutually monogamous relationship with a partner who does not have herpes
- Using condoms the right way every time you have sex

Be aware that not all herpes sores occur in areas that a condom can cover. Also, the skin can release the virus (shed) from areas that do not have a visible herpes sore. For these reasons, condoms may not fully protect you from getting herpes.

If your sex partner(s) has/have genital herpes, you can lower your risk of getting it if:
- Your partner takes an antiherpes medicine every day. This is something your partner should discuss with her or his healthcare provider.
- You avoid having vaginal, anal, or oral sex when your partner has herpes symptoms (i.e., during an "outbreak").

IS THERE A CURE OR TREATMENT FOR GENITAL HERPES?

There is no cure for genital herpes. However, there are medicines that can prevent or shorten outbreaks. A daily antiherpes medicine can make it less likely to pass the infection on to your sex partner(s).

WHAT HAPPENS IF YOU DO NOT RECEIVE TREATMENT

Genital herpes can cause painful genital sores and can be severe in people with suppressed immune systems.

If you touch your sores or fluids from the sores, you may transfer herpes to another body part like your eyes. Do not touch the sores or fluids to avoid spreading herpes to another part of your body. If you do touch the sores or fluids, quickly wash your hands thoroughly to help avoid spreading the infection.

If you are pregnant, there can be problems for you and your unborn fetus, or newborn baby.

YOU ARE PREGNANT. HOW COULD GENITAL HERPES AFFECT YOUR BABY?

If you are pregnant and have genital herpes, prenatal care visits are very important. Some research suggests that a genital herpes infection may lead to miscarriage or make it more likely to deliver your baby too early. You can pass herpes to your unborn child before birth, but it more commonly passes during delivery. This can lead to a deadly infection in your baby (called "neonatal herpes"). It is important that you avoid getting genital herpes during pregnancy. Tell your healthcare provider if you have ever had a genital herpes diagnosis or symptoms. Also, tell them about any possible exposure to genital herpes.

If you have genital herpes, you may need to take antiherpes medicine towards the end of your pregnancy. This medicine may reduce your risk of having signs or symptoms of genital herpes when you deliver. At the time of delivery, your healthcare provider should carefully examine you for herpes sores. If you have signs or symptoms of genital herpes at delivery, a 'C-section' is likely to occur.

CAN YOU STILL HAVE SEX IF YOU HAVE HERPES?

If you have herpes, you should talk to your sex partner(s) about their risk. Using condoms may help lower this risk but it will not get rid of the risk completely. Having sores or other symptoms of herpes can increase your risk of spreading the disease. Even if you do not have any symptoms, you can still infect your sex partners.

You may have concerns about how genital herpes will impact your health, sex life, and relationships. While herpes is not curable, it is important to know that it is manageable with medicine. Daily suppressive therapy (i.e., daily use of antiviral medication) can lower your risk of spreading the virus to others. Talk to a healthcare provider about your concerns and treatment options.

WHAT IS THE LINK BETWEEN GENITAL HERPES AND HIV?

Herpes infection can cause sores or breaks in the skin or lining of the mouth, vagina, and rectum. This provides a way for HIV to enter the body. Even without visible sores, herpes increases the number of immune cells in the lining of the genitals. HIV targets immune cells for entry into the body. Having both HIV and genital herpes increases the chance of spreading HIV to a HIV-negative partner during oral, vagina, or anal sex.

Section 42.3 | Herpes Zoster Virus

This section contains text excerpted from the following sources: Text under the heading "What Is Herpes Zoster Virus?" is excerpted from "Shingles," MedlinePlus, National Institutes of Health (NIH), March 15, 2017. Reviewed February 2022; Text beginning with the heading "Signs and Symptoms for Shingles (Herpes Zoster)" is excerpted from "Shingles (Herpes Zoster) – Signs and Symptoms," Centers for Disease Control and Prevention (CDC), June 26, 2019.

WHAT IS HERPES ZOSTER VIRUS?

Shingles is an outbreak of rash or blisters on the skin. It is caused by the varicella-zoster virus – the same virus that causes chickenpox. After you have chickenpox, the virus stays in your body. It may not cause problems for many years. But as you get older, the virus may reappear as shingles.

SIGNS AND SYMPTOMS OF HERPES ZOSTER

Before the rash appears, people often have pain, itching, or tingling in the area where it will develop. This may happen several days before the rash appears.

Most commonly, the rash occurs in a single stripe around either the left or the right side of the body. In other cases, the rash occurs on one side of the face. Shingles on the face can affect the eye and cause vision loss. In rare cases (usually in people with weakened immune systems), the rash may be more widespread on the body and look similar to a chickenpox rash.

Other symptoms of shingles can include:

- Fever
- Headache
- Chills
- Upset stomach

TRANSMISSION FOR HERPES ZOSTER

Shingles is caused by varicella zoster virus (VZV), the same virus that causes chickenpox. After a person recovers from chickenpox, the virus stays dormant (inactive) in their body. The virus can reactivate later, causing shingles.

Most people who develop shingles have only one episode during their lifetime. However, you can have shingles more than once.

If you have shingles, direct contact with the fluid from your rash blisters can spread VZV to people who have never had chickenpox or never received the chickenpox vaccine. If they get infected, they will develop chickenpox, not shingles. They could then develop shingles later in life.

The risk of spreading VZV to others is low if you cover the shingles rash. People with shingles cannot spread the virus before their rash blisters appear or after the rash crusts.

People with chickenpox are more likely to spread VZV than people with shingles.

To prevent spreading VZV to others:

- Cover the rash
- Avoid touching or scratching the rash

- Wash your hands often
- Avoid contact with the following people until your rash crusts:
  - Pregnant women who have never had chickenpox or the chickenpox vaccine
  - Premature or low birth weight infants and
  - People with weakened immune systems, such as people receiving immunosuppressive medications or undergoing chemotherapy, organ transplant recipients, and people with human immunodeficiency virus (HIV) infection

Some people have a greater risk of getting shingles. This includes people who:
- Have medical conditions that keep their immune systems from working properly, such as certain cancers such as leukemia and lymphoma, and human immunodeficiency virus (HIV)
- Receive drugs that keep their immune systems from working properly, such as steroids and drugs that are given after organ transplantation

COMPLICATIONS OF HERPES ZOSTER

The most common complication of shingles is long-term nerve pain called "postherpetic neuralgia" (PHN). PHN occurs in the areas where the shingles rash was, even after the rash clears up. It can last for months or years after the rash goes away. The pain from PHN can be so severe and debilitating that it interferes with daily life.

About 10 to 18 percent of people who get shingles will experience PHN. An older adult with shingles is more likely to develop PHN and have longer-lasting and more severe pain than a younger person with shingles. People younger than 40 rarely experience PHN.

Other Complications

Shingles may lead to serious complications involving the eye, including blindness. Very rarely, it can also lead to:

- Pneumonia
- Hearing problems
- Brain inflammation (encephalitis) or
- Death

TREATING HERPES ZOSTER

Several antiviral medicines – acyclovir, valacyclovir, and famciclovir – are available to treat shingles and shorten the length and severity of the illness. These medicines are most effective if you start taking them as soon as possible after the rash appears. If you think you have shingles, contact your healthcare provider as soon as possible to discuss treatment.

Pain medicine, either over-the-counter (OTC) or a prescription from your doctor, may help relieve the pain caused by shingles. Wet compresses, calamine lotion, and colloidal oatmeal baths (a lukewarm bath mixed with ground-up oatmeal) may help relieve itching.

Section 42.4 | Human Papillomavirus

This section includes text excerpted from "Genital HPV Infection – Fact Sheet," Centers for Disease Control and Prevention (CDC), January 3, 2022.

Human papillomavirus (HPV) is the most common sexually transmitted infection (STI) in the United States. HPV vaccines can prevent some of the health effects HPV causes.

WHAT IS HUMAN PAPILLOMAVIRUS?

There were about 43 million HPV infections in 2018, many among people in their late teens and early 20s. There are many different types of HPV. Some types can cause health problems, including genital warts and cancers. But, there are vaccines that can stop these health problems from happening. HPV is a different virus than HIV and HSV (herpes).

HOW IS HUMAN PAPILLOMAVIRUS SPREAD?

You can get HPV by having vaginal, anal, or oral sex with someone who has the virus. It is most commonly spread during vaginal or anal sex. It also spreads through close skin-to-skin touching during sex. A person with HPV can pass the infection to someone even when they have no signs or symptoms.

If you are sexually active, you can get HPV, even if you have had sex with only one person. You also can develop symptoms years after having sex with someone who has the infection. This makes it hard to know when you first got it.

DOES HUMAN PAPILLOMAVIRUS CAUSE HEALTH PROBLEMS?

In most cases (9 out of 10), HPV goes away on its own within two years without health problems. But when HPV does not go away, it can cause health problems such as genital warts and cancer.

Genital warts usually appear as a small bump or group of bumps in the genital area. They can be small or large, raised or flat, or shaped like a cauliflower. A healthcare provider can usually diagnose warts by looking at the genital area.

DOES HUMAN PAPILLOMAVIRUS CAUSE CANCER?

HPV can cause cervical and other cancers, including cancer of the vulva, vagina, penis, or anus. It can also cause cancer in the back of the throat (called "oropharyngeal cancer"). This can include the base of the tongue and tonsils.

Cancer often takes years, even decades, to develop after a person gets HPV. Genital warts and cancers result from different types of HPV.

There is no way to know who will develop cancer or other health problems from HPV. People with weak immune systems (including those with HIV) may be less able to fight off HPV. They may also be more likely to develop health problems from HPV.

HOW CAN YOU AVOID HPV AND THE HEALTH PROBLEMS IT CAN CAUSE?

You can do several things to lower your chances of getting HPV.

- **Get vaccinated**. The HPV vaccine is safe and effective. It can protect against diseases (including cancers) caused by HPV when given in the recommended age groups.
- **Get screened for cervical cancer**. Routine screening for women aged 21 to 65 years old can prevent cervical cancer.

If you are sexually active:
- Use condoms the right way every time you have sex. This can lower your chances of getting HPV. But HPV can infect areas the condom does not cover. So, condoms may not fully protect against getting HPV; and
- Be in a mutually monogamous relationship – or have sex only with someone who only has sex with you.

WHO SHOULD GET THE HUMAN PAPILLOMAVIRUS VACCINE?

The Centers for Disease Control and Prevention (CDC) recommends HPV vaccination for:
- All preteens (including boys and girls) at age 11 or 12 years (or can start at age 9 years).
- Everyone through age 26 years, if not vaccinated already.

Vaccination is not recommended for everyone older than age 26 years. However, some adults age 27 through 45 years who are not already vaccinated may decide to get the HPV vaccine after speaking with their healthcare provider about their risk for new HPV infections and the possible benefits of vaccination. HPV vaccination in this age range provides less benefit. Most sexually active adults have already been exposed to HPV, although not necessarily all of the HPV types targeted by vaccination.

At any age, having a new sex partner is a risk factor for getting a new HPV infection. People who are already in a long-term, mutually monogamous relationship are not likely to get a new HPV infection.

HOW TO KNOW IF YOU HAVE HUMAN PAPILLOMAVIRUS?

There is no test to find out a person's "HPV status." Also, there is no approved HPV test to find HPV in the mouth or throat.

There are HPV tests that can screen for cervical cancer. Healthcare providers only use these tests for screening women aged 30 years and older. HPV tests are not recommended to screen men, adolescents, or women under the age of 30 years.

Most people with HPV do not know they have the infection. They never develop symptoms or health problems from it. Some people find out they have HPV when they get genital warts. Women may find out they have HPV when they get an abnormal Pap test result (during cervical cancer screening). Others may only find out once they have developed more serious problems from HPV, such as cancers.

HOW COMMON IS HPV AND HEALTH PROBLEMS THAT DEVELOP FROM HPV?

- **HPV (the virus).** The CDC estimates that there were 43 million HPV infections in 2018. In that same year, there were 13 million new infections. HPV is so common that almost every sexually active person will get HPV at some point if they do not get vaccinated.
- Health problems related to HPV include genital warts and cervical cancer.
- **Genital warts.** Prior to HPV vaccines, genital warts caused by HPV affected roughly 340,000 to 360,000 people yearly.* About one in 100 sexually active adults in the U.S. has genital warts at any given time.
- **Cervical cancer.** Every year, nearly 12,000 women living in the United States will have cervical cancer. More than 4,000 women die from cervical cancer – even with screening and treatment.

There are other conditions and cancers caused by HPV that occur in people living in the United States. Every year, about 19,400 women and 12,100 men experience cancers caused by HPV.

*Note: *These figures only look at the number of people who sought care for genital warts. This could be less than the actual number of people who get genital warts.*

WILL HAVING HPV AFFECT YOUR PREGNANCY?

Pregnant people with HPV can get genital warts or develop abnormal cell changes on the cervix. Routine cervical cancer screening can help find abnormal cell changes. You should get routine cervical cancer screening even when you are pregnant.

IS THERE TREATMENT FOR HPV OR HEALTH PROBLEMS THAT DEVELOP FROM HPV?

There is no treatment for the virus itself. However, there are treatments for the health problems that HPV can cause:

- Genital warts can go away with treatment from your healthcare provider or with prescription medicine. If left untreated, genital warts may go away, stay the same, or grow in size or number.
- Cervical precancer treatment is available. Women who get routine Pap tests and follow up as needed can find problems before cancer develops. Prevention is always better than treatment.
- Other HPV-related cancers are also more treatable when found and treated early.

Section 42.5 | Progressive Multifocal Leukoencephalopathy

This section includes text excerpted from "Progressive Multifocal Leukoencephalopathy Information Page," National Institute of Neurological Disorders and Stroke (NINDS), July 29, 2019.

WHAT IS PROGRESSIVE MULTIFOCAL LEUKOENCEPHALOPATHY?

Progressive multifocal leukoencephalopathy (PML) is a disease of the white matter of the brain, caused by a virus infection that targets cells that make myelin – the material that insulates nerve cells (neurons). Polyomavirus JC (often called "JC virus") is carried by a majority of people and is harmless except among those with lowered immune defenses. The disease is rare and occurs in patients undergoing chronic corticosteroid or immunosuppressive therapy for organ transplant, or individuals with cancer (such as Hodgkin disease or lymphoma). Individuals with autoimmune conditions such as multiple sclerosis, rheumatoid arthritis, and systemic lupus erythematosus – some of whom are treated with biological therapies that allow JC virus reactivation – are at risk for PML as well. PML is most common among individuals with HIV-1 infection/acquired immunodeficiency syndrome (AIDS). Studies estimate that prior to effective antiretroviral therapy, as many as 5 percent of persons infected with HIV-1 eventually develop PML, which is an AIDS-defining illness. However, current HIV therapy using antiretroviral drugs (ART), which effectively restores immune system function, allows as many as half of all HIV-PML patients to survive, although they may sometimes have an inflammatory reaction in the regions of the brain affected by PML.

The symptoms of PML are diverse, since they are related to the location and amount of damage in the brain, and may evolve over the course of several weeks to months. The most prominent symptoms are clumsiness; progressive weakness; and visual, speech, and sometimes personality changes. The progression of deficits leads to life-threatening disability and (frequently) death. A diagnosis of PML can be made following brain biopsy or by combining observations of a progressive course of the disease, consistent white matter lesions visible on a magnetic resonance imaging (MRI) scan, and the detection of the JC virus in spinal fluid.

TREATMENT FOR PROGRESSIVE MULTIFOCAL LEUKOENCEPHALOPATHY

The best available therapy is reversal of the immune-deficient state, since there are no effective drugs that block virus infection without toxicity. Reversal may be achieved by using plasma exchange to accelerate the removal of the therapeutic agents that put patients at risk for PML. In the case of HIV-associated PML, immediately beginning antiretroviral therapy will benefit most individuals. Several new drugs that laboratory tests found effective against infection are being used in PML patients with special permission of the U.S. Food and Drug Administration (FDA). Hexadecyloxypropyl-Cidofovir (CMX001) is currently being studied as a treatment option for JVC because of its ability to suppress JVC by inhibiting viral DNA replication.

PROGNOSIS FOR PROGRESSIVE MULTIFOCAL LEUKOENCEPHALOPATHY

In general, PML has a mortality rate of 30–50 percent in the first few months following diagnosis but depends on the severity of the underlying disease and treatment received. Those who survive PML can be left with severe neurological disabilities.

Section 42.6 | Viral Hepatitis

This section includes text excerpted from "HIV and Hepatitis B," HIVinfo, U.S. Department of Health and Human Services (HHS), August 24, 2021.

WHAT IS HEPATITIS B?

Hepatitis B is a liver infection caused by the hepatitis B virus (HBV). The abbreviation HBV can stand for either the virus or the infection it causes.

HBV can be a short-term (acute) or a long-term (chronic) illness:

- Acute HBV occurs within 6 months after a person is exposed to HBV. In some people, acute HBV can lead to chronic HBV.

- Chronic HBV is a lifelong disease. Without treatment, chronic HBV can cause liver cancer or liver damage that leads to liver failure.

HBV is a contagious infection that can spread from person to person.

HOW DOES HBV SPREAD FROM PERSON TO PERSON?

HBV is spread through contact with the blood, semen, or other body fluid of a person who has HBV. Among adults in the United States, HBV is spread mainly through sexual contact.

HBV can also spread from person to person in the following ways:

- By sharing needles or other injection drug equipment (works) with someone who has HBV
- By sharing razors, toothbrushes, or similar personal items with someone who has HBV
- From contact with the blood or open sores of a person who has HBV
- From an accidental prick or cut from an HBV-contaminated needle or other sharp object
- From a mother who has HBV to her child during childbirth

WHAT IS THE CONNECTION BETWEEN HIV AND HBV?

Both HIV and HBV spread from person to person in semen, blood, or other body fluids. For this reason, the main risk factors for HIV and HBV are the same: having sex without a condom and injection drug use.

According to the Centers for Disease Control and Prevention (CDC), approximately 10 percent of people with HIV in the United States also have HBV. Infection with both HIV and HBV is called "HIV/HBV coinfection."

Chronic HBV advances faster to cirrhosis, end-stage liver disease, and liver cancer in people with HIV/HBV coinfection than in people with only HBV infection. But chronic HBV does not appear to cause HIV to advance faster in people with HIV/HBV coinfection.

SHOULD PEOPLE WITH HIV GET TESTED FOR HBV?

The CDC recommends that all people with HIV get tested for HBV. Testing can detect HBV even when a person has no symptoms of the infection.

There are several HBV blood tests. Results of different tests show different things. For example, a positive hepatitis B surface antigen (HBsAg) test result shows that a person has acute or chronic HBV and can spread the virus to others.

WHAT ARE THE SYMPTOMS OF HBV INFECTION?

Some people with acute HBV do not have symptoms. But some people can have signs of HBV soon after becoming infected. Symptoms of acute HBV can include the following:

- Loss of appetite
- Tiredness
- Nausea
- Vomiting
- Fever
- Abdominal pain
- Dark urine
- Clay-colored bowel movements
- Joint pain
- Jaundice (yellowing of the skin or the whites of the eyes)

Most people with chronic HBV do not have any symptoms and may not have symptoms for many years. Abnormal results on liver function tests may be the first sign of chronic HBV infection.

WHAT IS THE TREATMENT FOR HBV?

In general, HBV is treated with antiviral medicines. The medicines work to help limit damage to the liver.

People with HIV/HBV coinfection should be treated for both infections. Some HIV medicines are effective at treating both HIV and HBV.

The choice of medicines to treat HIV/HBV coinfection depends on the person. For example, some people may take HIV medicines that are also effective at treating HBV. Other people may take HIV medicines and an HBV antiviral medicine. If you have HIV/HBV coinfection, talk to your healthcare provider about the best medicines for you.

CAN HBV INFECTION BE PREVENTED?

Yes. The best way to prevent HBV is to get the hepatitis B vaccine.

The CDC recommends that people with HIV and people who are at risk for HIV get the HBV vaccine (or the combined hepatitis A virus/HBV vaccine). The housemates and sexual partners of people with HBV should get the HBV vaccine, too.

People, including people with HIV, can also take the following steps to reduce their risk of HBV infection:

- Use condoms during sex to reduce the risk of HBV infection and infection with other sexually transmitted diseases, such as gonorrhea and syphilis.
- Do not inject drugs. But if you do, do not share needles, syringes, or other drug injection equipment.
- Do not share toothbrushes, razors, or other personal items that may come in contact with another person's blood.
- If you get a tattoo or body piercing, make sure the instruments used are sterile.

Chapter 43 | **HIV/AIDS and Co-occurring Cancers**

Chapter Contents

Section 43.1 | **HIV Infection and Cancer Risk**

This section includes text excerpted from "HIV Infection and Cancer Risk," National Cancer Institute (NCI), September 14, 2017. Reviewed February 2022.

INCREASED RISK OF CANCER IN HIV AFFECTED PEOPLE

Yes. People infected with the human immunodeficiency virus (HIV) have a substantially higher risk of some types of cancer compared with uninfected people of the same age. The general term for these cancers is "HIV-associated cancers." Three of these cancers are known as "acquired immunodeficiency syndrome (AIDS)-defining cancers" or "AIDS-defining malignancies:" Kaposi sarcoma, aggressive B-cell non-Hodgkin lymphoma, and cervical cancer. A diagnosis of any of these cancers in someone infected with HIV confirms a diagnosis of AIDS.

Compared with the general population, people infected with HIV are currently about 500 times more likely to be diagnosed with Kaposi sarcoma, 12 times more likely to be diagnosed with non-Hodgkin lymphoma, and, among women, 3 times more likely to be diagnosed with cervical cancer.

In addition, people infected with HIV are at higher risk of several other types of cancer (collectively called "non–AIDS-defining cancers"). These other malignancies include cancers of the anus, liver, oral cavity/pharynx, lung, and Hodgkin lymphoma.

People infected with HIV are 19 times more likely to be diagnosed with anal cancer, 3 times as likely to be diagnosed with liver cancer, 2 times as likely to be diagnosed with lung cancer, about 2 times as likely to be diagnosed with oral cavity/pharynx cancer, and about 8 times more likely to be diagnosed with Hodgkin lymphoma compared with the general population.

In addition to being linked to an increased risk of cancer, HIV infection is associated with an increased risk of dying from cancer. HIV-infected people with a range of cancer types are more likely to die of their cancer than HIV-uninfected people with these cancers.

HIGH RISK CANCER TYPES FOR PEOPLE WITH HIV

Infection with HIV weakens the immune system and reduces the body's ability to fight viral infections that may lead to cancer. The viruses that are most likely to cause cancer in people with HIV are:

- Kaposi sarcoma-associated herpesvirus (KSHV), also known as "human herpesvirus 8" (HHV-8), which causes Kaposi sarcoma and some subtypes of lymphoma
- Epstein-Barr virus (EBV), which causes some subtypes of non-Hodgkin and Hodgkin lymphoma
- Human papillomaviruses (HPV), high-risk types of which cause cervical cancer, most anal cancers, and oropharyngeal, penile, vaginal, and vulvar cancer
- Hepatitis B virus (HBV) and hepatitis C virus (HCV), which both cause liver cancer

HIV-infected persons are more likely to be infected with these viruses than people in the general population.

In addition, the prevalence of some traditional risk factors for cancer, especially smoking (a known cause of lung and other cancers) and heavy alcohol use (which can increase the risk of liver cancer), is higher among people infected with HIV. Also, because people infected with HIV have compromised immune systems, both immunosuppression and inflammation may have direct or indirect roles in the development of some cancers that are elevated in people infected with HIV.

The poorer cancer survival of HIV-infected people may result, at least in part, from the weakened immune system in such individuals. The increased risk of death could also result from the cancer being more advanced at diagnosis, delays in cancer treatment, or poorer access to appropriate cancer treatment.

ANTIRETROVIRAL THERAPY

The introduction of highly active antiretroviral therapy (HAART), also called "combination antiretroviral therapy" (cART), starting in the mid-1990s greatly reduced the incidence of certain cancers in HIV-infected patients, especially Kaposi sarcoma and non-Hodgkin lymphoma. The likely explanation for this reduced incidence is that cART lowers the amount of HIV circulating in the blood, thereby allowing partial restoration of immune system function to fight the viruses that cause many of these cancers.

Although the risk of these AIDS-defining cancers among people infected with HIV is lower than in the past, it is still much higher than among people in the general population. This persistently high risk may reflect the fact that cART does not completely restore immune system functioning. Also, many people infected with HIV are not aware they are infected, have had difficulty in accessing medical care, or for other reasons are not receiving adequate antiretroviral therapy.

The introduction of cART has not reduced the incidence of all HIV-related cancers, and in fact there has been an increase in non–AIDS-defining cancers. For example, the incidence of liver and anal cancer may be increasing among HIV-infected individuals.

An important factor contributing to the increase in non-AIDS-defining cancers is that as cART has reduced the number of deaths from AIDS, the HIV-infected population has grown in size and become older. The fastest growing proportion of HIV-infected individuals is the over-40 age group. These individuals are now developing cancers common in older age and also have an increased cumulative risk of developing HIV-associated cancers.

REDUCING CANCER RISK IN HIV AFFECTED PEOPLE

Taking cART as indicated based on current HIV treatment guidelines lowers the risk of Kaposi sarcoma and non-Hodgkin lymphoma and increases overall survival.

The risk of lung, oral, and other cancers can be reduced by quitting smoking. Because HIV-infected people have a higher risk of lung cancer, it is especially important that they do not smoke.

The higher incidence of liver cancer among HIV-infected people appears to be related to more frequent infection with hepatitis virus (particularly HCV in the United States) than among HIV-uninfected people. Therefore, HIV-infected individuals should know their hepatitis status.

In addition, if HIV-infected people currently have viral hepatitis, they should discuss with their healthcare provider whether antiviral treatment is an option for them. Some drugs may be used for both HBV-suppressing therapy and cART.

Because HIV-infected women have a higher risk of cervical cancer, it is important that they be screened regularly for this disease. In addition, the Centers for Disease Control and Prevention (CDC) recommends vaccination against human papillomavirus (HPV) for women and men with HIV infection up to age 26 years. Cervical cancer screening guidelines that incorporate results of a Pap test and an HPV deoxyribonucleic Acid (DNA) test are evolving, and women should discuss screening options with their healthcare provider.

Some researchers recommend anal Pap test screening to detect and treat early lesions before they progress to anal cancer. However, it is not clear if this type of screening benefits all HIV-infected people or if treating such lesions prevents anal cancer. These questions are being addressed in an NCI-funded trial called the "Anal Cancer/HSIL Outcomes Research (ANCHOR) Study." This study is currently enrolling women and men with HIV to undergo anal Pap testing and then be randomly assigned to receive either treatment or observation (no treatment). The goal is to determine whether treatment of anal lesions prevents anal cancer in HIV-infected people with anal lesions.

KSHV is secreted in saliva, and transmission of this virus may occur through deep kissing, through the use of saliva as a lubricant in sex, or through oral – anal sex. Reducing contact through these routes may reduce the chance of being infected with KSHV.

Section 43.2 | Kaposi Sarcoma

This section includes text excerpted from "Kaposi Sarcoma Treatment (PDQ®) – Patient Version," National Cancer Institute (NCI), August 23, 2021.

WHAT IS KAPOSI SARCOMA?

Kaposi sarcoma is a disease in which malignant lesions (cancer) can form in the skin, mucous membranes, lymph nodes, and other organs.

Kaposi sarcoma is a cancer that causes lesions (abnormal tissue) to grow in the skin; the mucous membranes lining the mouth, nose, and throat; lymph nodes; or other organs. The lesions are usually purple and are made of cancer cells, new blood vessels, red blood cells, and white blood cells. Kaposi sarcoma is different from other cancers in that lesions may begin in more than one place in the body at the same time.

Human herpesvirus-8 (HHV-8) is found in the lesions of all patients with Kaposi sarcoma. This virus is also called "Kaposi sarcoma herpesvirus" (KSHV). Most people with HHV-8 do not get Kaposi sarcoma. People with HHV-8 are more likely to develop Kaposi sarcoma if their immune system is weakened by disease, such as human immunodeficiency virus (HIV), or by drugs given after an organ transplant.

There are several types of Kaposi sarcoma. The two types discussed in this section include:

- Classic Kaposi sarcoma
- Epidemic Kaposi sarcoma (HIV-associated Kaposi sarcoma)

CLASSIC KAPOSI SARCOMA

Classic Kaposi sarcoma is found most often in older men of Italian or Eastern European Jewish origin.

Classic Kaposi sarcoma is a rare disease that gets worse slowly over many years.

Signs of Classic Kaposi Sarcoma

Patients may have one or more red, purple, or brown skin lesions on the legs and feet, most often on the ankles or soles of the feet.

Over time, lesions may form in other parts of the body, such as the stomach, intestines, or lymph nodes. The lesions usually do not cause any symptoms, but may grow in size and number over a period of 10 years or more. Pressure from the lesions may block the flow of lymph and blood in the legs and cause painful swelling. Lesions in the digestive tract may cause gastrointestinal (GI) bleeding.

EPIDEMIC KAPOSI SARCOMA

Patients with human immunodeficiency virus (HIV) are at risk of developing epidemic Kaposi sarcoma (HIV-associated Kaposi sarcoma).

Acquired immunodeficiency syndrome (AIDS) is caused by HIV, which attacks and weakens the body's immune system. A weakened immune system is unable to fight infection and disease. People with HIV have an increased risk of infection and cancer.

A person with HIV and certain types of infection or cancer, such as Kaposi sarcoma, is diagnosed as having AIDS. Sometimes, a person is diagnosed with AIDS and epidemic Kaposi sarcoma at the same time.

The use of drug therapy called "highly active antiretroviral therapy" (HAART) reduces the risk of epidemic Kaposi sarcoma in patients with HIV.

HAART is a combination of several drugs used to lessen the damage to the immune system caused by HIV infection. Treatment with HAART reduces the risk of epidemic Kaposi sarcoma, although it is possible for a person to develop epidemic Kaposi sarcoma while taking HAART.

Signs of Epidemic Kaposi Sarcoma

The signs of epidemic Kaposi sarcoma can include lesions in different parts of the body, including any of the following:

- Skin
- Lining of the mouth
- Lymph nodes
- Stomach and intestines

- Lungs and lining of the chest
- Liver
- Spleen

Kaposi sarcoma is sometimes found in the lining of the mouth during a regular dental checkup.

In most patients with epidemic Kaposi sarcoma, the disease will spread to other parts of the body over time.

TREATMENT OPTIONS FOR KAPOSI SARCOMA

Different types of treatments are available for patients with Kaposi sarcoma. Some treatments are standard (the currently used treatment), and some are being tested in clinical trials. A treatment clinical trial is a research study meant to help improve current treatments or obtain information on new treatments for patients with cancer. When clinical trials show that a new treatment is better than the standard treatment, the new treatment may become the standard treatment. Patients may want to think about taking part in a clinical trial. Some clinical trials are open only to patients who have not started treatment.

Standard Treatments Used for Kaposi Sarcoma

Treatment of epidemic Kaposi sarcoma combines treatment for Kaposi sarcoma with treatment for acquired immunodeficiency syndrome (AIDS). The six types of standard treatment used to treat Kaposi sarcoma include:

HAART

Highly active antiretroviral therapy (HAART) is a combination of several drugs used to lessen the damage to the immune system caused by human immunodeficiency virus (HIV) infection. For many patients, HAART alone may be enough to treat epidemic Kaposi sarcoma. For other patients, HAART may be combined with other standard treatments to treat epidemic Kaposi sarcoma.

RADIATION THERAPY

Radiation therapy is a cancer treatment that uses high-energy x-rays or other types of radiation to kill cancer cells or keep them from growing. There are two types of radiation therapy:

- **External radiation therapy**. It uses a machine outside the body to send radiation toward the area of the body with cancer.
- **Internal radiation therapy**. It uses a radioactive substance sealed in needles, seeds, wires, or catheters that are placed directly into or near the cancer.

The way the radiation therapy is given depends on the type of the cancer being treated. Certain types of external radiation therapy are used to treat Kaposi sarcoma lesions. Photon radiation therapy treats lesions with high-energy light. Electron beam radiation therapy uses tiny negatively charged particles called "electrons."

SURGERY

The following surgical procedures may be used for Kaposi sarcoma to treat small, surface lesions:

- **Local excision**. The cancer is cut from the skin along with a small amount of normal tissue around it.
- **Electrodesiccation and curettage**. The tumor is cut from the skin with a curette (a sharp, spoon-shaped tool). A needle-shaped electrode is then used to treat the area with an electric current that stops the bleeding and destroys cancer cells that remain around the edge of the wound. The process may be repeated one to three times during the surgery to remove all of the cancer.

CRYOSURGERY

Cryosurgery is a treatment that uses an instrument to freeze and destroy abnormal tissue. This type of treatment is also called "cryotherapy."

CHEMOTHERAPY

Chemotherapy is a cancer treatment that uses drugs to stop the growth of cancer cells, either by killing the cells or by stopping them from dividing. When chemotherapy is taken by mouth or injected into a vein or muscle, the drugs enter the bloodstream and can reach cancer cells throughout the body (systemic chemotherapy). When chemotherapy is placed directly into the cerebrospinal fluid, an organ, tissue, or a body cavity such as the abdomen, the drugs mainly affect cancer cells in those areas (regional chemotherapy).

In electrochemotherapy, intravenous chemotherapy is given and a probe is used to send electric pulses to the tumor. The pulses make an opening in the membrane around the tumor cell and allow the chemotherapy to get inside.

The way the chemotherapy is given depends on where the Kaposi sarcoma lesions occur in the body. In Kaposi sarcoma, chemotherapy may be given in the following ways:

- For local Kaposi sarcoma lesions, such as in the mouth, anticancer drugs may be injected directly into the lesion (intralesional chemotherapy).
- For local lesions on the skin, a topical agent may be applied to the skin as a gel. Electrochemotherapy may also be used.
- For widespread lesions on the skin, intravenous chemotherapy may be given.

Liposomal chemotherapy uses liposomes (very tiny fat particles) to carry anticancer drugs. Liposomal doxorubicin is used to treat Kaposi sarcoma. The liposomes build up in Kaposi sarcoma tissue more than in healthy tissue, and the doxorubicin is released slowly. This increases the effect of the doxorubicin and causes less damage to healthy tissue.

IMMUNOTHERAPY

Immunotherapy is a treatment that uses the patient's immune system to fight cancer. Substances made by the body or made in a laboratory are used to boost, direct, or restore the body's natural defenses against cancer. This cancer treatment is a type of biologic therapy. Interferon alfa and interleukin-12 are biologic agents used to treat Kaposi sarcoma.

Section 43.3 | AIDS-Related Lymphoma

This section includes text excerpted from "AIDS-Related Lymphoma Treatment (PDQ®) – Patient Version," National Cancer Institute (NCI), December 3, 2021.

WHAT IS AIDS-RELATED LYMPHOMA?

Acquired immunodeficiency syndrome (AIDS)-related lymphoma is a disease in which malignant (cancer) cells form in the lymph system of patients who have AIDS.

AIDS is caused by the human immunodeficiency virus (HIV), which attacks and weakens the body's immune system. A weakened immune system is unable to fight infection and disease. People with HIV disease have an increased risk of infection and lymphoma or other types of cancer. A person with HIV and certain types of infection or cancer, such as lymphoma, is diagnosed as having AIDS. Sometimes, people are diagnosed with AIDS and AIDS-related lymphoma at the same time.

AIDS-related lymphoma is a type of cancer that affects the lymph system. The lymph system is part of the immune system. It helps protect the body from infection and disease.

The lymph system is made up of the following:

- **Lymph**. The colorless, watery fluid travels through the lymph vessels and carries T and B lymphocytes. Lymphocytes are a type of white blood cell.
- **Lymph vessels**. A network of thin tubes that collect lymph from different parts of the body and return it to the bloodstream.
- **Lymph nodes**. Small, bean-shaped structures filter lymph and store white blood cells that help fight infection and disease. Lymph nodes are found along a network of lymph vessels throughout the body. Groups of lymph nodes are found in the neck, underarm, mediastinum, abdomen, pelvis, and groin.

- **Spleen**. An organ that makes lymphocytes, stores red blood cells and lymphocytes, filters the blood and destroys old blood cells. The spleen is on the left side of the abdomen near the stomach.
- **Thymus**. An organ in which T lymphocytes mature and multiply. The thymus is in the chest behind the breastbone.
- **Tonsils**. Two small masses of lymph tissue at the back of the throat. There is one tonsil on each side of the throat.
- **Bone marrow**. The soft, spongy tissue in the center of certain bones, such as the hip bone and breastbone. White blood cells, red blood cells, and platelets are made in the bone marrow.

Lymph tissue is also found in other parts of the body such as the brain, stomach, thyroid gland, and skin.

Sometimes AIDS-related lymphoma occurs outside the lymph nodes in the bone marrow, liver, meninges (thin membranes that cover the brain) and gastrointestinal tract. Less often, it may occur in the anus, heart, bile duct, gingiva, and muscles.

DIFFERENT TYPES OF LYMPHOMA

Lymphomas are divided into two general types:
- Hodgkin lymphoma
- Non-Hodgkin lymphoma

Both non-Hodgkin lymphoma and Hodgkin lymphoma may occur in patients with AIDS, but non-Hodgkin lymphoma is more common. When a person with AIDS has non-Hodgkin lymphoma, it is called "AIDS-related lymphoma." When AIDS-related lymphoma occurs in the central nervous system (CNS), it is called "AIDS-related primary CNS lymphoma."

Non-Hodgkin lymphomas are grouped by the way their cells look under a microscope. They may be indolent (slow-growing) or aggressive (fast-growing). AIDS-related lymphomas are aggressive. There are two main types of AIDS-related non-Hodgkin lymphoma:

515

- Diffuse large B-cell lymphoma (including B-cell immunoblastic lymphoma).
- Burkitt or Burkitt-like lymphoma.

SIGNS OF AIDS-RELATED LYMPHOMA

These and other signs and symptoms may be caused by AIDS-related lymphoma or by other conditions. Check with your doctor if you have any of the following:
- Weight loss or fever for no known reason
- Drenching night sweats
- Painless, swollen lymph nodes in the neck, chest, underarm, or groin
- A feeling of fullness below the ribs

DIAGNOSIS OF AIDS-RELATED LYMPHOMA

The following tests and procedures may be used:
- **Physical exam and health history**. An exam of the body to check general signs of health, including checking for signs of disease, such as lumps or anything else that seems unusual. A history of the patient's health, including fever, drenching night sweats, weight loss, health habits, and past illnesses and treatments will also be taken.
- **Complete blood count (CBC)**. A procedure in which a sample of blood is drawn and checked for the following:
  - The number of red blood cells, white blood cells, and platelets.
  - The amount of hemoglobin (the protein that carries oxygen) in the red blood cells.
  - The portion of the sample is made up of red blood cells.
- **Blood chemistry studies**. A procedure in which a blood sample is checked to measure the amounts of certain substances released into the blood by organs and tissues in the body. An unusual (higher or lower

than normal) amount of a substance can be a sign of disease.

- **Lactate dehydrogenase (LDH) test**. A procedure in which a blood sample is checked to measure the amount of lactic dehydrogenase. An increased amount of LDH in the blood may be a sign of tissue damage, lymphoma, or other diseases.
- **Hepatitis B and hepatitis C test**. A procedure in which a sample of blood is checked to measure the amounts of hepatitis B virus-specific antigens and/ or antibodies and the amounts of hepatitis C virus-specific antibodies. These antigens or antibodies are called "markers." Different markers or combinations of markers are used to determine whether a patient has a hepatitis B or C infection, has had a prior infection or vaccination, or is susceptible to infection.
- **HIV test**. A test to measure the level of HIV antibodies in a sample of blood. Antibodies are made by the body when it is invaded by a foreign substance. A high level of HIV antibodies may mean the body has been infected with HIV.
- **CT scan (CAT scan)**. A procedure that makes a series of detailed pictures of areas inside the body, such as the neck, chest, abdomen, pelvis, and lymph nodes, taken from different angles. The pictures are made by a computer linked to an x-ray machine. A dye may be injected into a vein or swallowed to help the organs or tissues show up more clearly. This procedure is also called "computed tomography" (CT), computerized tomography, or computerized axial tomography.
- **Positron emission tomography (PET) scan**. A procedure to find malignant tumor cells in the body. A small amount of radioactive glucose (sugar) is injected into a vein. The PET scanner rotates around the body and makes a picture of where glucose is being used in the body. Malignant tumor cells show up brighter in

the picture because they are more active and take up more glucose than normal cells do.

- **Bone marrow aspiration and biopsy**. The removal of bone marrow and a small piece of bone by inserting a hollow needle into the hipbone or breastbone. A pathologist views the bone marrow and bone under a microscope to look for signs of cancer.
- **Lymph node biopsy**. The removal of all or part of a lymph node. A pathologist views the tissue under a microscope to look for cancer cells. One of the following types of biopsies may be done:
  - **Excisional biopsy**. The removal of an entire lymph node.
  - **Incisional biopsy**. The removal of part of a lymph node.
  - **Core biopsy**. The removal of tissue from a lymph node using a wide needle.

Other areas of the body, such as the liver, lung, bone, bone marrow, and brain, may also have a sample of tissue removed and checked by a pathologist for signs of cancer.

If cancer is found, the following tests may be done to study the cancer cells:

- **Immunohistochemistry**. A laboratory test that uses antibodies to check for certain antigens (markers) in a sample of a patient's tissue. The antibodies are usually linked to an enzyme or a fluorescent dye. After the antibodies bind to a specific antigen in the tissue sample, the enzyme or dye is activated, and the antigen can then be seen under a microscope. This type of test is used to help diagnose cancer and to help tell one type of cancer from another type of cancer.
- **Cytogenetic analysis**. A laboratory test in which the chromosomes of cells in a sample of blood or bone marrow are counted and checked for any changes, such as broken, missing, rearranged, or extra chromosomes. Changes in certain chromosomes may be a sign of cancer. Cytogenetic analysis is used to help diagnose

cancer, plan treatment, or find out how well treatment is working.

- **Fluorescence in situ hybridization (FISH).** A laboratory test is used to look at and count genes or chromosomes in cells and tissues. Pieces of DNA that contain fluorescent dyes are made in the laboratory and added to a sample of a patient's cells or tissues. When these dyed pieces of DNA attach to certain genes or areas of chromosomes in the sample, they light up when viewed under a fluorescent microscope. The FISH test is used to help diagnose cancer and help plan treatment.
- **Immunophenotyping.** A laboratory test that uses antibodies to identify cancer cells based on the types of antigens or markers on the surface of the cells. This test is used to help diagnose specific types of lymphoma.

TREATMENT FOR AIDS-RELATED LYMPHOMAS
Peripheral/Systemic Lymphoma

Lymphoma that starts in the lymph system or elsewhere in the body, other than the brain, is called "peripheral" or "systemic lymphoma." It may spread throughout the body, including to the brain or bone marrow. It is often diagnosed in an advanced stage.

Primary CNS Lymphoma

Primary central nervous system (CNS) lymphoma starts in the central nervous system (brain and spinal cord). It is linked to the Epstein-Barr virus. Lymphoma that starts somewhere else in the body and spreads to the central nervous system is not primary CNS lymphoma.

Chapter 44 |
Other AIDS-Related Health Concerns

Chapter Contents

This section includes text excerpted from "Neuromuscular Diseases Associated with HIV-1 Infection," National Center for Biotechnology Information (NCBI), December 1, 2010. Reviewed February 2022.

In resource-rich environments, highly active antiretroviral therapy (HAART) has led to improved longevity in patients living with human immunodeficiency virus (HIV). In many patients, HIV has become one of a number of chronic illnesses. Some of the comorbid conditions now frequently seen in HIV patients are the same as those that affect the general population such as hypertension, diabetes, and obesity. Others, like HIV-associated nephropathy, are consequences of long-term exposure to HIV. Unfortunately, either due to lack of access to care, treatment failure, or medication nonadherence, there are still patients with advanced acquired immunodeficiency syndrome (AIDS) who are at risk for the neurologic complications seen commonly in the pre-HAART era. Over the past decade, there have also been significant demographic shifts in the epidemic. In the United States, African-Americans, Hispanics, and women, often of lower socioeconomic status, account for a growing number of new infections, and the overall population of people living with HIV/AIDS is aging. The effects of HAART, comorbidities, aging and racial, ethnic, and socioeconomic disparity add new complexity to HIV and its related conditions.

Neurologic disorders are common in HIV. They occur at all stages of the disease and at all levels of the neuraxis. The etiologies of these disorders are variable and include HIV itself and the resulting immunosuppression and dysregulation; other comorbid illnesses and infections; and side effects of HAART and other medications.

DISTAL SYMMETRIC POLYNEUROPATHY

Distal symmetric polyneuropathy (DSP) is the most common neurologic complication of HIV. It is estimated that currently more than 50 percent of patients with advanced HIV have evidence of DSP on neurologic examination. Of these, many are symptomatic with numbness, pain or paresthesias. Although DSP usually occurs as a consequence of HIV itself, toxic neuropathy due to the antiretrovirals stavudine (d4T), didanosine (ddI), and zalcitabine (ddC), commonly referred to as d-drugs, is clinically indistinguishable. These agents, which are thought to cause neuropathy via mitochondrial toxicity, are now uncommonly used in resource-rich environments, although they are still in use in the developing world.

Early studies recognized markers of advanced HIV infection, such as low CD4 count and high viral load, as well as exposure to d-drugs, as predictors of DSP. However, since the introduction of HAART, these risk factors have not been consistently reproduced. Some HAART-era studies have shown no increased risk of HIV-DSP in patients receiving d-drugs, others have found demographic factors including older age, male gender, and white race to be associated with increased risk of HIV-DSP. It is logical that comorbid conditions such as diabetes mellitus, alcohol abuse, vitamin B^{12} deficiency, poor nutritional status and perhaps hepatitis C would also increase the risk of DSP, although this has not been proven.

INFLAMMATORY DEMYELINATING POLYNEUROPATHY

Inflammatory demyelinating polyneuropathy (IDP) may occur in its acute form, acute inflammatory demyelinating polyradiculoneuropathy (AIDP) or Guillain-Barre syndrome (GBS), early in the course of the disease as part of the acute retroviral syndrome. In this setting, its manifestations are similar to those seen in HIV-negative patients with AIDP, and due to the absence of data specific to HIV, treatment recommendations are derived from experience in HIV-negative patients. Most patients presenting with AIDP are initially managed in an inpatient setting to begin treatment and monitor for dangerous complications such as autonomic instability and respiratory failure. First-line treatment of AIDP is either plasmapheresis or intravenous immunoglobulin (IVIg).

The chronic form, Chronic inflammatory demyelinating polyneuropathy (CIDP), is more common in HIV. HIV-positive patients, especially those with high CD4 count, may present similarly to their HIV-negative counterparts, with relapsing motor and sensory symptoms that require ongoing immunomodulatory treatment. However atypical phenotypes are not uncommon. Such cases may fall into the overlap between mononeuropathy multiplex and IDP described by some authors.

MONONEUROPATHIES

Mononeuropathies are relatively common in patients with HIV infection. This is in part due to the high prevalence of the common entrapment neuropathies, such as median neuropathy at the wrist and ulnar neuropathy at the elbow, in the general population. It is also logical to presume that HIV may have a deleterious effect on the peripheral nerves that may predispose patients to entrapment neuropathies even in the absence of an observable polyneuropathy. In general, these focal neuropathies are treated no differently than they are in the HIV-negative population. Focal cranial neuropathies warrant special mention. Unilateral and bilateral facial palsies may occur in HIV-positive patients.

FACIAL PALSIES

Facial palsies have been described in the context of seroconversion with aseptic HIV-associated meningitis, but can occur at any stage of the disease. In most cases, a specific etiology cannot be found and so the facial palsy is classified as idiopathic or Bell's palsy. Specific etiologies of facial palsies in HIV reported in the literature include the varicella-zoster virus (VZV) and meningeal lymphomatosis. Syphilis and tuberculosis (TB) are other potential causes. All of these etiologies have the potential to cause multiple cranial neuropathies. VZV typically causes a facial palsy as part of the Ramsay Hunt syndrome, which is caused by reactivation of latent VZV in the geniculate ganglion causing polyneuritis that may involve cranial nerves V (Trigeminal nerve), VII (Facial nerve), VIII (Vestibulocochlear nerve) and IX (Glossopharyngeal nerve). Ramsay Hunt syndrome is characterized by a herpetic eruption in the cutaneous distribution of the trigeminal nerve accompanied by facial nerve palsy and ear pain. Other symptoms may include tinnitus, vertigo, and loss of hearing or taste. Ramsay Hunt syndrome in the general population is typically treated with antivirals and corticosteroids, although a recent Cochrane review found insufficient evidence to recommend these treatments. Despite the lack of evidence specific to Ramsay Hunt syndrome, some have justified this approach in light of the more complete data available for the treatment of herpes zoster in other parts of the body. This will be addressed in greater detail as part of the discussion of polyradiculopathies. In the HIV-positive patient with Ramsay Hunt syndrome, the antiviral treatment seems prudent. The potential risks and benefits of adjunctive corticosteroids must be weighed for each individual patient, taking into account the degree of immunocompromise.

TB can lead to cranial neuropathies by causing basilar meningitis.

In the general population idiopathic facial palsy, or Bell's palsy, has been attributed to vascular, inflammatory, and viral etiologies, especially herpes viruses. This has led to the common practice of empiric treatment with corticosteroids and antivirals such as acyclovir. Recently, data from a large clinical trial have indicated that in the general population corticosteroids are effective in the treatment of Bell palsy, but antivirals are not. The implication of these findings for the HIV-positive population is unclear. Clinicians may choose to treat these patients with antivirals anyway with the rationale that herpes viruses are often more active in HIV, and therefore more likely to be causative of Bell palsy.

MONONEUROPATHY MULTIPLEX

Classic mononeuropathy multiplex, with painful, stepwise, multifocal deficits due to nerve infarction associated with vasculitis, appears to be rare in HIV. This dramatic syndrome is clinically and pathologically well described in the early literature in patients with advanced AIDS and Cytomegalovirus (CMV) infection. In these patients mononeuropathy multiplex may be rapidly progressive, quickly involving multiple nerve distributions, and even becoming confluent. Decreased motor and sensory potentials consistent with axonal degeneration are most often seen on nerve conduction studies. Electromyography may show denervation. A positive CMV polymerase chain reaction (PCR) in cerebrospinal fluid (CSF), evidence of CMV on nerve biopsy or evidence of CMV infection in other organs such as retinitis, pneumonia, and gastroenteritis, is helpful in diagnosis, but the clinician may choose to treat empirically even in the absence of clearly demonstrable CMV. Treatment is with antivirals such as ganciclovir, foscarnet, and cidofovir. In addition, immune reconstitution with HAART should be attempted whenever possible. The prognosis for recovery is poor, which is at least in part due to the overall health status of these patients. A milder form of mononeuropathy multiplex, involving one or a few nerves, occurs in HIV patients with a high CD4+ count. This syndrome is probably immune-mediated and may be a variant of intrinsically disordered protein (IDP) with more prominent axonal features. Deficits are most often self-limited, resolving after several months. However, in patients with inadequate spontaneous recovery, immunomodulatory treatment such as corticosteroids, plasmapheresis, or IVIg may provide benefit.

AUTONOMIC NEUROPATHY

In other systemic conditions associated with high rates of DSP, such as diabetes, autonomic neuropathy is also common. Early reports from the pre-HAART era suggested that autonomic neuropathy was also common in HIV-positive patients, but these results have not been consistently reproduced in the HAART era. There are several studies from the cardiac literature that demonstrate cardiac autonomic dysfunction in HIV as reflected by decreased heart rate variability. An Indian study assessing the autonomic nervous system in the context of the hypothalamic-pituitary-adrenal axis also demonstrated attenuated autonomic function. However, two recent studies, performed in India and Mozambique, failed to demonstrate autonomic abnormalities using a standard battery of autonomic testing. The African study did find more autonomic symptoms in HIV-positive patients. Further research is needed to determine the prevalence and impact of autonomic neuropathy in HIV.

RADICULOPATHIES

In addition to causing mononeuropathy multiplex, in the patient with advanced AIDS, CMV can infect the cauda equina leading to inflammation and necrosis of the lumbosacral nerve roots and a progressive polyradiculopathy. Patients present with a rapidly evolving cauda equina syndrome, with weakness and numbness in the lower extremities and sphincter dysfunction. Neurological examination reveals a flaccid paraparesis and lower extremity areflexia. The upper extremities and cranial nerves may be involved in advanced cases. Management and prognosis is similar to that described above for CMV-related mononeuropathy multiplex. Although rarer, a similar clinical picture can be caused by neurosyphilis or lymphomatous meningitis. In addition, a patient was observed with a CD4+ count of above 200 who presented with asymmetric weakness of the lower extremities that progressed over one year. Nerve root biopsy revealed Epstein-Barr virus (EBV)-associated neurolymphomatosis of the cauda equina.

Gadolinium enhanced magnetic resonance imaging (MRI) of the lumbosacral spine is usually the first diagnostic step in patients with suspected progressive polyradiculopathy. Although the study may be normal or show only meningeal enhancement in the cauda equina, it is necessary to exclude focal compressive lesions of the cauda equina. Lumbar puncture is also essential, as the diagnosis of CMV-related polyradiculitis is confirmed by detection of CMV in CSF with the polymerase chain reaction (PCR). Low glucose, elevated protein, and a prominent polymorphonuclear pleocytosis in the CSF are considered classical findings, but a relatively normal CSF does not exclude the diagnosis. Electrodiagnostic studies show evidence of severe axonal polyradiculopathy, including low amplitude or absent responses with nerve conduction studies and extensive denervation of lower extremity muscles on needle electromyography (EMG).

MYOPATHY

Several disorders of muscle have been reported in patients with HIV. These disorders range in severity from myalgia and asymptomatically elevated (CK) to rhabdomyolysis. Although these muscle disorders are all rare, the most common is HIV-associated myopathy, also known as "HIV-associated polymyositis." HIV-associated myopathy is clinically and pathologically similar to autoimmune polymyositis in HIV-negative patients. It occurs at all stages of HIV disease and is characterized by slowly progressive, proximal, and symmetric weakness. Myalgias are often present but are not specific. The diagnostic criteria used to define polymyositis in HIV-negative patients are also useful in the diagnosis of HIV-associated myopathy. These include objective muscle weakness, elevated serum CK, myopathic findings on EMG, and a myopathic muscle biopsy. The presence of all four criteria leads to a definitive diagnosis; if three are met the diagnosis is probable. Pathologic characteristics include inflammatory infiltrates of T-cells and macrophages primarily in the endomysial parenchyma. Fiber necrosis may also be seen.

Due to the rarity of HIV-associated myopathy, the prognosis and best course of treatment are not well established. The largest case series found that over half of those treated with corticosteroids attained complete remission and were able to discontinue therapy after a mean of 9 months. The remainder of the patients improved over months to years. Our experience has been more variable. While several of our patients have responded to immunomodulatory therapy with corticosteroids or IVIg, we follow several patients with HIV-myopathy who have had a significant weakness for many years with only a modest response to these treatments. Other immunosuppressive therapies that are used in the treatment of polymyositis, such as methotrexate and azathioprine, may be considered in HIV-associated myopathy, but there is little evidence of efficacy, and concern over their immunosuppressant toxicity. The mechanism by which HIV leads to inflammatory myopathy is not fully understood, but a T-cell mediated and MHC-I-restricted cytotoxic process triggered by HIV has been proposed. HIV-associated myopathy has also been described as part of an immune reconstitution inflammatory syndrome (IRIS).

Certain antiretrovirals may lead to toxic myopathy, presumably through impairment of mitochondrial function. Zidovudine (AZT) myopathy can manifest as fixed weakness or exercise intolerance which resolves within months of withdrawing the drug. CK level is normal or mildly elevated and muscle biopsy reveals ragged red fibers. Stavudine (d4T), which is now used uncommonly in resource-rich nations, can cause HIV-associated neuromuscular weakness syndrome (HANWS). HANWS is characterized by rapidly progressive weakness, resembling Guillain-Barre syndrome, associated with lactic acidosis, nausea, vomiting, weight loss, abdominal distension, hepatomegaly, and lipoatrophy. Electrodiagnostic studies and pathologic specimens reported in a study of 69 patients, revealed heterogeneous etiologies of weakness. Severe axonal polyneuropathy was the most common, however demyelinating and mixed neuropathies as well as myopathy also occurred. Muscle biopsy specimens revealed evidence of mitochondrial dysfunction, including ragged red fibers and depletion of mitochondrial DNA. These findings, together with lactic acidosis, support a mitochondrial mechanism.

There are reports of various other forms of myopathy in HIV-positive patients. Infectious myopathy, or pyomyositis, has been described in patients with advanced AIDS. Infections are usually bacterial with staphylococcus aureus cultured most commonly. Other possible causative organisms include toxoplasmosis, cryptococcus, and mycoplasma avium intracellulare. The wasting syndrome seen in AIDS may be a myopathy in some cases. Acute rhabdomyolysis with myalgia, weakness and markedly elevated CK level has been reported either as an effect of HIV itself or as a side effect of medications including didanosine. Dermatomyositis, nemaline rod myopathy, and inclusion body myositis have also been reported.

Section 44.2 | Oral Health Issues

This section includes text excerpted from "HIV/AIDS & Oral Health," National Institute of Dental and Craniofacial Research (NIDCR), July 2018. Reviewed February 2022.

People with human immunodeficiency virus (HIV), the virus that causes acquired immunodeficiency syndrome (AIDS), are at special risk for oral health problems. Some of the most common oral problems for people with HIV/AIDS are: chronic dry mouth, gingivitis, bone loss around the teeth (periodontitis), canker sores, oral warts, fever blisters, oral candidiasis (thrush), hairy leukoplakia (which causes a rough, white patch on the tongue), and dental caries. Combination antiretroviral therapy (cART), which is used to treat the HIV condition and restore immune system function, has made some oral problems less common. Oral conditions can be painful, annoying, and can lead to other problems.

CAUSES OF ORAL HEALTH ISSUES

People with HIV/AIDS have an increased risk for oral health problems because HIV/AIDS weakens the immune system and makes it harder to fight off infection.

SYMPTOMS OF ORAL HEALTH ISSUES

Oral health problems are listed in the Table 44.1.

TREATMENT FOR ORAL HEALTH ISSUES

The most common oral problems linked with HIV can be treated. So talk with your doctor or dentist about what treatment might work for you.

PREVENTION TIPS FOR ORAL HEALTH ISSUES

In addition to the problems listed in Table 44.1, you may experience dry mouth. Dry mouth happens when you do not have enough saliva, or spit, to keep your mouth wet. Saliva helps you chew and digest food, protects teeth from decay, and prevents infections by controlling bacteria and fungi in the mouth. Without enough saliva, you could develop tooth decay or other infections and might have trouble chewing and swallowing. Your mouth might also feel sticky or dry and have a burning feeling, and you may have cracked, chapped lips.

To help with a dry mouth, try these things:
- Sip water or sugarless drinks often.
- Chew sugarless gum or suck on sugarless hard candy.
- Avoid tobacco.
- Avoid alcohol.
- Avoid salty foods.
- Use a humidifier at night.

Table 44.1. Symptoms of Oral Health Issues

Description	It Could Be:	What and Where?	Painful?	Contagious?	Treatment
Red sores ulcers	Aphthous. Also known as "Canker Sores"	Red sores that might also have a yellow-gray film on top. They are usually on the moveable parts of the mouth such as the tongue or inside of the cheeks and lips.	Yes	No	Mild cases – Over-the-counter (OTC) cream or prescription mouthwash that contains corticosteroids; More severe cases – corticosteroids in a pill form
Red sores ulcers	Herpes. A viral infection	Red sores usually on the roof of the mouth. They are sometimes on the outside of the lips, where they are called "fever blisters."	Sometimes	Yes	Prescription pill can reduce healing time and frequency of outbreaks.
White hairlike growth	Hairy Leukoplakia caused by the Epstein-Barr virus	White patches that do not wipe away; sometimes very thick and "hairlike." Usually appear on the side of the tongue or sometimes inside the cheeks and lower lip.	Not usually	No	Mild cases – not usually required; More severe cases – a prescription pill that may reduce severity of symptoms. In some severe cases, a pain reliever might also be required.
White creamy or bumpy patches like cottage cheese	Candidiasis, a fungal (yeast) infection – Also known as "thrush"	White or yellowish patches (or can sometimes be red). If wiped away, there will be redness or bleeding underneath. They can appear anywhere in the mouth.	Sometimes, a burning feeling	No	Mild cases – prescription antifungal lozenge or mouthwash; More severe cases – prescription antifungal pills.

Table 44.1. Continued

Description	It Could Be:	What and Where?	Painful?	Contagious?	Treatment
Warts		Small, white, gray, or pinkish rough bumps that look like cauliflower. They can appear inside the lips and on other parts of the mouth.	Not usually	Possibly	Inside the mouth – a doctor can remove them surgically or use "cryosurgery" – a way of freezing them off. On the lips – a prescription cream that will wear away the wart. Warts can return after treatment.

Talk to your doctor or dentist about prescribing artificial saliva, which may help keep your mouth moist.

Section 44.3 | Kidney Disease

This section includes text excerpted from "HIV and Kidney Disease," HIVinfo, U.S. Department of Health and Human Services (HHS), August 19, 2021.

WHAT ARE THE KIDNEYS AND WHAT DO THEY DO?

The kidneys are two fist-sized organs in the body. They are located near the middle of the back on either side of the spine.

The main job of the kidneys is to filter harmful waste and extra water from the blood. The waste and water become urine, which is flushed from the body. The kidneys also release hormones that help control blood pressure, make red blood cells, and keep bones strong.

Kidney function declines as people age. Injury or disease, including HIV infection, can damage the kidneys. Damage to the kidneys can lead to kidney disease (also called "renal disease"). Kidney disease can advance to kidney failure known as "end-stage renal disease."

WHAT ARE THE CAUSES OF KIDNEY DISEASE?

Diabetes and high blood pressure are the leading causes of kidney disease. Other factors that increase the risk of kidney disease include heart disease and a family history of kidney failure.

A person's risk of kidney disease increases as they get older. The longer a person has diabetes, high blood pressure, or heart disease, the greater their risk of kidney disease.

The risk of kidney failure is especially high among African Americans, Hispanics, and American Indians, partially because these communities have high rates of diabetes and high blood pressure.

ARE PEOPLE WITH HIV AT RISK FOR KIDNEY DISEASE?

The risk factors for kidney disease in people with human immuno-deficiency virus (HIV) include all those listed above. In addition, poorly controlled HIV infection and coinfection with the hepatitis C virus (HCV) increase the risk of kidney disease in people with HIV.

Antiretroviral therapy (ART) is the use of HIV medicines to treat HIV. People on ART take a combination of HIV medicines (called an "HIV treatment regimen") every day. HIV medicines are recommended for everyone who has HIV. Some HIV medicines can affect the kidneys. Healthcare providers carefully consider the risk of kidney damage when recommending specific HIV medi-cines to include in an HIV treatment regimen. If a person with HIV shows signs of kidney disease, their healthcare provider may adjust the dose of their HIV medicines or change which HIV medicines are included in their treatment regimen.

WHAT ARE THE SYMPTOMS OF KIDNEY DISEASE?

Kidney disease can advance very slowly. Slowly worsening kid-ney disease is called "chronic kidney disease." As kidney disease gets worse, a person may have swelling of the legs, feet, or ankles (called "edema"). Symptoms of advanced chronic kidney disease can include:

- Increased or decreased urination
- Feeling tired or having trouble sleeping
- Nausea and vomiting
- Itching or numbness

Blood and urine tests are used to detect kidney disease. Care for people with HIV includes testing for kidney disease.

WHAT IS THE TREATMENT FOR KIDNEY DISEASE?

People with kidney disease can take steps to protect their kidneys from further damage. For example, many people with kidney dis-ease take medicines to control high blood pressure. They may also reduce the amount of salt and protein in their diet to manage their kidney disease. Some people live with kidney disease for many years; in others, kidney disease progresses to kidney failure. The treatments for kidney failure are dialysis and a kidney transplant. Both treatments take over the job of the failed kidneys.

- There are two main types of dialysis. Like the kidneys, both types filter harmful waste and extra water out of the blood. In hemodialysis, a machine outside of the body is used to filter the blood. In peritoneal dialysis, the lining of the abdomen filters the blood inside the body.
- A kidney transplant is surgery to place a healthy kidney from a donor into the body of a person with kidney failure. The donated kidney can be from a person who just died or from a living person.

Both dialysis and a kidney transplant are used to treat kidney failure in people with HIV.

HOW CAN PEOPLE WITH HIV REDUCE THEIR RISK OF KIDNEY DISEASE?

People with HIV can take the following steps to reduce their risk of kidney disease:

- Take HIV medicines every day to keep HIV under control.
- Eat a healthy diet that includes fresh fruits, fresh or frozen vegetables, whole grains, and low-fat or fat-free dairy products.
- Cut back on foods high in salt and sugar.
- Be physically active for 30 minutes or more on most days.
- Keep all medical appointments. During medical visits, talk to a healthcare provider about the risk of kidney disease.

Section 44.4 | Heart Disease

This section includes text excerpted from "HIV and Heart Disease," HIVinfo, U.S. Department of Health and Human Services (HHS), August 10, 2021.

WHAT IS HEART DISEASE?

There are many different types of heart diseases. Coronary heart disease (also called "coronary artery disease") is the most common type of heart disease. It is the leading cause of death in the United States.

WHAT CAUSES HEART DISEASE

Heart disease is caused by the buildup of plaque inside the blood vessels (called the "coronary arteries") that carry blood to the heart. Plaque is a waxy substance made up of fat, cholesterol, calcium, and other substances found in the blood. Over time, plaque buildup in the coronary arteries (called "atherosclerosis") reduces the blood flow to the heart, which can cause chest pain (called "angina") or a heart attack.

WHAT ARE THE RISK FACTORS FOR HEART DISEASE?

Some risk factors for heart disease can be changed or controlled by lifestyle changes or medicines, while other risk factors cannot. Risk factors that can be controlled to prevent or delay heart disease include the following:

- High blood pressure (also known as "hypertension")
- High blood cholesterol levels
- Diabetes
- Eating an unhealthy diet
- A lack of physical activity
- Smoking
- Being overweight or obese
- Stress

Risk factors for heart disease that cannot be changed include having a family history of early heart disease and older age.

ARE PEOPLE WITH HIV AT RISK FOR HEART DISEASE?

Yes. The risk factors for heart disease are the same for people with human immunodeficiency virus (HIV) and people without HIV. However, HIV and some HIV medicines may increase the risk of heart disease in people with HIV.

WHAT ARE THE SYMPTOMS OF HEART DISEASE?

Some people who have heart disease have no symptoms. However, some people may have chest pain, shortness of breath, fatigue, or weakness. If you have any of these symptoms, contact your health-care provider.

Chest pain that does not go away or occurs while a person is resting may be a sign of a heart attack.

WHAT IS THE TREATMENT FOR HEART DISEASE?

Treatment for heart disease often includes lifestyle changes. For example, people with heart disease may change their eating habits, exercise more to lose weight, or quit smoking.

Medicines and surgery are also used to treat heart disease.

Medicines

Medicines used to treat heart disease include drugs to lower blood pressure, reduce cholesterol levels, or prevent or relieve chest pain. Some of these medicines may interact with HIV medicines. Healthcare providers carefully consider potential drug-drug interactions between HIV medicines and any other medicines a person may be taking.

Surgery

Coronary artery bypass grafting (CABG) is the most common type of surgery to treat heart disease in adults. During CABG, a healthy artery or vein from the body is used to bypass (go around) the blocked part of a coronary artery.

HOW CAN PEOPLE WITH HIV REDUCE THEIR RISK OF HEART DISEASE?

People with HIV can take the following steps to reduce their risk of heart disease:

- Take HIV medicines every day to keep HIV under control.
- Eat a healthy diet that includes lots of vegetables, fruits, and whole grains, and is low in saturated fats, added sugars, and salt.
- Be physically active on a regular basis.
- Quit smoking.
- Keep all medical appointments. During medical visits, talk to a healthcare provider about the risk of heart disease.

Section 44.5 | Wasting Syndrome

This section includes text excerpted from "HIV Wasting Syndrome," U.S. Department of Veterans Affairs (VA), December 27, 2019.

The wasting syndrome refers to an unwanted weight loss of more than 10 percent of a person's body weight, with either diarrhea or weakness and fever that have lasted at least 30 days. For a 150-pound man, this means a weight loss of 15 pounds or more. Weight loss can result in loss of both fat and muscle. Once lost, the weight is difficult to regain.

The condition may occur in people with advanced HIV disease and can be caused by many things: HIV, inflammation, or opportunistic infections. The person may get full easily or have no appetite at all.

The most important treatment for wasting syndrome is the effective treatment of HIV with antiretroviral medications. In addition, the condition may be controlled, to some degree, by eating a good diet. A "good diet" for a person with HIV may not be the low-fat, low-calorie diet recommended for healthy people. Compared with other people, you may need to take in more calories and protein to keep from losing muscle mass. To do this, you can add to your meals:

- Peanut butter
- Legumes (dried beans and peas)
- Cheeses
- Eggs
- Instant breakfast drinks
- Milkshakes
- Sauces

You can also maintain or increase muscle mass through exercise, especially with progressive strength-building exercises. These include resistance and weight-lifting exercise.

Part 6 | Living with HIV Infection

Chapter 45 | **Coping with an HIV/AIDS Diagnosis**

Finding out that you have human immunodeficiency virus (HIV) can be scary and overwhelming. If you feel overwhelmed, try to remember that you can get help and that these feelings will get better with time.

Testing positive for HIV is a serious matter but one that you can deal with. Starting HIV medications early is one of the best ways to take care of your health. This chapter will take you through the steps you need to take to protect your health:

- Understand your diagnosis
- Find support
- Work with your provider
- Monitor your health
- Be aware of possible complications
- Protect others
- Start treatment
- Move forward with your life

UNDERSTAND YOUR DIAGNOSIS

When your provider tells you that you have HIV, it means that you have been infected with HIV. However, the HIV test does not tell you if you have acquired immunodeficiency syndrome (AIDS), how long you have been infected, or how sick you might be. Soon after your diagnosis, your provider will run other tests to determine your overall health, and the condition of your immune system.

This chapter includes text excerpted from "Getting an HIV Diagnosis – Your Next Steps: Entire Lesson," U.S. Department of Veterans Affairs (VA), June 3, 2019.

LEARN ABOUT HIV

The more you learn about HIV, the better you will be at making decisions about your health. You do not have to learn everything all at once. It is important to go at a pace that is comfortable for you.

There are many ways to learn about HIV:

- Read information online. Remember that there is a lot of internet information that can be inaccurate or misleading. Be sure to look for reputable sites whose content can be trusted. Check out government or nonprofit educational organizations that deal with HIV issues.
- Use your local library. The most current information may be in the library's collection of newspapers, journals, and magazines.
- Check with your local medical center to see if there is an on-site library where you can find patient materials on HIV. Your provider will also likely have handouts to share with you.

TELLING OTHERS

Deciding to tell others that you are living with HIV is an important personal choice. It can make a big difference in how you cope with the disease. It can also affect your relationships with people.

If you decide to share information about your diagnosis, it is best to tell people you trust and people who are directly affected. These include:

- Family members
- People you spend a lot of time with, such as good friends
- All your healthcare providers, such as doctors, nurses, and dentists
- Sex partner(s)

You do not have to tell everyone about your HIV status right away. You might want to talk with a counselor or social worker first.

FIND SUPPORT

Talk with others who are living with HIV. Ask your provider if they know of any support groups. Or you can search the internet for virtual groups to join. Always discuss what you learn from these sources with your provider. The information may not be accurate; and even if it is, it may not be right for your particular situation.

Finding support means finding people who are willing to help you through the emotional and physical issues you are facing. If you let the right people in your life know that you are living with HIV, they can:

- Offer you support and understanding
- Provide you with assistance, such as helping with child care, or making medical visits
- Learn about prevention

SUPPORT RESOURCES

Joining a group of people who are facing the same challenges you are facing can have important benefits. These include making new friendships, improving your mood, and better understanding your needs and those of your family. People in support groups often help each other deal with common experiences associated with HIV.

Support groups are especially helpful if you live alone or do not have family and friends nearby.

There are different types of support available, from hotlines to face-to-face groups. Here are descriptions of some of the most popular types, and suggestions about how to find them.

Hotlines or Chats

Hotlines or chats can provide information, support, or link you with local/national services. Search online for hotlines or websites with a chat feature.

Self-Help Organizations

Self-help groups enable people to share experiences and pool their knowledge to help each other and themselves. They are run by members, not by professionals (though professionals are involved).

You may, for example, be able to find groups specifically for women, people of color, gay men, transgender individuals, or other specific groups of people. These groups are typically volunteer, nonprofit organizations, with no fees (though sometimes there are small dues).

WORK WITH YOUR PROVIDER

It is so important to get medical care and start treatment as soon as you find out you have HIV. Please see a provider with experience treating people with HIV. Most VA providers who treat HIV are specialists in infectious disease. They work with a team of other health professionals who focus on HIV as a chronic, or lifelong, disease.

Treatments for HIV are not perfect (no medicine is), but are very tolerable and extremely effective for most people. They also work very well to minimize the chance that you may transmit HIV to sex partners (for pregnant women they also decrease the risk of infecting the baby). A healthcare provider can explain the best options for you.

Before Appointments

Start a list or notebook of your questions or concerns so you do not forget anything. Prepare for your appointment with your provider by writing down:

- Any symptoms or problems you want to tell your provider about (including things such as poor sleep, trouble concentrating, feeling tired)
- A list of the medications, herbs, and vitamins that you are taking, including a list of any HIV medications you have taken in the past and any problems you had when taking them.
- Upcoming tests or new information you have heard about
- Changes in your living situation, such as a job change

You may want to ask a friend or family member to come with you and take notes.

During Appointments

Go over your lab results, and keep track of them. If your provider wants you to have some medical tests, make sure you understand what the test is for and what your provider will do with the results. If you do not understand what your provider is saying, ask them to explain it in everyday terms.

If you feel your provider has forgotten something during the appointment, it is better to ask about it than to leave wondering about it. It is your right to ask questions of your provider. You also have a legal right to see your medical records.

Be open. Your provider is not there to judge you, but to help make decisions based on your particular circumstances. Tell your provider about your sexual and drug use history. These behaviors can put you at risk of getting other sexually transmitted diseases (STDs). If your body is fighting off these other diseases, it will not be able to fight off HIV as effectively.

MONITOR YOUR HEALTH

Once you have been diagnosed with HIV, you need to pay close attention to your health.

You can keep track of your health in two ways. First, have regular lab tests done. Lab tests can often show signs of illness before you have any noticeable symptoms.

Second, listen to what your body is telling you, and be on the alert for signs that something is not right. Note any change in your health – good or bad. And do not be afraid to call your provider.

Have Regular Lab Tests

Your provider will use laboratory tests to check your health. Some of these tests will be done soon after you learn you have HIV.

The lab tests look at several things:

- How well your immune system is functioning
- How well your medications are controlling the HIV
- Certain basic body functions (tests look at your kidneys, liver, cholesterol, and blood cells)
- Whether you have other diseases that are associated with HIV

For your first few provider visits, be prepared to have a lot of blood drawn. Do not worry, you are not going to have so much blood drawn at every appointment.

BE AWARE OF POSSIBLE COMPLICATIONS

By weakening your immune system, HIV can leave you vulnerable to certain cancers and infections. These infections are called "opportunistic" because they take the opportunity to attack when your immune system is weak. But the good news is that taking your HIV medications can help prevent these infections.

HIV also is an inflammatory disease that affects many parts of the body, not just the immune system. That means that HIV can affect organs such as the brain, kidneys, liver, and heart and may increase the risk of some cancers.

HIV medicines can sometimes have side effects. Sometimes these can raise the risk of heart disease or kidney disease. It is important that you let your providers know if you notice any concerning symptoms.

Know When to Call Your Provider

You do not need to panic every time you have a headache or get a runny nose. But if a symptom is concerning you or is not going away, it is always best to have a provider check it out.

The following symptoms may or may not be serious, but do not wait until your next appointment before calling your provider if you are experiencing them.

Breathing problems:
- Persistent cough
- Wheezing or noisy breathing
- Sharp pain when breathing
- Difficulty catching your breath

Skin problems:
- The appearance of brownish, purple, or pink blotches on the skin
- New or worsening rash – especially important if you are taking medication

Eye or vision problems:
- Blurring, wavy lines, sudden blind spots
- Eye pain
- Sensitivity to light

Aches and pains:
- Numbness, tingling, or pain in hands and feet
- Headache, especially when accompanied by a fever
- Stiffness in neck
- Severe or persistent cough
- Persistent cramps
- Pain in lower abdomen, often during sex (women in particular)

Other symptoms:
- Mental changes – confusion, disorientation, loss of memory or balance
- The appearance of swollen lymph nodes (glands), especially when larger on one side of the body
- Diarrhea – when severe, accompanied by fever, or lasting more than 3 days
- Weight loss
- High or persistent fever
- Fatigue
- Frequent urination

PROTECT OTHERS

When you are living with HIV, it is important that you take measures so you do not pass the virus to sex partners, to injection drug partners, or (for women who wish to become pregnant) to a baby during pregnancy or delivery, or by breast-feeding. Starting and staying on HIV medications (antiretroviral therapy, or ART) is a hugely effective way to minimize the risk of transmitting the HIV virus. Using condoms and clean injection equipment also can prevent HIV from passing to other people. Condoms can also protect you from getting other STDs. Partners who do not have

HIV can use pre-exposure prophylaxis (PrEP) a daily pill that can prevent HIV infection.

Sometimes it can be difficult to explain that you have HIV to people you have had sex with or shared syringes with in the past. However, it is important that they know so they can get tested. If you need help telling people that you may have exposed them to HIV, many city or county health departments will tell them for you, without using your name. Ask your provider about this service.

Before telling your partner that you are living with HIV, take some time alone to think about how you want to bring up the subject.

- Decide when and where would be the best time and place to have a conversation. Choose a time when you expect that you will both be comfortable, rested, and as relaxed as possible.
- Think about how your partner may react to stressful situations. If there is a history of violence in your relationship, consider your safety first and make a plan with a case manager or counselor.

START TREATMENT

When or whether to start treatment for HIV is a decision that each person must make with their providers. In general, experts recommend starting HIV treatment very soon after your diagnosis; this can help prevent some of the damage that HIV causes in many parts of the body. HIV treatment (known as "antiretroviral therapy," or "ART") is strongly recommended for all people with HIV, and more urgently for anyone who has evidence of immune suppression (a CD4+ cell count that is below normal) or an AIDS diagnosis (an infection or cancer associated with HIV). It is also urgently recommended for anyone who has a sex partner who does not have HIV, and for women who may become pregnant.

MOVE FORWARD WITH YOUR LIFE

Life does not end with a diagnosis of HIV. In fact, with proper treatment, people with HIV usually live long healthy lives. HIV can be a manageable chronic disease, such as diabetes or heart disease. Taking care of your overall health can help you deal with HIV:

- Take your medicines every day
- Get regular medical and dental checkups
- Eat a healthy diet
- Exercise regularly
- Avoid smoking and recreational drug use
- Go easy on alcohol
- Use condoms during sex (it can protect others from getting HIV, prevent unintended pregnancy, and protect you from other STDs)

Chapter 46 | Staying Healthy When You Have HIV/AIDS

Section 46.1 | **Nutrition and Food Safety**

This section includes text excerpted from "HIV and Nutrition and Food Safety," HIVinfo, U.S. Department of Health and Human Services (HHS), August 23, 2021.

WHY IS GOOD NUTRITION IMPORTANT FOR PEOPLE LIVING WITH HIV?

Good nutrition is about finding and maintaining a healthy eating style. Good nutrition supports overall health and helps maintain the immune system. It also helps people with human immunodeficiency virus (HIV) maintain a healthy weight and absorb HIV medicines.

HIV attacks and destroys the immune system, which makes it harder for the body to fight off infections. People with HIV take a combination of HIV medicines (called an "HIV treatment regimen") every day. The medicines prevent HIV from destroying the immune system. A healthy diet also helps strengthen the immune system and keep people with HIV healthy.

WHAT IS A HEALTHY DIET FOR PEOPLE LIVING WITH HIV?

In general, the basics of a healthy diet are the same for everyone, including people with HIV.

- Eat a variety of foods from the five food groups: fruits, vegetables, grains, protein foods, and dairy.
- Eat the right amount of food to maintain a healthy weight.
- Choose foods low in saturated fat, sodium (salt), and added sugars.

CAN HIV OR HIV MEDICINES CAUSE NUTRITION-RELATED PROBLEMS?

HIV and HIV medicines can sometimes cause nutrition-related problems. For example, some HIV-related infections can make it hard to eat or swallow. Side effects from HIV medicines, such as loss of appetite, nausea, or diarrhea, can make it hard to stick to an HIV regimen. If you have HIV and are having a nutrition-related problem, talk to your healthcare provider.

555

To avoid nutrition-related problems, people with HIV must also pay attention to food safety.

WHAT IS FOOD SAFETY?

Food and water can be contaminated with germs that cause illnesses (called "foodborne illnesses" or "food poisoning"). Food safety is about how to select, handle, prepare, and store food to prevent foodborne illnesses.

WHY IS FOOD SAFETY IMPORTANT FOR PEOPLE LIVING WITH HIV?

Because HIV damages the immune system, foodborne illnesses are likely to be more serious and last longer in people with HIV than in people with a healthy immune system. Following food safety guidelines reduces the risk of foodborne illnesses.

WHAT STEPS CAN PEOPLE WITH HIV TAKE TO PREVENT FOODBORNE ILLNESSES?

If you have HIV, follow these food safety guidelines to reduce your risk of foodborne illnesses:
- Do not eat or drink the following foods:
  - Raw eggs or foods that contain raw eggs, for example, homemade cookie dough
  - Raw or undercooked poultry, meat, and seafood
  - Unpasteurized milk or dairy products and fruit juices

Follow the four basic steps to food safety: clean, separate, cook, and chill.
- **Clean**. Wash your hands, cooking utensils, and countertops often when preparing foods.
- **Separate**. Separate foods to prevent the spread of any germs from one food to another. For example, keep raw meat, poultry, seafood, and eggs separate from foods that are ready to eat, including fruits, vegetables, and breads.

- **Cook**. Use a food thermometer to make sure that foods are cooked to safe temperatures.
- **Chill**. Refrigerate or freeze meat, poultry, eggs, seafood, or other foods that are likely to spoil within 2 hours of cooking or purchasing.

Section 46.2 | Exercise and Physical Activity

This section contains text excerpted from the following sources: Text beginning with the heading "Should People Living with HIV Exercise?" is excerpted from "Exercise and Physical Activity," HIV.gov, U.S. Department of Health and Human Services (HHS), November 4, 2020; Text under the heading "Exercise for People with HIV" is excerpted from "Exercise for People with HIV," U.S. Department of Veterans Affairs (VA), November 20, 2020.

SHOULD PEOPLE LIVING WITH HIV EXERCISE?

Yes! Being HIV-positive is no different from being HIV-negative when it comes to exercise. Regular physical activity and exercise are part of a healthy lifestyle for everyone, including people living with HIV.

WHAT ARE THE BENEFITS OF PHYSICAL ACTIVITY?

Physical activity has many important benefits. It can:
- Boost your mood
- Sharpen your focus
- Reduce your stress
- Improve your sleep

Physical activity can also help you reduce your risk of developing cardiovascular disease, high blood pressure, type 2 diabetes, and several types of cancer. These are all health conditions that can affect people living with HIV.

HOW MUCH ACTIVITY SHOULD YOU DO?

According to the evidence-based Physical Activity Guidelines (2018), adults need at least 150 to 300 minutes per week of moderate-intensity aerobic activity, such as biking, brisk walking, or fast dancing. Adults also need muscle-strengthening activity, like lifting weights or doing push-ups, at least 2 days per week.

If you are living with HIV or have another chronic health condition, talk to your healthcare provider or a physical activity specialist to make sure these guidelines are right for you.

The most important thing is to move more and sit less!

WHAT TYPES OF ACTIVITY ARE RIGHT FOR PEOPLE LIVING WITH HIV?

People living with HIV can do the same types of physical activity and exercise as individuals who do not have HIV.

Physical activity is any body movement that works your muscles and requires more energy than resting. Brisk walking, running, biking, dancing, jumping rope, and swimming are a few examples of physical activity.

Exercise is a type of physical activity that is planned and structured with the goal of improving your health or fitness. Taking an aerobics class and playing on a sports team are examples of exercise.

Both are part of living healthy.

Take time to find a fitness routine that you enjoy. You may consider taking part in a group activity that allows you to engage with others. Make it fun, and commit to being physically active regularly.

EXERCISE FOR PEOPLE WITH HIV

Regular exercise is part of a healthy lifestyle when you are living with HIV.

Benefits of exercise include:
- Maintains or builds muscle mass
- Reduces cholesterol and triglyceride levels (less risk of heart disease)
- Increases energy
- Regulates bowel function
- Strengthens bones (less risk of osteoporosis)
- Improves blood circulation
- Increases lung capacity

- Helps with sound, restful sleep
- Lowers stress
- Improves appetite

Before Starting

Before starting an exercise program, talk to your healthcare provider. Consider your current health status and other medical conditions that may affect the type of exercise you can do.

Make sure you can set aside time for your exercise program. Experts recommend about 150 minutes (2-1/2 hours) of moderate aerobic activity per week. That means about 30 minutes of brisk walking, bicycling, or working around the house, 5 days a week. This amount of exercise can reduce the risks of developing coronary heart disease, high blood pressure, colon cancer, and diabetes.

If this amount of time seems too much, consider starting with 3 times a week. The important thing is consistency. This is an ongoing program and you will not benefit without consistency.

Types of Exercise

Two types of exercise are resistance training and aerobic exercise. Resistance training, sometimes called "strength training," helps to build muscle strength and mass. Aerobic exercise is important because it strengthens your lungs and your heart.

Section 46.3 | Mental Health

This section includes text excerpted from "HIV and Mental Health," HIVinfo, U.S. Department of Health and Human Services (HHS), August 13, 2021.

WHAT IS MENTAL HEALTH?

Mental health refers to a person's overall emotional, psychological, and social well-being. Mental health affects how people think, feel, and act. Good mental health helps people make healthy choices, reach personal goals, develop healthy relationships, and cope with stress.

Poor mental health means people find it difficult to manage how they feel, think, act, or cope with stress. Poor mental health is not the same as mental illness. Mental illnesses are mental, behavioral, or emotional disorders that may not result in any impairment or may result in mild, moderate, or severe impairment that may limit or interfere with function in one or more areas of life. Mental illnesses include many different conditions, such as posttraumatic stress disorder (PTSD), bipolar disorder, and schizophrenia.

A person can have poor mental health and not have a diagnosed mental illness. Likewise, a person with a mental illness can still enjoy mental well-being.

If you are living with the human immunodeficiency virus (HIV), it is important to take care of both your physical health and your mental health.

ARE PEOPLE WITH HIV AT RISK FOR MENTAL-HEALTH CONDITIONS?

Anyone can have mental-health problems. Mental-health conditions are common in the United States. According to the National Institute of Mental Health (NIMH), in 2019, about one in five American adults experienced a mental-health issue.

People with HIV are at high risk of some mental-health conditions because of the stress associated with living with HIV. For example, people living with HIV are twice as likely to have depression as people who do not have HIV.

It is important to remember that mental-health conditions are treatable and that people who have mental-health problems can recover.

WHAT CAN CAUSE MENTAL-HEALTH PROBLEMS IN PEOPLE WITH HIV?

The following factors can increase the risk of mental-health problems in anyone:
- Major life changes, such as the death of a loved one or the loss of a job
- Negative life experiences, such as abuse or trauma

- Biological factors, such as genes or brain chemistry
- A family history of mental-health problems

In addition to these factors, the stress of having a serious medical illness or condition, like HIV, may also negatively affect a person's mental health. Situations that can contribute to mental-health problems in people with HIV include:

- Difficulty in telling others about an HIV diagnosis
- Stigma and discrimination associated with HIV
- Loss of social support and isolation
- Difficulty in getting mental-health services

In people with HIV, HIV infection and related opportunistic infections can affect the brain and the rest of the nervous system. This may lead to changes in how a person thinks and behaves. In addition, some medicines used to treat HIV may have side effects that affect a person's mental health.

WHAT ARE THE WARNING SIGNS OF A MENTAL-HEALTH PROBLEM?

Changes in how a person feels or acts can be a warning sign of a mental-health problem. For example, potential signs of depression include:

- Losing interest in activities that are usually enjoyable
- Experiencing persistent sadness or feeling empty
- Feeling anxious or stressed
- Having suicidal thoughts

If you have any signs of a mental-health problem, it is important to get help.

WHAT SHOULD PEOPLE WITH HIV DO IF THEY NEED HELP FOR A MENTAL-HEALTH PROBLEM?

People with HIV can talk to their healthcare provider about how they are feeling. They can also tell their healthcare providers if they are having any problems with drugs or alcohol.

Healthcare providers will consider whether any HIV medicines may be affecting the person's mental health. They can also help people with HIV find a mental healthcare provider, such as a psychiatrist or therapist.

Here are additional ways that people with HIV can improve their mental health:

- Join a support group
- Try meditation, yoga, or deep breathing to relax
- Get enough sleep, eat healthy meals, and stay physically active

Section 46.4 | HIV, Alcohol, and Drugs

This section includes text excerpted from "Drugs, Alcohol, and HIV," U.S. Department of Veterans Affairs (VA), April 30, 2019.

If you have just found out that you are human immunodeficiency virus (HIV) positive, you might be wondering what alcohol and other "recreational" drugs will do to your body. (Recreational drugs are drugs that are not being used for medical purposes, such as cocaine, amphetamines, and pot; this also includes prescription medicines that are being used for pleasure.)

You may be wondering whether these drugs are bad for your immune system. And what about your HIV medications – can recreational drugs affect those?

Each person is different, and a lot depends on which drugs you use, how much you use, and how often you use them.

However, most experts would agree that, in large amounts, drugs and alcohol are bad for your immune system and your overall health. Remember, when you have HIV, your immune system is already weakened.

In this series, you can read about what alcohol and drugs can do to your overall health.

DRUGS AND ALCOHOL: EFFECTS ON YOUR IMMUNE SYSTEM

Drinking too much alcohol can weaken your immune system. A weaker immune system will have a harder time fighting off common infections (such as a cold), as well as HIV-related infections. A weaker immune system also increases the chance that you will experience more side effects from your HIV medications.

Smoking marijuana (pot) or any other drug irritates the lungs. You may be more likely to get serious lung infections, such as pneumonia.

Other common recreational drugs, such as cocaine or crystal methamphetamine ("meth," "speed"), can leave your body dehydrated and exhausted, as well as lead to skin irritation. All of these things can make it easier for you to get infections.

Alcohol and other drugs affect your liver the most. The liver rounds up waste from chemicals that you put in your body. Those chemicals include recreational drugs as well as prescription drugs, such as your HIV medications. A weaker liver means it is less efficient.

If you also have hepatitis C (or any other kind of hepatitis), your liver is already working very hard to fight the disease itself and deal with the strong drugs that you may be taking for your hepatitis treatment.

DRUGS AND ALCOHOL: INTERACTIONS WITH YOUR HIV MEDS

HIV medications can be hard on your body. When you are taking these medications, it is important that your liver works as well as possible. The liver is responsible for getting rid of waste products from the medications.

When you are HIV positive, your body may react differently to alcohol and drugs. Many people find that it takes longer to recover from using pot, alcohol, or other recreational drugs than it did before they had HIV.

Remember that having HIV means a major change has taken place in your body. You may choose to use alcohol and drugs in moderation, but be sure to respect your body. Pay attention to what and how much you eat, drink, smoke, and take into your body.

Certain HIV medications can boost the level of recreational drugs in your system in unexpected and potentially dangerous ways. For example, amphetamines (such as crystal meth) can be present at 3 to 22 times their normal levels in the bloodstream when mixed with an HIV drug called "ritonavir" (Norvir). That Is because ritonavir affects the body's ability to break down these other drugs.

If you are going to take a recreational drug while you are on HIV medication, it is better to start with a very low amount of the recreational drug (as low as 1/4 the normal amount) and allow time to see how it affects you before increasing the amount. Keep in mind that recreational drugs are not regulated, so you never know exactly how much you are getting.

Although you may feel uncomfortable at first, you should tell your doctor what drugs you are using. That way, your doctor will know how the substances you are using affect your HIV drugs and your overall health.

DRUGS, ALCOHOL, AND SAFER SEX

Many drugs, including alcohol and methamphetamine, may affect your ability to make decisions.

Even if you take your HIV medications regularly and practice safer sex when you are not high, when you are under the influence of methamphetamine or other drugs you may be willing to take more risks. For example, you might not use a condom or take your HIV medications.

Alcohol also can affect the decisions you make about safer sex. For example, if you have too much to drink, you may not remember where you put the condoms, and decide simply not to use them. These are decisions you probably would not make if you were sober.

These actions put your partner at risk for HIV and put you at risk for other sexually transmitted diseases or for pregnancy.

Remember to take your HIV medications every day, and to keep condoms handy in places where you might have sex. Also, try to limit the amount of drugs you use or alcohol you drink if you know you are going to have sex.

HIV AND INJECTION DRUG USE

Sharing a needle or any equipment when injecting drugs is dangerous for you and for your sharing partners. They could get HIV from you, and you could get another disease, such as hepatitis, from them.

The safest option is not to share. Use clean needles and syringes each time, and keep your own equipment to yourself. There are sterile syringe programs that can help provide clean needles. Because of the dangers of injection drug use, the best way to lower your risk is to stop injecting drugs.

If you do inject drugs, follow these reminders:

- Never reuse or "share" syringes, water, or drug preparation equipment
- Use only syringes obtained from a reliable source (such as pharmacies and needle or syringe services programs)
- Use a new, sterile syringe each time to prepare and inject drugs. If this is not possible, sterilize your syringe or disinfect your syringe and other equipment with bleach
- If possible, use sterile water to prepare drugs; otherwise, use clean water from a reliable source (such as fresh tap water)
- Use a new or disinfected container ("cooker") and a new filter ("cotton") to prepare drugs
- Clean the injection site with a new alcohol swab prior to injection
- Safely dispose of syringes after one use

DRUGS AND ALCOHOL: POINTS TO REMEMBER

- Before you drink or use drugs, it is important to think about risks.
- If you would like to cut back on your use of alcohol or other drugs, talk to your healthcare provider about getting help and finding the treatment you need.

Section 46.5 | Smoking: A Health Threat

This section includes text excerpted from "Smoking," HIV.gov, U.S. Department of Health and Human Services (HHS), November 9, 2020.

HOW DOES SMOKING AFFECT PEOPLE WITH HIV?

Smoking is dangerous for everyone. It harms nearly every organ of the body, causes many diseases, and affects the health of smokers in general. The risks of serious health consequences are much higher for people with human immunodeficiency virus (HIV), who smoke at twice the rate of the general population.

Smokers with HIV are more likely than nonsmokers with HIV to develop:

- Lung cancer, head and neck cancers, cervical and anal cancers, and other cancers
- Heart disease and stroke
- Chronic obstructive pulmonary disease (COPD) and
- Serious HIV-related infections, including bacterial pneumonia

Smokers with HIV are also more likely to have a poorer response to HIV treatment, a greater chance of developing a life-threatening illness that leads to an acquired immunodeficiency syndrome (AIDS) diagnosis, and a shorter lifespan than people with HIV who do not smoke. In fact, one study found that people with HIV who adhere to antiretroviral therapy (ART), but smoke are substantially more likely to die from lung cancer than from AIDS-related causes.

WHY SHOULD YOU QUIT SMOKING?

Quitting smoking has major and immediate health benefits for all tobacco users. In fact, quitting smoking may be one of the most important steps toward better health that a person with HIV can take.

The benefits include:

- Lowering your risk of lung cancer and many other types of cancer
- Reducing your risk of heart disease, stroke, and COPD

- Reducing HIV-related symptoms such as fatigue, nausea, and body pain
- Improving your quality of life and
- Increasing your life expectancy.

According to the Centers for Disease Control and Prevention (CDC), quitting smoking is beneficial to your health at any age. Every people who have smoked for many years or has smoked heavily will benefit from quitting.

In addition to quitting smoking, do your best to avoid second-hand smoke, which is smoke from the burning end of a cigarette, and smoke that is breathed out from other people smoking. There is no risk-free level of exposure to secondhand smoke. It has immediate harmful effects on your heart and blood vessels and causes heart disease, stroke, and lung cancer.

GET HELP TO QUIT SMOKING

Talk with your healthcare provider about programs and products that can help you quit smoking. There is not one right way to quit. Explore your options and find a quit method that is right for you.

Get tips for quitting from Tips From Former Smokers (www.cdc. gov/tobacco/campaign/tips), the CDC's national tobacco education campaign. The campaign features the real stories of people who are living with smoking-related health conditions, including HIV.

WHAT ABOUT E-CIGARETTES

E-cigarettes are devices that heat liquid into an aerosol that the user breathes in and out. They are considered tobacco products because most of them contain nicotine, which comes from tobacco. Scientists are still learning about their long-term health effects. But they know that nicotine is highly addictive and harmful for youth, young adults, and pregnant woman, and that e-cigarettes can also contain cancer-causing chemicals and tiny particles that get into your lungs. E-cigarettes are not currently approved by the U.S. Food and Drug Administration (FDA) as a quit smoking aid. Talk to your healthcare provider and use proven-effective methods to quit.

Section 46.6 | **HIV and Substance Use**

This section includes text excerpted from "HIV and Substance Use," HIVinfo, U.S. Department of Health and Human Services (HHS), August 13, 2021.

WHAT IS THE CONNECTION BETWEEN HIV AND SUBSTANCE USE?

Substance use is the use of drugs and alcohol and includes the misuse of prescription drugs and over-the-counter medicines. Substance use is related to human immunodeficiency virus (HIV) in the following ways:

- The use of alcohol and recreational drugs can lead to risky behaviors that increase the chances of getting HIV or passing it on to others (called "HIV transmission"). Recreational drugs include injection and noninjection drugs, such as opioids (including heroin), methamphetamine (meth), crack cocaine, and inhalants (poppers). Some prescription drugs and over-the-counter medicines contain stimulants that when used inappropriately can also lead to risky behaviors.
- Substance use can harm the health of a person with HIV. Specifically, drug and alcohol use can weaken the immune system and damage the liver.

HOW DOES SUBSTANCE USE INCREASE THE RISK OF GETTING HIV?

Drugs and alcohol use affects the brain, making it hard to think clearly. This includes the use of prescription drugs and over-the-counter medicines for purposes other than prescribed, in excessive amounts, or over a longer period than was intended. People using drugs or alcohol may make poor decisions and take risks.

Some risky behaviors can increase the risk of getting or transmitting HIV. For example, a person using drugs or alcohol may have sex without a condom or share needles when injecting drugs.

In the United States, HIV is spread mainly by:

- Having anal or vaginal sex with someone who has HIV without using a condom or taking medicines to prevent or treat HIV

- Sharing injection drug equipment (works), such as needles, with someone who has HIV

HOW CAN SUBSTANCE USE AFFECT A PERSON WITH HIV?

Substance use can harm the health of a person with HIV in several ways.

- **Drugs and alcohol can weaken the immune system.** HIV damages the immune system, making it harder for the body to fight infections and certain cancers. Drug or alcohol use can further damage the immune system and cause HIV infection to worsen.
- **Drugs and alcohol can damage the liver and cause liver disease.** One of the main functions of the liver is to remove harmful substances (toxins) from the blood. Toxins are produced when the liver breaks down the chemicals in drugs or alcohol. Drug and alcohol use can damage the liver, making it work harder to remove toxins from the body. The buildup of toxins can weaken the body and lead to liver disease.
- **Some recreational drugs can interact with HIV medicines.** Drug interactions between HIV medicines and recreational drugs can increase the risk of dangerous side effects. For example, overdoses due to interactions between some HIV medicines and drugs, such as ecstasy (MDMA) or GHB, have been reported.
- **Drug and alcohol use can make it hard to take HIV medicines every day.** People with HIV take a combination of HIV medicines (called an "HIV treatment regimen") every day to stay healthy. Drug or alcohol use can make it hard to focus and stick to a daily HIV treatment regimen. Skipping HIV medicines allows HIV to multiply and damage the immune system.

IF YOU USE DRUGS OR DRINK ALCOHOL, TAKE THE FOLLOWING STEPS TO PROTECT YOUR HEALTH

If you use drugs or alcohol:

- Do not have sex if you are high
- Use a condom correctly every time you have sex

If you drink alcohol:
- Drink in moderation. Moderate drinking is up to 1 drink per day for women and up to 2 drinks per day for men. One drink is a 12-oz bottle of beer, a 5-oz glass of wine, or a shot of liquor.
- Visit Rethinking Drinking, a website from the National Institute on Alcohol Abuse and Alcoholism (NIAAA) (www.rethinkingdrinking.niaaa.nih.gov). This website can help you evaluate your drinking habits and consider how alcohol may be affecting your health.

If you inject drugs:
- Use only new, sterile needles and drug injection equipment (works) each time you inject
- Never share needles and works

Therapy, medicines, and other methods are also available to help you stop or cut down on drinking alcohol or using drugs. You can talk with a counselor or a healthcare provider about options that might be right for you.

Section 46.7 | Vaccinations

This section includes text excerpted from "Vaccines and People with HIV," HIV.gov, U.S. Department of Health and Human Services (HHS), November 12, 2021.

SHOULD PEOPLE WITH HIV GET VACCINES?

Yes. Vaccines play an important role in keeping people healthy. They protect you against serious and sometimes deadly diseases.

Vaccines are especially important for people with chronic health conditions such as human immunodeficiency virus (HIV), which can make it harder to fight off vaccine-preventable diseases such as pneumococcal disease or the flu. HIV can also make it more likely that you will have serious complications from those diseases, which is why getting recommended vaccines is an important part of your overall HIV medical care.

Vaccines are very effective and they do not just protect individuals from disease. They also protect communities. When most people in a community get vaccinated and become immune to a disease, there is little chance of a disease outbreak. Eventually, the disease becomes rare – and sometimes, it is wiped out altogether.

WHAT ARE VACCINES?

Vaccines protect your body from diseases and infections such as COVID-19, human papillomavirus (HPV), influenza (flu), hepatitis B, and polio. They are given by needle injection (a shot), by mouth, or sprayed into the nose.

Vaccines help your immune system fight infections faster and more effectively. When you get a vaccine, it sparks an immune response, helping your body fight off and remember the germ so it can attack it if the germ ever invades again. And since vaccines are made of very small amounts of weak or dead germs, they will not make you sick.

Vaccines often provide long-lasting immunity to serious diseases without the risk of serious illness.

ARE ALL TYPES OF VACCINES SAFE FOR PEOPLE LIVING WITH HIV?

Vaccines are generally safe for people with HIV. However, some types of vaccines may not be recommended. For example, live attenuated vaccines (LAV) – like the chickenpox vaccine – contain a weakened but, live form of the germ that causes the disease. LAVs can potentially cause an infection for people with HIV. However, depending on age, health, previous vaccinations, or other factors, some LAVs may be recommended. Talk to your healthcare provider about what is recommended for you.

CAN HIV AFFECT HOW WELL A VACCINE WORKS?

Yes. HIV can weaken your body's immune response to a vaccine, making the vaccine less effective. In general, vaccines work best when your CD4 count is above 200 copies/mm3.

Also, by stimulating your immune system, vaccines may cause your HIV viral load to increase temporarily.

IS THERE A VACCINE AGAINST HIV?

No. There is currently no vaccine that has been approved by the U.S. Food and Drug Administration (FDA) to prevent HIV infection or treat those who have it. However, scientists are working to develop both types.

Section 46.8 | Staying Healthy While Traveling

This section includes text excerpted from "Traveling with HIV," Centers for Disease Control and Prevention (CDC), May 20, 2021.

WHY DO YOU NEED TO TAKE PRECAUTIONS WHEN T RAVELING ABROAD?

Traveling outside the United States can be risky for anyone. However, it may require special precautions for people with human immunodeficiency virus (HIV). For example, travel to some developing countries can increase the risk of getting an opportunistic infection. For some destinations, you may need certain vaccines. Your healthcare provider can review your medical record to ensure the vaccines are safe for you.

BEFORE YOU TRAVEL
Talk to Your Healthcare Provider at Least 4–6 Weeks before You Travel

- Learn about the health risks in the places you plan to visit.
- Learn about specific measures you need to take to stay healthy.

- Gather the names of HIV healthcare providers or clinics in the area you plan to visit.

Learn about Your Insurance
- Review your medical insurance to see what travel coverage it provides.
- Take proof of insurance. Copy or scan your policy and send the image to an email address you can access when traveling.
- Leave a copy of your insurance at home and tell your friends or family where you left it.
- Consider purchasing additional travel insurance if your insurance does not cover emergency transportation to a healthcare facility, or the cost of care received in other countries.

Learn about Your Destination
- Find out if the countries you plan to visit have special health rules for visitors, especially visitors with HIV.

DURING TRAVEL
Stick to Safe Eating and Drinking Habits
- Food and water in some developing countries may contain germs that could make you sick.
- Eat only hot foods.
- Drink bottled water or drinks, hot coffee or tea, wine, beer, or other alcoholic beverages.
- Avoid raw fruit or vegetables that you do not peel yourself.
- Avoid eating raw or undercooked seafood or meat or unpasteurized dairy products.
- Tap water and drinks or ice made with the tap water could make you sick.

Take Care of Yourself and Protect Others
- Take all your medications on schedule

- Stick to your special diet if you are on one.
- Take the same precautions you take at home to prevent transmitting HIV to others.

Avoid Direct Contact with Animal Waste

- Animal waste (stool) in soil or on sidewalks can be harmful to people with HIV.
- Wear shoes to protect yourself from direct contact with animal waste.
- Use towels to protect yourself from animal waste when lying on a beach or in parks.
- Wash your hands with soap and water after physical contact with animals.

Avoid Hospitals and Clinics Where Coughing Tuberculosis Patients Are Treated

- Tuberculosis (TB) is very common worldwide and can be severe in people with HIV.
- See your healthcare provider when you return to discuss whether you should be tested for TB.

Chapter 47 | Life Issues When You Have HIV/AIDS

Chapter Contents

Section 47.1 | Standing Up to HIV-Related Stigma

This section contains text excerpted from the following sources: Text beginning with the heading "What Is HIV Stigma?" is excerpted from "Standing Up to Stigma," HIV.gov, U.S. Department of Health and Human Services (HHS), February 24, 2020; Text under the heading "Ways to Stop HIV Stigma and Discrimination" is excerpted from "Ways to Stop HIV Stigma and Discrimination," Centers for Disease Control and Prevention (CDC), February 2, 2021.

WHAT IS HIV STIGMA?

Human immunodeficiency virus (HIV) stigma refers to irrational or negative attitudes, behaviors, and judgments towards people living with or at risk of HIV. It can negatively affect the health and well-being of people living with HIV by discouraging some individuals from learning their HIV status, accessing treatment, or staying in care. HIV stigma can also affect those at risk of HIV by discouraging them from seeking HIV prevention tools and testing, and from talking openly with their sex partners about safer sex options.

Populations disproportionately affected by HIV are also often affected by stigma due to, among other things, their gender, sexual orientation, gender identity, race/ethnicity, drug use, or sex work.

HIV stigma drives acts of discrimination in all sectors of society, including healthcare, education, the workplace, the justice system, families, and communities.

Breaking down HIV stigma is a critical part of ending the HIV epidemic.

WHAT IS INTERNALIZED STIGMA FOR PEOPLE WITH HIV?

Internalized stigma is when a person with HIV experiences negative feelings or thoughts about themselves due to their HIV status. Almost 8 in 10 adults with HIV receiving HIV medical care in the United States report feeling internalized HIV-related stigma, according to a Centers for Disease Control and Prevention (CDC) study. Internalized stigma can lead to depression, isolation, and feelings of shame, and can affect individuals' ability to stay adherent to their HIV medication.

HOW CAN YOU STAND UP TO HIV-RELATED STIGMA?

You can play an important role in reducing stigma and discrimination by offering support and speaking out to correct myths and stereotypes about HIV that you hear from others.

Learn which words have negative meanings for people at risk for or living with HIV and which are empowering. Be intentional when you choose your words and mindful of how they can affect those around you.

WAYS TO STOP HIV STIGMA AND DISCRIMINATION

You might be wondering how you can address an issue as complex as HIV stigma. But there are many small things you can do that will make a big difference.

If each of us commits to making positive changes in our families and communities, we can help end HIV stigma and work to stop HIV together.

Section 47.2 | Employment

This section contains text excerpted from the following sources: Text begins with excerpts from "Employment and Health," HIV.gov, U.S. Department of Health and Human Services (HHS), May 15, 2017. Reviewed February 2022; Text beginning with the heading "Guidance for Employees with HIV and Their Coworkers" is excerpted from "Guidance for Employees with HIV and Their Coworkers," Centers for Disease Control and Prevention (CDC), June 15, 2020.

With proper care and treatment, many people living with human immunodeficiency virus (HIV) lead normal, healthy lives, including having a job. Most people living with HIV can continue working at their current jobs or look for a new job in their chosen field. Your overall well-being and financial health can be more stable when you are gainfully employed.

GETTING A NEW JOB OR RETURNING TO WORK

Working will affect a lot of your life: your medical status, your finances, your social life, the way you spend your time, and perhaps even your housing or transportation needs. Before taking action on getting a new job or returning to work, you may want to get information and perspectives from:

- Your HIV case manager or counselor, if you have one
- Benefits counselors at an HIV service organization or other community organization
- The Social Security Administrations Work Incentives Planning and Assistance Program (WIPA)
- Other people living with HIV who are working, or have returned to work
- Providers of any of your housing, medical, or financial benefits
- Public and nonprofit employment and training service providers

Here are some questions to discuss with them:
- What are my goals for employment?
- What kind of work do I want to do?
- What are the resources that can help me set and achieve a new career goal?
- Are there state or local laws that further strengthen anti-discrimination protections in the American Disabilities Act (ADA)?
- How do I access training or education that will help me achieve my goals?
- How can I plan to take care of my health if I go to work?
- How will my going to work impact the benefits I am receiving?

REQUESTING REASONABLE ACCOMMODATIONS

Qualified individuals with disabilities, including people living with HIV, have the right to request reasonable accommodations in the workplace. A reasonable accommodation is any modification or adjustment to a job or work environment that enables a qualified person with a disability to apply for or perform a job.

An accommodation may be tangible (e.g., a certain type of chair) or nontangible (e.g., a modified work schedule for someone with a medical condition requiring regular appointments with a healthcare provider). You are qualified if you are able to perform the essential functions of the job, with or without reasonable accommodation.

Your supervisor may not be trained in reasonable accommodations or know how to negotiate them. For that reason, often it is best to go directly to the person responsible for human resources at your employer, even if that person works in a different location. In a small business, that person may well be the owner.

When you request an accommodation, state clearly what you need (e.g., time off for a clinic visit every third Tuesday of the month, a certain type of chair, or a change in your work hours) and be ready to supply a doctors note supporting your request. The initial note need not contain your diagnosis, but it should verify that you are under that doctors care and that he/she believes you need the accommodation to maintain your health or to be able to fulfill essential functions of your job.

Many people living with HIV do not want to give a lot of details about their health. If you prefer not to provide a lot of information, you may want to limit the medical information you initially give to your employer. However, if your need for accommodation is not obvious, your employer may require that you provide medical documentation to establish that you have a disability as defined by the ADA, to show that the employee needs the requested accommodation, and to help determine effective accommodation options. This can, but often does not, include disclosing your specific medical condition.

Be aware that not all people with HIV or AIDS will need accommodations to perform their jobs and many others may only need a few or simple accommodations. The U.S. Department of Labors (DOL) Job Accommodation Network (JAN) provides free, expert, and confidential technical assistance to both employees and employers on workplace accommodations and disability employment issues, which includes resources for employees living with HIV or AIDS.

GUIDANCE FOR EMPLOYEES WITH HIV AND THEIR COWORKERS

As an employer or human resources (HR) professional, you may be seeking guidance on how to provide a positive and productive work environment for employees with HIV and their coworkers. Here are common questions, along with guidance, to offer employees with HIV.

Disclosing Your Status as an Employee

If you have HIV, in most cases, the decision to disclose your HIV status at work is a personal choice.

One benefit of disclosing at work is that it can create supportive relationships with your coworkers. On the other hand, telling people that you have HIV may have the opposite effect and cause your colleagues to treat you differently. You have to be the judge of which outcome is more likely.

If you decide to disclose to one or more of your coworkers, think carefully about which individuals to tell and how to tell them. Should you tell your boss or the human resources department before you talk to your coworkers? Should you tell your entire work team about your diagnosis or just disclose to individuals? It is good to have a plan in mind before you start telling your colleagues.

Your Rights as an Employee with HIV

As an employee with HIV, you have a right to remain in the workforce to the fullest extent possible, and a right to equal employment opportunities. Several federal, state, and local laws determine how employers design workplace programs pertaining to employees with HIV.

Employees with HIV are protected from discrimination in employment by law under the ADA. This law prohibits most private employers, state and local governments, employment agencies, joint labor management committees, and labor unions from discriminating against qualified individuals with disabilities. These provisions include, but are not limited to:

- Job application procedures
- Hiring and firing

- Advancement
- Compensation
- Job training

The ADA applies to employers with 15 or more employees for each working day in each of 20 or more calendar weeks.

GUIDANCE FOR COWORKERS OF AN EMPLOYEE WITH HIV

Here is guidance to offer those who work with employees with HIV.

Working with an Employee Who Has HIV

When you learn that a coworker has HIV, you may be surprised, and unsure of what to do. Although this may be an initial reaction, you should treat all of your coworkers in a respectful and equal manner.

People with HIV want to continue to live and work to the fullest extent possible. If you are unsure of what to do when responding to a coworker who has HIV, the best advice is to maintain professionalism and respect. There are many ways to respond when learning a coworker has HIV:

- **Be compassionate.** Try to empathize with the difficult circumstances and uncertainties that your coworker is experiencing. Be there to listen and help if needed.
- **Be supportive.** Be the workplace friend and coworker you have always been. Include your coworker in the same work and social activities as always, whenever possible. Extend your support just as you would to other coworkers.
- **Protect the right to privacy and confidentiality.** If your coworker tells you that they have HIV, it is illegal for you to tell others without their permission.
  - If you hear a rumor that a coworker has HIV, do not repeat it.
  - Even if a person has told others that they have HIV, do not tell your other coworkers. Allow your coworker the right to tell others.

582

- Once a coworker has told you that they have HIV, you may be curious and want to know more. First, ask if they want to talk about it. Do not pressure your coworker with questions. Let your coworker decide how much or how little they want to share.

Section 47.3 | Sex and Sexuality and HIV

This section includes text excerpted from "Sex and Sexuality for People with HIV," U.S. Department of Veterans Affairs (VA), May 28, 2019.

When you are first diagnosed with human immunodeficiency virus (HIV), you may not want to think about having sex. Some people may be afraid of infecting a partner and decide sex is too risky. These are common reactions, especially if you got HIV through sex. Chances are, however, that you will want to have sex again. The good news is that there is no reason why you cannot. People living with HIV enjoy sex and fall in love, just like other people. And there are many ways to have satisfying and safe sexual relationships.

One of the most effective ways to prevent HIV from passing to an HIV-negative sex partner is to take your own HIV medications (antiretroviral therapy, or ART) every day – these not only protect your health but can prevent transmission of HIV.

If you are having a hard time dealing with negative feelings like anger or fear, you can get help. Talk to your healthcare provider about support groups or counseling. Sex is a difficult topic for many people living with HIV – you are not alone.

By reading this information, you are already taking a good first step toward a healthy sex life. Having good information will help you make good decisions.

TALKING TO YOUR HEALTHCARE PROVIDER

Your provider or other members of your healthcare team may ask you about your sexual practices each time you go in for a checkup.

It may feel embarrassing at first to be honest and open. But they are trying to help you stay healthy.

Your healthcare provider and staff will still give you care if you have had sex with someone of the same sex or someone other than your spouse.

Make sure you set aside time to ask questions about safer sex, sexually transmitted diseases (STDs), or any other questions you might have. If you feel that you need help dealing with your feelings, ask about support groups or counseling.

Many people living with HIV ask their provider to talk with them and their partners about HIV and how it is transmitted. They can answer technical questions and address the specifics of your situation. If you live with someone, they may have questions about everyday contact as well as sexual contact.

TELLING YOUR SEX PARTNERS

This may be one of the hardest things you have to do. But you need to tell your sex partner(s) that you are living with HIV, whether you have a primary partner such as a spouse or girlfriend or boyfriend, have more than one partner, or are single or casually dating.

What follows are tips for talking to your main partner, other partners, and former partners.

Talking to Your Main Partner

If you are in a relationship, one of the first things you will probably think about after learning that you have HIV is telling your partner or partners. For some couples, a positive HIV test may have been expected. For others, the news will be a surprise that can be difficult.

Your partner may not be prepared to offer you support during a time when you need it. Your partner may be worrying about their own HIV status. On the other hand, if you think you may have contracted HIV from your partner, you are probably dealing with your own feelings.

Unless your partner is known to have HIV infection, they should get an HIV test right away. Do not assume that the results will come back positive, even if you have been having unprotected sex or sharing needles. Your partner may assume the worst and may blame you for possibly spreading the disease. It is important that you discuss these feelings with each other in an open and honest way, perhaps with a licensed counselor.

Talking to New Partners

Talking about HIV with someone you are dating casually or someone you met recently may be difficult. You might not know this person very well or know what kind of reaction to expect. When telling a casual partner or someone you are dating, each situation is different and you might use a different approach each time. Sometimes you may feel comfortable being direct and saying, "Before we have sex, I want you to know that I have HIV."

Other times, you may want to bring it up by saying something like, "Let's talk about safer sex." Whichever approach you choose, you should tell the person that you have HIV before you have sex the first time. Otherwise, there may be hurt feelings or mistrust later. Also, be sure to take your HIV medications every day (this is very effective in protecting partners from infection) and practice safer sex.

Talking to Former Partners

With people you had sex with in the past or people you have shared needles with, it can be very difficult to explain that you have HIV. However, it is important that they know so that they can get tested.

If you need help telling people that you may have been exposed to HIV, most city or county health departments will tell them for you, without using your name. Ask your provider about this service.

Remember Some of the Points

Before telling your partner that you have HIV, take some time to think about how you want to bring it up.

- Decide when and where would be the best time and place to have a conversation. Choose a time when you expect that you will both be comfortable and as relaxed as possible.

- Think about how your partner may react to stressful situations. If there is a history of violence in your relationship, consider your safety first and make a plan with a social worker or counselor.
- Imagine several ways in which your partner might react to the news. Write down what they might say, and then think about what you might say in response.

WHAT IS "SAFER SEX"?

We know a lot about how HIV is transmitted from person to person. Having safer sex means you take this into account and avoid risky practices.

There are two reasons to practice safer sex: to protect yourself and to protect others.

Protecting Yourself

If you have HIV, you need to protect your health. When it comes to sex, this means practicing safer sex (like using condoms) to avoid sexually transmitted diseases like herpes and hepatitis. HIV makes it harder for your body to fight off diseases. What might be a small health problem for someone without HIV could be big health problem for you. Your healthcare provider can prescribe condoms for you if you need them.

Protecting Your Partner

Taking care of others means making sure that you do not pass HIV or any other sexually transmitted infections to them.

"Being safe" usually means protecting yourself and others by using condoms for the highest-risk sex activities, specifically for anal and vaginal sex. When done correctly, condom use is very effective at preventing HIV transmission. In recent years, "being safe" has come to include two other important strategies for reducing HIV infections: 1. HIV treatment (ART medications) for people with HIV and, 2. PrEP for HIV negative people. Both are very effective at reducing the risk of HIV infection. One or more of them is likely to be appropriate for your situation – be sure to ask your healthcare provider for more information.

What about Antiretroviral Therapy for HIV Prevention

One of the most effective ways you can prevent HIV from passing to an HIV-negative sex partner is to take your ART (HIV medications) every day. If they are working well to suppress the HIV in your body they also will prevent transmission of HIV to others.

What about Pre-exposure Prophylaxis

HIV-negative individuals may, under the supervision of their healthcare provider, take a pill every day to prevent HIV infection. We call this pre-exposure prophylaxis, or PrEP. Usually these are persons who are at relatively high risk of becoming infected with HIV (e.g., because they have a partner with HIV, they have risky sexual exposures, or they share injection drug equipment). The medications used for PrEP are Truvada and Descovy. PrEP appears to be extremely effective if it is taken every day, and is not effective if it is taken irregularly.

WHAT IS RISKY SEX?

Risky sex is sex that may lead to infection of an HIV-negative individual. There are many ways to decrease the risk of HIV infection, like (for the partner living with HIV) taking HIV medications (ART) every day, or (for the HIV-negative partner) using PrEP, or (for partners of any HIV status) using condoms or other latex barriers during sex.

HIV is passed through body fluids such as semen, vaginal, or anal fluid, or blood. The less contact you have with these, the lower the risk. The most sensitive areas where these fluids are risky are in the vagina or anus and rectum (ass). The protective tissue there is thin, and is easily torn, which makes it easier for the virus to enter your body. Saliva (spit) and tears are not as risky.

In general, vaginal or anal sex without a condom is the most risky.

Here is a list of sexual activities organized by level of risk to help you and your partner make decisions:

- High risk
  - Anal sex without a condom (penis in the anus)
  - Vaginal sex without a condom (penis in the vagina)
- Low risk
  - Sex with a condom when you use it correctly
  - Oral sex, but do not swallow semen (cum)
  - Deep kissing (French kissing or tongue kissing)
  - Sharing sex toys that have been cleaned or covered with a new condom between uses
- No risk
  - Hugging, massage
  - Masturbation
  - Fantasizing
  - Dry kissing
  - Phone sex
  - Cyber sex
  - Using sex toys that you do not share

TALKING ABOUT SAFER SEX

You and your partners will have to decide what you are comfortable doing sexually.

Here are some tips:

- Find a time and place outside the bedroom to talk.
- Decide your own boundaries, concerns and desires before you start to talk.
- Make sure you clearly state what you want. Use only "I" statements, for example: "I want to use a condom when we have sex."
- Make sure you do not do, or agree to do, anything that you are not 100 percent comfortable with.
- Listen to what your partner is saying. Acknowledge your partner's feelings and opinions. You will need to come up with solutions that work for both of you.

- Be positive. Use reasons for safer sex that are about you, not your partner.

Of course, only you and your partner can decide what level of risk you are willing to take.

BIRTH CONTROL AND HIV

The only forms of birth control that will protect against HIV are abstinence and using condoms while having sex. Other methods of birth control offer protection against unplanned pregnancy, but do not protect against HIV or other sexually transmitted diseases.

Birth control options that DO protect against HIV:
- Abstinence (not having sex)
- Male condom
- Internal or female condom

Birth control options that DO NOT protect against HIV:
- Oral contraceptive ("the pill")
- Injectable contraceptive (shot)
- Contraceptive implant
- IUD (intrauterine device)
- Emergency contraception ("morning-after pill")
- Diaphragm, cap, and shield
- Vasectomy (getting your tubes tied if you are a man)
- Tubal ligation (getting your tubes tied if you are a woman)

Considerations for Women with HIV

If you are in a monogamous relationship and your partner also has HIV, you may decide to use a birth control method other than condoms. (These methods would not protect against other STDs or re-infection.)

Safe methods of birth control for a woman with HIV with a partner who also has HIV include:
- Using a diaphragm
- Tubal ligation (getting your tubes tied)

- IUD (intrauterine device)

Use only after checking with your provider (these may interact with your HIV medications):
- Birth control pills
- Contraceptive injection (e.g., Depo-Provera)
- Contraceptive implant (e.g., Norplant)

TIPS FOR USING CONDOMS AND DENTAL DAMS

If you need condoms, you can ask your healthcare provider for a prescription for condoms at your next visit. If you are not used to using condoms: practice, practice, practice.

Male condom dos and don'ts:
- **Shop around**. Use lubricated latex condoms. Always use latex, because lambskin condoms do not block HIV and STDs, and polyurethane condoms break more often than latex (if you are allergic to latex, polyurethane condoms are an option). There is a lot of variety – one will work for you!
- **Keep it fresh**. Store condoms loosely in a cool, dry place (not your wallet). Check the expiration date. Throw away condoms that have expired, were exposed to very hot temperatures, or were washed in the washer. If you think the condom might not be good, get a new one.
- **Take it easy**. Open the package carefully, so that you do not rip the condom and make sure that the condom package has not been punctured (there should be a pocket of air). Check the condom for damaged packaging and signs of aging such as brittleness, stickiness, and discoloration.
- **Keep it hard**. Put on the condom after the penis is erect and before it touches any part of a partner's body. If a penis is uncircumcised (uncut), the foreskin must be pulled back before putting on the condom.
- **Heads up**. Make sure the condom is right-side out. Before you put it on the penis, unroll the condom

about half an inch to see which direction it is unrolling. Then put it on the head of the penis and hold the tip of the condom between your fingers as you roll it all the way down the shaft of the penis from head to base. This keeps out air bubbles that can cause the condom to break. It also leaves a space for semen to collect after ejaculation.

- **Slippery when wet**. If you use a lubricant (lube), it should be a water-soluble lubricant (e.g., ID Glide, K-Y Jelly, Slippery Stuff, Foreplay, Wet, Astroglide) in order to prevent breakdown of the condom. Put lubricant on after you put on the condom, not before- it could slip off. Add more lube often. Dry condoms break more easily. Products such as petroleum jelly, massage oils, butter, Crisco, Vaseline, and hand creams are not considered water-soluble lubricants and should not be used.
- **Come and go**. Withdraw the penis immediately after ejaculation, while the penis is still erect; grasp the rim of the condom between your fingers and slowly withdraw the penis (with the condom still on) so that no semen is spilled.
- **Clean up**. Throw out the used condom right away. Tie it off to prevent spillage or wrap it in bathroom tissue and put it in the garbage. Condoms can clog toilets. Use a condom only once. Never use the same condom for vaginal and anal intercourse. Never use a condom that has been used by someone else.

Do You Have to Use a Condom for Oral Sex?

It is possible for oral sex to transmit HIV, whether the infected partner is performing or receiving oral sex. But the risk is very low compared with unprotected vaginal or anal sex, however other sexually transmitted infections can be transmitted through oral sex.

If you choose to perform oral sex, you may:

- Use a latex condom on the penis; or
- Use a latex barrier (such as a natural rubber latex sheet, a dental dam, or a cut-open condom that makes a

square) between your mouth and the vagina. A latex
Barrier such as a dental dam reduces the risk of blood
or vaginal fluids entering your mouth. Plastic food
wrap also can be used as a barrier.
- If either you or your partner are allergic to latex, plastic
(polyurethane) condoms can be used.

If you perform oral sex and this sex includes oral contact with
your partner's anus (anilingus or rimming),
- Use a latex barrier (such as a natural rubber latex sheet,
a dental dam, or a cut-open condom that makes a
square) between your mouth and the anus. Plastic food
wrap also can be used as a barrier.

If you share sex toys, such as dildos or vibrators, with your
partner,
- Each partner should use a new condom on the sex toy,
and be sure to clean sex toys between each use.

Internal condom

Internal condom (also called "female condom"), this type of condom was originally designed to be inserted into the vagina before
sex. It also can be used in the anus, by either men or women,
though its effectiveness in preventing HIV transmission via anal
sex has not been studied.

The internal condom is a large condom fitted with larger and
smaller flexible rings at each end. The rings help keep it inside the
vagina during sex; for anal sex, the inner ring usually is removed
before it is inserted. It is made of nitrile, so any lubricant can
be used without damaging it. It may seem a little awkward at
first, but can be a useful alternative to the traditional "male" condom. Female condoms generally cost more than male condoms.
Remember to:
- Store the condom in a cool dry place, not in direct heat
or sunlight.
- Throw away any condoms that have expired – the date
is printed on the wrappers.

- Check the package for damage and check the condom for signs of aging such as brittleness, stickiness, and discoloration. The internal condom is lubricated, so it will be somewhat wet.
- Before inserting the condom, you can squeeze lubricant into the condom pouch and rub the sides together to spread it around.
- Put the condom in before sex play because pre-ejaculatory fluid, which comes from the penis, may contain HIV. The condom can be inserted up to 8 hours before sex.
- The internal condom has a firm but flexible ring at each end of it. To insert the condom in the vagina, squeeze the ring at the closed end between the fingers (like a diaphragm), and push it up into the back of the vagina. The open ring must stay outside the vagina at all times, and it will partly cover the lip area. For use in the anus, most people remove the internal ring before insertion.
- Do not use a male condom with the internal condom.
- Do not use an internal condom with a diaphragm.
- If the penis is inserted outside the condom pouch or if the outer ring (open ring) slips into the vagina, stop and take the condom out. Use a new condom before you start sex again.
- Do not tear the condom with fingernails or jewelry.
- Use a condom only once and properly dispose of it in the trash (not the toilet).

Section 47.4 | Aging with HIV/AIDS

This section includes text excerpted from "Aging with HIV," HIV.gov, U.S. Department of Health and Human Services (HHS), May 17, 2021.

GROWING OLDER WITH HIV

Nowadays, thanks to improvements in the effectiveness of treatment with HIV medicine (called "antiretroviral therapy" or "ART"), people with HIV who are diagnosed early and who get and stay on ART can keep the virus suppressed and live long and healthy lives. For this reason, nearly half of people living with diagnosed HIV in the United States are aged 50 and older. Many of them have been living with HIV for many years; others were diagnosed with HIV later in life.

That is a significant change from the early years of the epidemic when people who were diagnosed with HIV or AIDS could expect to live only 1–2 years after their diagnosis. This meant that the issues of aging were not a major focus for people with HIV disease.

According to the Centers for Disease Control and Prevention (CDC), in 2018, over half (51 percent) of people in the United States and dependent areas with diagnosed HIV were aged 50 and older. In addition, people aged 50 and older accounted for 17 percent of the 37,968 new HIV diagnoses in 2018 in the United States and dependent areas. Though new HIV diagnoses are declining among people aged 50 and older, around 1 in 6 HIV diagnoses in 2018 were in this group.

People over age 50 with HIV make up 46.8 percent of the over half a million clients served by the Ryan White HIV/AIDS Program (RWHAP). In 2019, 92.2 percent of clients aged 50 and older receiving RWHAP HIV medical care were virally suppressed, which was higher than the national RWHAP average (88.1 percent).

HEALTH ISSUES AND AGING WITH HIV

People aging with HIV share many of the same health concerns as the general population aged 50 and older: multiple chronic diseases or conditions, the use of multiple medications, changes in physical and cognitive abilities, and increased vulnerability to stressors. In addition, while effective HIV treatment has decreased the likelihood of AIDS-defining illnesses among people aging with HIV, many HIV-associated non-AIDS conditions occur frequently in older persons with HIV, such as cardiovascular disease, diabetes, renal disease, and cancer. These conditions are likely related to a number of interacting factors, including chronic inflammation caused by HIV. Researchers are working to better understand what causes chronic inflammation, even when people are being treated with ART.

HIV and its treatment can also have effects on the brain. Researchers estimate that between 25 and 50 percent of people with HIV have HIV-Associated Neurocognitive Disorder (HAND), a spectrum of cognitive, motor, and/or mood disorders categorized into three levels: asymptomatic, mild, and HIV-associated dementia. Researchers are studying how HIV and its treatment affect the brain, including the effects on older people living with HIV.

LATE HIV DIAGNOSIS

Older Americans are more likely than younger Americans to be diagnosed with human immunodeficiency virus (HIV) late in the course of their disease, meaning they get a late start receiving the benefits of HIV treatment and possibly incur more damage to their immune system. This can lead to poorer prognoses and shorter survival after an HIV diagnosis. Late diagnoses can occur because healthcare providers may not always test older people for HIV infection, and older people may mistake HIV symptoms for signs of normal aging and do not consider HIV as a possible cause they should discuss with their provider.

According to Centers for Disease Control and Prevention (CDC), in 2018, 35 percent of people aged 50 and older already had late-stage HIV infection (AIDS) when they received a diagnosis (i.e., they received a diagnosis later in the course of their disease.)

COVID-19 AND OLDER ADULTS WITH HIV

Researchers are still learning about COVID-19 and how it affects people with HIV. Based on limited data, scientists believe people with HIV who are on effective HIV treatment have the same risk for COVID-19 as people who do not have HIV.

Older adults and people of any age who have serious underlying medical conditions might be at increased risk for severe illness. This includes people who have weakened immune systems. The risk for people with HIV getting very sick is greatest in people with a low CD4 cell count and people not on effective HIV treatment (antiretroviral therapy or ART).

THE IMPORTANCE OF SUPPORT SERVICES

Living with HIV presents certain challenges, no matter what your age. But older people with HIV may face different issues than their younger counterparts, including greater social isolation and loneliness. Stigma is also a particular concern among older people with HIV. Stigma negatively affects people's quality of life, self-image, and behaviors, and may prevent them from disclosing their HIV status or seeking the healthcare or social services that many aging adults may require. HIV care.

Therefore, it is important for older people with HIV to get linked to HIV care and have access to mental health and other support services to help them stay healthy and remain engaged in HIV care. You can find support services through your healthcare provider, your local community center, or an HIV service organization.

Chapter 48 | **HIV/AIDS Status Disclosure**

SHOULD YOU TELL OTHER PEOPLE ABOUT YOUR POSITIVE TEST RESULT?

It is important to share your status with your sex partner(s) and/or people with whom you inject drugs. Whether you disclose your status to others is your decision.

Partners

It is important to disclose your human immunodeficiency virus (HIV) status to your sex partner(s) and anyone you share needles with, even if you are not comfortable doing it. Communicating with each other about your HIV status means you can take steps to keep both of you healthy.

The more practice you have disclosing your HIV status, the easier it will become. Many resources can help you learn ways to disclose your status to your partners.

If you are nervous about disclosing your test result, or you have been threatened or injured by a partner, you can ask your doctor or the local health department to help you tell your partner(s) that they might have been exposed to HIV. This type of assistance is called "partner notification" or "partner services." Health departments do not reveal your name to your partner(s). They will only tell your partner(s) that they have been exposed to HIV and should get tested.

This chapter includes text excerpted from "Talking about Your HIV Status," HIV.gov, U.S. Department of Health and Human Services (HHS), May 15, 2017. Reviewed February 2022.

Many states have laws that require you to tell your sexual partners if you are HIV-positive before you have sex (anal, vaginal, or oral) or tell your drug-using partners before you share drugs or needles to inject drugs. In some states, you can be charged with a crime if you do not tell your partner your HIV status, even if you used a condom or another type of protection and the partner does not become infected.

Healthcare Providers

Your healthcare providers (doctors, clinical workers, dentists, etc.) have to know about your HIV status in order to be able to give you the best possible care. It is also important that healthcare providers know your HIV status so that they do not prescribe medication for you that may be harmful when taken with your HIV medications.

Some states require you to disclose your HIV-positive status before you receive any healthcare services from a physician or dentist. For this reason, it is important to discuss the laws in your state about disclosure in medical settings with the healthcare provider who gave you your HIV test results.

Your HIV test result will become part of your medical records so that your doctor or other healthcare providers can give you the best care possible. All medical information, including HIV test results, falls under strict confidentiality laws such as the Health Insurance Portability and Accountability Act's (HIPAA) Privacy Rule and cannot be released without your permission. There are some limited exceptions to confidentiality. These come into play only when not disclosing the information could result in harm to the other person.

Family and Friends

In most cases, your family and friends will not know your test results or HIV status unless you tell them yourself. While telling your family that you have HIV may seem hard, you should know that disclosure actually has many benefits – studies have shown that people who disclose their HIV status respond better to treatment than those who do not.

If you are under 18, however, some states allow your healthcare provider to tell your parent(s) that you received services for HIV if they think doing so is in your best interest.

Employers

In most cases, your employer will not know your HIV status unless you tell them. But, your employer does have a right to ask if you have any health conditions that would affect your ability to do your job or pose a serious risk to others. (An example might be a healthcare professional, like a surgeon, who does procedures where there is a risk of blood or other body fluids being exchanged.)

If you have health insurance through your employer, the insurance company cannot legally tell your employer that you have HIV. But, it is possible that your employer could find out if the insurance company provides detailed information to your employer about the benefits it pays or the costs of insurance.

All people with HIV are covered under the Americans with Disabilities Act (ADA). This means that your employer cannot discriminate against you because of your HIV status as long as you can do your job.

Chapter 49 | **HIV/AIDS Patients and Legal Rights**

Chapter Contents

Section 49.1 | Your Rights in the Workplace

This section includes text excerpted from "Living with HIV Infection Your Legal Rights in the Workplace Under the ADA," U.S. Equal Employment Opportunity Commission (EEOC), December 1, 2015. Reviewed February 2022.

If you have human immunodeficiency virus (HIV) infection or acquired immunodeficiency syndrome (AIDS), you have workplace privacy rights, you are protected against discrimination and harassment at work because of your condition, and you may have a legal right to reasonable accommodations that can help you to do your job. The following questions briefly explain these rights, which are provided under the Americans with Disabilities Act (ADA). You may also have additional rights under other laws, such as the Family and Medical Leave Act (FMLA) and various medical insurance laws, not discussed here.

ARE YOU ALLOWED TO KEEP YOUR CONDITION PRIVATE?

In most situations, you can keep your condition private. Generally, employers cannot ask you whether you are HIV-positive, or whether you have any other medical condition, before making a job offer. An employer is allowed to ask medical questions in four situations:

- When it is engaging in affirmative action for people with disabilities, in which case you may choose whether to respond.
- When you ask for reasonable accommodation.
- After it has made you a job offer, but before employment begins, as long as everyone entering the same job category is asked the same questions.
- On the job, when there is objective evidence that you may be unable to do your job or that you may pose a safety risk because of your condition. Your employer cannot rely on myths or stereotypes about your condition to conclude that you are unable to do your job or pose a safety risk.

You may also need to discuss your condition to establish eligibility for benefits under other laws, such as the FMLA.

If you need to talk about your condition in order to answer a nonmedical question (e.g., if you are asked why there are gaps in your résumé), you may choose whether to respond. However, you should know that the employer could reject you for not answering the question, or for lying. If you do talk about your condition, the employer cannot discriminate against you, and it must keep the information confidential, even from co-workers. (If you wish to discuss your condition with coworkers, you may choose to do so.)

WHAT IF YOUR CONDITION COULD AFFECT YOUR JOB PERFORMANCE?

If your job performance could be affected by HIV infection, the side effects of HIV medication, or another medical condition that has developed because of HIV, you may be entitled to a reasonable accommodation that will help to solve the problem.

A reasonable accommodation is some type of change in the way things are done that you need because of a disability. Possible reasonable accommodations include altered break and work schedules (e.g., frequent breaks to rest or use the restroom or modified schedules to accommodate medical appointments), changes in supervisory methods (e.g., written instructions from a supervisor who usually does not provide them), accommodations for visual impairments (e.g., magnifiers, screen reading software, and qualified readers), ergonomic office furniture, unpaid time off (e.g., for treatment or recuperation), permission to work from home, and reassignment to a vacant position if you can no longer do your job because of your condition. These are only examples – you are free to request any change that you need because of your condition. However, your employer does not have to remove the essential functions (fundamental duties) of your job, let you do less work for the same amount of pay, or let you do lower-quality work.

Because an employer does not have to excuse poor job performance, even if it was caused by a medical condition or the side effects of medication, it may be better to ask for accommodation before any problems occur or become worse.

HOW CAN YOU GET A REASONABLE ACCOMMODATION?

Ask for one. Tell a supervisor, HR manager, or another appropriate person that you need a change to the way things are normally done because of a medical condition. You may ask for accommodation at any time. (However, many people choose to wait at least until they receive a job offer because it is very hard to prove illegal discrimination that takes place before a job offer.)

WHAT WILL HAPPEN AFTER YOU ASK FOR A REASONABLE ACCOMMODATION?

Your employer may ask you to put your request in writing and to describe your condition and how it affects your work. You may also be asked to submit a letter from your doctor documenting that you have a medical condition and that you need accommodation. If you do not want the employer to know your specific diagnosis, it may be enough to provide documentation that describes your condition more generally (by stating, e.g., that you have an "immune disorder"). The doctor may also be asked whether particularly reasonable accommodations would meet your needs.

If a reasonable accommodation would help you do your job, the employer must give you one unless it involves significant difficulty or expense. The employer cannot legally fire you or refuse to hire or promote you, because you asked for a reasonable accommodation, or because you need one. The employer also cannot charge you for the costs of accommodation. However, if more than one accommodation would work, your employer can choose which one to give you.

IF YOUR EMPLOYER KNOWS THAT YOU HAVE HIV INFECTION, COULD YOU GET FIRED?

Employers are not allowed to discriminate against you simply because you have an HIV infection. This includes firing you, rejecting you for a job or promotion, and forcing you to take leave.

Although employers do not have to keep employees who are unable to do the job, or who pose a "direct threat" to safety (a significant risk of substantial harm to yourself or others), they cannot rely on myths or stereotypes about HIV infection when deciding what you can safely or effectively do. Before an employer can reject you based on your condition, it must have objective evidence that you are unable to perform your job duties, or that you would create a significant safety risk, even with reasonable accommodation.

WHAT IF YOU ARE BEING HARASSED BECAUSE OF YOUR CONDITION?

Harassment based on a disability is not allowed under the ADA. You should tell your employer about any harassment if you want the employer to stop the problem. Follow your employer's reporting procedures if there are any. If you report the harassment, your employer is legally required to take action to prevent it from occurring in the future.

WHAT SHOULD YOU DO IF YOU THINK THAT YOUR RIGHTS HAVE BEEN VIOLATED?

The Equal Employment Opportunity Commission (EEOC) will help you to decide what to do next and conduct an investigation if you decide to file a charge of discrimination. Because you must file a charge within 180 days of the alleged violation in order to take further legal action (or 300 days if the employer is also covered by a state or local employment discrimination law), it is best to begin the process early. It is illegal for your employer to retaliate against you for contacting the EEOC or filing a charge.

Section 49.2 | Laws for Your Welfare

This section contains text excerpted from the following sources: Text under the heading "The Americans with Disabilities Act and Persons with HIV/AIDS" is excerpted from "Questions and Answers: The Americans with Disabilities Act and Persons with HIV/AIDS," ADA.gov, U.S. Department of Justice (DOJ), February 25, 2020; Text under the heading "Family and Medical Leave Act (FMLA)" is excerpted from "Family and Medical Leave (FMLA)," U.S. Department of Labor (DOL), March 31, 2016. Reviewed February 2022; Text under the heading "Health Insurance Portability and Accountability (HIPAA)" is excerpted from "FAQs on HIPAA Portability and Nondiscrimination Requirements for Employers and Advisers," U.S. Department of Labor (DOL), September 15, 2014. Reviewed February 2022; Text under the heading "COBRA: 7 Important Facts" is excerpted from "COBRA: Seven Important Facts," Centers for Medicare & Medicaid Services (CMS), November 18, 2019.

THE AMERICANS WITH DISABILITIES ACT AND PERSONS WITH HIV/AIDS
What Is the ADA?

The Americans with Disabilities Act (ADA) gives federal civil rights protections to individuals with disabilities similar to those provided to individuals on the basis of race, color, sex, national origin, age, and religion. It guarantees equal opportunity for individuals with disabilities in public accommodations, employment, transportation, State and local government services, and telecommunications.

Are People Living with HIV or AIDS Protected by the ADA?

Yes. An individual has a "disability" under the ADA if he or she has a physical or mental impairment that substantially limits one or more major life activities, including major bodily functions such as the functions of the immune system; has a record of such an impairment, or has an actual or perceived mental or physical impairment that is not transitory and minor and is subjected to an action prohibited under the ADA. Persons with HIV, both symptomatic and asymptomatic, have physical impairments that substantially limit one or more major life activities or major bodily functions and are, therefore, protected by the law.

Persons who are discriminated against because they are regarded as having HIV are also protected. For example, a person who was fired on the basis of a rumor that he had AIDS, even if he did not, would be protected by the law.

Moreover, the ADA protects persons who are discriminated against because they have a known association or relationship with an individual who has HIV. For example, the ADA would protect a woman (who does not have HIV) who was denied a job because her roommate had AIDS.

FAMILY AND MEDICAL LEAVE ACT (FMLA)

The Family and Medical Leave Act (FMLA) provides certain employees with up to 12 weeks of unpaid, job-protected leave per year. It also requires that their group health benefits be maintained during the leave.

FMLA is designed to help employees balance their work and family responsibilities by allowing them to take reasonable unpaid leave for certain family and medical reasons. It also seeks to accommodate the legitimate interests of employers and promote equal employment opportunities for men and women.

FMLA applies to all public agencies, all public and private elementary and secondary schools, and companies with 50 or more employees. These employers must provide an eligible employee with up to 12 weeks of unpaid leave each year for any of the following reasons:

- For the birth and care of the newborn child of an employee
- For placement with the employee of a child for adoption or foster care
- To care for an immediate family member (i.e., spouse, child, or parent) with a serious health condition or
- To take medical leave when the employee is unable to work because of a serious health condition

Employees are eligible for leave if they have worked for their employer at least 12 months, at least 1,250 hours over the past 12 months, and work at a location where the company employs 50 or more employees within 75 miles. Whether an employee has worked a minimum of 1,250 hours of service is determined according to The Fair Labor Standards Act (FLSA) principles for determining compensable hours or work.

Time taken off work due to pregnancy complications can be counted against the 12 weeks of family and medical leave.

Military family leave provisions, first added to the FMLA in 2008, afford FMLA protections specific to the needs of military families.

Special rules apply to employees of local education agencies. The U.S. Department of Labor (DOL) administers FMLA; however, the Office of Personnel Management administers FMLA for most federal employees.

HEALTH INSURANCE PORTABILITY AND ACCOUNTABILITY (HIPAA)

The Health Insurance Portability and Accountability Act of 1996 (HIPAA) includes provisions of Federal law governing health coverage portability, health information privacy, administrative simplification, medical savings accounts, and long-term care insurance. The responsibility of the U.S. Department of Labor (DOL) is the law's portability and nondiscrimination requirements. HIPAA's provisions affect group health plan coverage in the following ways:

- Provide certain individuals special enrollment rights in group health coverage when specific events occur, e.g., the birth of a child (regardless of any open season)
- Prohibit discrimination in group health plan eligibility, benefits, and premiums based on specific health factors and
- While HIPAA previously provided for limits with respect to preexisting condition exclusions, new protections under the Affordable Care Act now prohibit preexisting condition exclusions for plan years beginning on or after January 1, 2014. For plan years beginning on or after January 1, 2014, plans are no longer required to issue the general notice of preexisting condition exclusion and individual notice of period of preexisting condition exclusion. Plans are also no longer required to issue certificates of creditable coverage after December 31, 2014. These amendments were made because plans are prohibited from imposing

preexisting condition exclusions for plan years beginning on or after January 1, 2014.

COBRA: 7 IMPORTANT FACTS

The Consolidated Omnibus Budget Reconciliation Act (COBRA) is a federal law that may let you keep your employer group health plan. This is called "continuation coverage." coverage for a limited time after your employment ends or you lose coverage as a dependent of the covered employee.

In general, COBRA only applies to employers with 20 or more employees. However, some states require insurers covering employers with fewer than 20 employees to let you keep your coverage for a limited time.

In most situations that give you COBRA rights (other than a divorce), you should get a notice from your employer's benefits administrator or the group health plan. The notice will tell you your coverage is ending and offer you the right to elect COBRA continuation coverage.

COBRA coverage generally is offered for 18 months (36 months in some cases). Ask the employer's benefits administrator or group health plan about your COBRA rights if you find out your coverage has ended and you do not get a notice, or if you get divorced.

The employer must tell the plan administrator if you qualify for COBRA because the covered employee died, lost their job, or became entitled to Medicare. Once the plan administrator is notified, the plan must let you know you have the right to choose COBRA coverage.

You or the covered employee needs to tell the plan administrator if you qualify for COBRA because you got divorced or legally separated (court-issued separation decree) from the covered employee, or you were a dependent child or dependent adult child who is no longer a dependent.

You will need to tell the plan administrator about your change in the situation within 60 days of the change.

Before you elect COBRA, talk with your State Health Insurance Assistance Program (SHIP) about Part B and Medigap.

Chapter 50 | Public Benefits and Housing Options for Persons with HIV

Chapter Contents

Section 50.1 | Social Security for People Living with HIV/AIDS

This section includes text excerpted from "Social Security for People Living with HIV/AIDS," U.S. Social Security Administration (SSA), December 1, 2019.

If you have human immunodeficiency virus (HIV)/acquired immunodeficiency syndrome (AIDS) and cannot work, you may qualify for disability benefits from the Social Security Administration (SSA). Your condition must be expected to last at least a year or end in death and must be serious enough to prevent you from doing substantial gainful work. The number of earnings we consider substantial and gainful changes each year.

If your child has HIV/AIDS, she or he may be able to get Supplemental Security Income (SSI) if your household income is low enough.

BENEFITS PAID UNDER TWO PROGRAMS

Disability benefits are offered under two programs: the Social Security Disability Insurance (SSDI) program for people who paid Social Security taxes; and the Supplemental Security Income program for people who have little income and few resources. If your Social Security benefits are very low and you have limited income and resources, you may qualify for benefits from both programs.

HOW DO YOU QUALIFY FOR SOCIAL SECURITY DISABILITY BENEFITS?

When you work and pay Social Security taxes, you earn Social Security credits. (Most people earn the maximum of four credits a year.) The number of years of work needed for disability benefits depends on how old you are when you become disabled. Generally, you need five years of work in the 10 years before the year you become disabled. Younger workers need fewer years of work. If your application is approved, your first Social Security disability benefit will be paid for the sixth full month after the date your disability began.

WHAT WILL YOU GET FROM SOCIAL SECURITY?

The amount of your monthly benefit depends on how much you earned while you were working. You will also qualify for Medicare after you have been getting disability benefits for 24 months. Medicare helps pay for hospital and hospice care, lab tests, home healthcare, and other medical services.

HOW DO YOU QUALIFY FOR SSI DISABILITY PAYMENTS?

If you have not worked long enough to get Social Security or your Social Security benefits are low, you may qualify for SSI payments, if your total income and resources are low enough. If you get SSI, you will most likely be eligible for the Supplemental Nutrition Assistance Program (SNAP) and Medicaid. Medicaid takes care of your medical bills while you are in the hospital or receiving outpatient care. In some states, Medicaid pays for hospice care, a private nurse, and prescription drugs used to fight HIV disease.

HOW DO YOU FILE FOR BENEFITS?

You can apply for Social Security disability benefits online or through a phone call to make an appointment to file a disability claim at your local Social Security office or to set up an appointment for someone to take your claim over the telephone. The disability claims interview lasts about one hour.

HOW IS YOUR CLAIM DECIDED?

All applications received from people with HIV/AIDS are processed as quickly as possible. Social Security works with an agency in each state called the Disability Determination Services. The state agency will look at the information you and your doctor provide and decide if you qualify for benefits. You are paid the SSI benefits right away for up to six months before a final decision is made on your claim if:
- You are not working
- You meet the SSI rules about income and resources and

- Your doctor or other medical source certifies that your HIV infection meets certain criteria based on medical eligibility rules

HOW CAN YOU HELP SPEED UP YOUR CLAIM?

You can help speed up the processing of your claim by having certain information when you apply. This includes:

- Your Social Security number and birth certificate and the Social Security numbers and birth certificates of any family members who may be applying for benefits; and
- A copy of your most recent W-2 form. (If you are applying for SSI, you need to provide information about your income and resources; for example, bank statements, unemployment records, rent receipts, and car registration.)

Other required information includes:

- The names and addresses of any doctors, hospitals, or clinics you have been to for treatment;
- How HIV/AIDS has affected your daily activities, such as cleaning, shopping, cooking, taking the bus, etc.; and
- The kinds of jobs you have had during the past 15 years.

WHAT HAPPENS IF YOU GO BACK TO WORK

If you return to work, there are special rules that let your benefits continue while you work. These rules are important for people with HIV/AIDS who may be able to go back to work when they are feeling better.

Section 50.2 | Affordable Care Act for People Living with HIV/AIDS

This section includes text excerpted from "The Affordable Care Act and HIV/AIDS," HIV.gov, U.S. Department of Health and Human Services (HHS), January 17, 2022.

IMPROVING ACCESS TO COVERAGE

The Affordable Care Act (ACA) provides Americans – including those with and at risk for HIV – better access to healthcare coverage and more health insurance options. Health insurance gives people with HIV access to appropriate HIV medical care, particularly antiretroviral therapy (ART), which helps people with HIV stay healthy and prevent transmitting HIV to others.

Here are just some of the ways the ACA has improved access to coverage for people with or at risk for HIV:

- **Coverage for people with preexisting conditions.** Thanks to the ACA, no American can ever again be dropped or denied coverage because of a preexisting health condition, such as asthma, cancer, or HIV. Insurers also are prohibited from canceling or rescinding coverage because of mistakes made on an application, and can no longer impose lifetime caps on insurance benefits. These changes are significant because prior to the ACA, many people living with HIV or other chronic health conditions experienced obstacles in getting health coverage, were dropped from coverage or avoided seeking coverage for fear of being denied. Now they can get covered and get the care they need.
- **Broader Medicaid eligibility.** Under the ACA, states have the option, which is fully Federally funded for the first three years, to expand Medicaid to generally include those with incomes at or below 138 percent of the Federal poverty line, including single adults without children who were previously not generally eligible for Medicaid. As of October 2021, 39 states (including DC) have adopted the Medicaid expansion. Medicaid is the largest payer for HIV care in the United

States, and the expansion of Medicaid to low-income childless adults is particularly important for many gay, bisexual, and other men who have sex with men (MSM) who were previously ineligible for Medicaid, and yet remain the population most affected by the HIV epidemic. Further, in states that opt for Medicaid expansion, people with HIV who meet the income threshold no longer have to wait for an AIDS diagnosis in order to become eligible for Medicaid. That means they can get into life-extending care and treatment before the disease has significantly damaged their immune system.

- **More affordable coverage.** The ACA requires most Americans to have qualifying health insurance. To help people access quality, affordable coverage, the ACA created the Healthcare.gov Marketplace (and some state-run Marketplaces, sometimes called "exchanges") that help consumers compare different health plans and determine what savings they may qualify for. The ACA also provides financial assistance for people with low and middle incomes in the form of tax credits that lower the cost of their monthly premiums and lower their out-of-pocket costs. These tax credits depend on a family's household size and income. In addition, Americans can apply for free or low-cost coverage through Medicaid and Children's Health Insurance Program (CHIP) at any time, all year. If you qualify, coverage can begin immediately.
- **Lower prescription drug costs for Medicare recipients.** In the past, as many as one in four seniors went without a prescription drug every year because they could not afford it. The ACA closed, over time, the Medicare Part D prescription drug coverage gap once known as the donut hole – the gap between when a person's initial Medicare drug coverage ended and when they qualified for catastrophic coverage. Previously, when people reached the donut hole, they

had to pay the full cost for their prescription drugs until they reached the catastrophic coverage level and many struggled to pay for their medications. Under the ACA, the donut hole began shrinking in 2011 and closed in 2020. Now, people in the coverage gap will pay no more than 25 percent of the cost of their covered medications. Also, as a result of the ACA, AIDS Drug Assistance Program (ADAP) spending is now counted as part of Medicare Part D's True Out-of-Pocket ("TrOOP") costs, allowing ADAP clients who are Medicare Part D enrollees to reach the catastrophic coverage level faster, when Medicare starts covering the full cost of medications.

ENSURING QUALITY COVERAGE

The Affordable Care Act also helps all Americans, including those with or at risk for HIV, have access to the best quality coverage and care. This includes:

- **Preventive services.** Under the ACA, most new health insurance plans must cover certain recommended preventive services including HIV testing for everyone age 15 to 65 and other ages at increased risk without additional cost-sharing, such as copays or deductibles. Since about one in eight people with HIV in the United States (13%) are unaware of their HIV status, improving access to HIV testing will help more people learn their status so they can be connected to care and treatment. Pre-exposure prophylaxis (PrEP) to prevent HIV is also covered for HIV-negative adults at high risk for getting HIV through sex or injection drug use. This coverage of PrEP includes medications as well as necessary clinic visits and lab tests. Other preventive health services related to HIV risk and/or health outcomes are also covered, such as sexually transmitted infection counselling, syphilis screening, hepatitis B and hepatitis C screening, and hepatitis A and hepatitis B immunizations.

- **Comprehensive coverage**. The law establishes a minimum set of benefits (called "essential health benefits") that must be covered under health plans offered in the individual and small group markets, both inside and outside of the Health Insurance Marketplace. These include many health services that are important for people with HIV, including prescription drug services, hospital inpatient care, lab tests, services and devices to help you manage a chronic disease, and mental health and substance use disorder services, as well as HIV screening, PrEP, and other preventive services for those at risk for HIV.
- **Coordinated care for those with chronic health conditions**. The law recognizes the value of patient-centered medical homes as an effective way to strengthen the quality of care, especially for people with complex chronic conditions such as HIV. The patient-centered medical home model of care can foster greater patient retention and higher quality HIV care because of its focus on treating the many needs of the patient at once and better coordination across medical specialties and support services. The Ryan White HIV/AIDS Program has been a pioneer in the development of this model in the HIV healthcare system. The ACA also authorized an optional Medicaid State Plan benefit for states to establish Health Homes to coordinate care for Medicaid beneficiaries with certain chronic health conditions. HIV/AIDS is one of the chronic health conditions that states may request approval to cover.

ENHANCING THE CAPACITY OF THE HEALTHCARE DELIVERY SYSTEM

The ACA expands the capacity of the healthcare delivery system to better serve all Americans, including those with and at risk for HIV. For example:

- **Expansion of community health centers**. The ACA has made a major investment in expanding the network of community health centers that provide preventive and primary care services to nearly 29 million Americans every year, regardless of their ability to pay. Health centers provide high-quality primary care services and support public health priorities such as responding to the opioid crisis, the implementation of the National HIV/AIDS Strategy, the Ending the HIV Epidemic in the United States initiative (EHE), and the response to COVID-19.

- **Delivering culturally competent care**. The ACA expands initiatives to strengthen cultural competency training for all healthcare providers and ensure all populations are treated equitably. It also bolsters the Federal commitment to reducing health disparities. One effort underway to expand the capacity of health centers to deliver culturally competent care to populations heavily impacted by HIV is the National LGBTQIA+ Health Education Center, funded by Health Resources and Services Administration (HRSA). This center helps healthcare organizations better address the needs of lesbian, gay, bisexual, transgender, queer, intersex, asexual, and all sexual and gender minority people, including individuals' needs for HIV prevention, testing, and treatment.

- **Increasing the healthcare workforce for underserved communities**. Thanks to the ACA, the National Health Service Corps (NHSC) is providing loans and scholarships to more doctors, nurses, and other healthcare providers, a critical healthcare workforce expansion to better serve vulnerable populations. This is in line with a key recommendation of the National HIV/AIDS Strategy to increase the number and diversity of available providers of clinical care and related services for people living with HIV, many of whom live in underserved communities.

LEARN MORE ABOUT THE AFFORDABLE CARE ACT

Here are several resources to help you stay informed about the Affordable Care Act and its impact on people with HIV:

- HealthCare.gov (www.healthcare.gov) is the U.S. Department of Health and Human Services (HHS) website to help you understand your health coverage options and compare health plans so you can enroll in a plan that works for you and your family.
- The Ryan White TARGETHIV Center's Health Coverage Library (targethiv.org/library/topics/health-coverage) is a collection of resources to help Ryan White agencies and consumers better understand healthcare coverage.
- The Ryan White Access, Care, & Engagement (ACE) TA Center (targethiv.org/ace) helps Ryan White HIV/AIDS Program grantees and subgrantees enroll diverse clients, especially people of color, in health insurance and build provider cultural competence.
- Formerly the National Alliance for State and Territorial AIDS Directors (NASTAD) offers resources about health reform efforts and how they may affect people living with HIV/AIDS.
- Greater Than AIDS. Health Coverage, HIV and You (www.greaterthan.org/campaigns/health-coverage-hiv-you) is a site developed by the Kaiser Family Foundation to help people living with HIV learn about their coverage options and how the law could affect their care and treatment.

Section 50.3 | Housing Options for People with HIV

This section includes text excerpted from "Housing and Health," HIV.gov, U.S. Department of Health and Human Services (HHS), August 21, 2019.

WHY DO PEOPLE WITH HIV NEED STABLE HOUSING?

Stable housing is closely linked to successful human immunodeficiency virus (HIV) outcomes. With safe, decent, and affordable housing, people with HIV are better able to access medical care and supportive services, get on HIV treatment, take their HIV medication consistently, and see their healthcare provider regularly. In short: the more stable your living situation, the better you do in care.

Individuals with HIV who are homeless or lack stable housing, on the other hand, are more likely to delay HIV care and less likely to access care consistently or to adhere to their HIV treatment.

Throughout many communities, people with HIV risk losing their housing due to such factors as stigma and discrimination, increased medical costs and limited incomes or reduced ability to keep working due to HIV-related illnesses.

WHAT FEDERAL HOUSING ASSISTANCE PROGRAMS ARE AVAILABLE FOR PEOPLE WITH HIV?

To help take care of the housing needs of low-income people living with HIV and their families, the U.S. Department of Housing and Urban Development's (HUD) Office of HIV/AIDS Housing manages the Housing Opportunities for Persons With AIDS (HOPWA) program. The HOPWA program is the only Federal program dedicated to addressing the housing needs of people living with HIV. Under the HOPWA Program, HUD makes grants to local communities, States, and nonprofit organizations for projects that benefit low-income people living with HIV and their families. Many local HOPWA programs and projects provide short-term and long-term rental assistance, operate community residences, or provide other supportive housing facilities that have been created to address the needs of people with HIV.

ARE PEOPLE WITH HIV ELIGIBLE FOR OTHER HUD PROGRAMS?

In addition to the HOPWA program, people living with HIV are eligible for any HUD program for which they might otherwise qualify (such as by being low-income or homeless). Programs include public housing, the Section 8 Housing Choice Voucher Program, housing opportunities supported by Community Development Block Grants, the HOME Investment Partnerships Program, and the Continuum of Care Homeless Assistance Program.

- **Find Housing Assistance**. If you are homeless, at risk of becoming homeless or know someone who is, help is available.
- **Access Other Housing Information**. Find resources for homeless persons, including, youth, veterans, and the chronically homeless, as well as rental, homebuyer, and homeowner assistance.

Chapter 51 | Caring for Someone with HIV/AIDS

HOW CAN YOU HELP SOMEONE WHO HAS BEEN NEWLY DIAGNOSED WITH HIV?

There are many things that you can do to help a friend or loved one who has been recently diagnosed with human immunodeficiency virus (HIV):

- **Talk**. Be available to have open, honest conversations about HIV. Follow the lead of the person who is diagnosed with HIV. They may not always want to talk about it, or may not be ready. They may want to connect with you in the same ways they did before being diagnosed. Do things you did together before their diagnosis; talk about things you talked about before their diagnosis. Show them that you see them as the same person and that they are more than their diagnosis.
- **Listen**. Being diagnosed with HIV is life-changing news. Listen to your loved one and offer your support. Reassure them that HIV is a manageable health condition. There are medicines that can treat HIV and help them stay healthy.
- **Learn**. Educate yourself about HIV: what it is, how it is transmitted, how it is treated, and how people can stay healthy while living with HIV. Having a solid understanding of HIV is a big step forward in supporting your loved one. This website is a good place

This chapter includes text excerpted from "Supporting Someone Living with HIV," HIV.gov, U.S. Department of Health and Human Services (HHS), May 15, 2017. Reviewed February 2022.

to begin to familiarize yourself with HIV. Have these resources available for your newly diagnosed friend if they want them. Knowledge is empowering, but keep in mind that your friend may not want the information right away.

- **Encourage treatment.** Some people who are recently diagnosed may find it hard to take that first step to HIV treatment. Your support and assistance may be helpful. By getting linked to HIV medical care early, starting treatment with HIV medication, called "antiretroviral therapy" (ART), adhering to medication, and staying in care, people with HIV can keep the virus under control, and prevent their HIV infection from progressing to AIDS. HIV treatment is recommended for all people with HIV and should be started as soon as possible after diagnosis. Encourage your friend or loved one to see a doctor and start HIV treatment as soon as possible. If they do not have an HIV care provider, you can help them find one. There are programs that can provide HIV medical care or help with paying for HIV medications. Use HIV.gov's HIV Testing Sites and Care Services Locator to find a provider.

- **Support medication adherence.** It is important for people living with HIV to take their HIV medication every day, exactly as prescribed. Ask your loved ones what you can do to support them in establishing a medication routine and sticking to it. Also, ask what other needs they might have and how you can help them stay healthy.

- **Get support.** Take care of yourself and get support if you need it. Turn to others for any questions, concerns, or anxieties you may have so that the person who is diagnosed can focus on taking care of their own health.

If you are the sexual partner of someone who has been diagnosed with HIV, you should also get tested so that you know your own HIV status. If you test negative, talk to your healthcare provider about pre-exposure prophylaxis (PrEP), taking HIV medicine daily to prevent HIV infection. PrEP is recommended for people at high risk of HIV infection, including those who are in a long-term relationship with a partner who has HIV. If you test positive, get connected to HIV treatment and care as soon as possible.

WHAT IF YOUR FRIEND TELLS YOU THAT THEY HAVE HIV?

More than a million people in the United States are living with HIV, so you may know someone who has the virus. If your friend, family member, or coworker has been HIV-positive for some time and has just told you, here is how you can be supportive:

- **Acknowledge**. If someone has disclosed their HIV status to you, thank them for trusting you with their private health information.
- **Ask**. If appropriate, ask if there is anything that you can do to help them. One reason they may have chosen to disclose their status to you is that they need an ally or advocate, or they may need help with a particular issue or challenge. Some people are public with this information; other people keep it very private. Ask whether other people know this information, and how private they are about their HIV status.
- **Reassure**. Let the person know, through your words or actions, that their HIV status does not change your relationship and that you will keep this information private if they want you to.
- **Learn**. Educate yourself about HIV. Lots of people living with HIV are on ART and have the virus under control. Others are at different stages of treatment and care. Do not make assumptions and look to your friend for guidance.

HOW CAN YOU HELP END HIV?

Want to get involved in HIV-related efforts? Here are some ideas:

- **Reach out to a local HIV service organization**. Many HIV service organizations have opportunities for people living with HIV and others to share their time and talents. Depending on the organization, volunteer opportunities may include:

- Assisting with onsite or mobile testing events by being a greeter, registrar, health educator, or HIV tester
- Providing administrative support, such as filing, data entry, or answering phones
- Helping out with special events
- Participating in fundraising or advocacy activities
- Providing language skills
- Offering professional services, such as legal assistance or medical care, if licensed

- **Engage with others.** Social media tools like Facebook, Twitter, Instagram, and Snapchat offer many opportunities to connect with others who are interested and involved in HIV issues. You can also share information about HIV via these channels to help others learn more.
- **Get involved in HIV awareness days.** Check out our HIV awareness days page to see how you can support national observances to raise awareness and encourage people to get tested for HIV, seek, or return to care.
- **Learn.** Stay abreast of changes in HIV prevention, care, treatment, and research and learn about new tools or resources. Check out our learning opportunities page to find webinars, conferences, Twitter chats, and other events.
- **Share what you know.** You can make a difference by learning more about HIV and sharing that knowledge with others. Talk to others about testing, how to prevent HIV, the effectiveness of treatment, and the importance of getting and staying in medical care. Use our Basics pages to find answers to questions you or others may have. You can easily share those pages on social media or via email using the buttons at the top right side of each page.

Chapter 52 | Coronavirus (COVID-19) and People with HIV

If you have symptoms of COVID-19, get tested and stay home and away from others except to get medical care. Most people have mild illnesses and can recover at home. If you have an emergency warning sign (including trouble breathing), call 911. Keep taking your HIV medicine as prescribed. This will help keep your immune system healthy. If you have been diagnosed with HIV but are not currently taking HIV medicine, talk to your healthcare provider about the benefits of getting on treatment. If you do not have a healthcare provider, contact your nearest community health center or health department.

COVID-19 VACCINES AND PEOPLE WITH HIV

- **Get vaccinated.** The U.S. Department of Health and Human Services (HHS) Guidance for COVID-19 and with HIV recommends that people with HIV should receive COVID-19 vaccines, regardless of their CD4 or viral load, because the potential benefits outweigh the potential risks.

This chapter contains text excerpted from the following sources: Text in this chapter begins with excerpts from "Coronavirus (COVID-19) and People with HIV," HIV.gov, U.S. Department of Health and Human Services (HHS), February 4, 2021; Text under the heading "What to Know about HIV and COVID-19" is excerpted from "What to Know about HIV and COVID-19," Centers for Disease Control and Prevention (CDC), February 4, 2022; Text under the heading "COVID-19 and Travel" is excerpted from "Travel," Centers for Disease Control and Prevention (CDC), January 27, 2022.

- **Additional primary shot**. The Centers for Disease Control and Prevention (CDC) recommends that, after completing the COVID-19 vaccine primary series, some people who have advanced HIV (including an AIDS diagnosis) or untreated HIV should get an additional primary shot to make sure they have enough protection against COVID-19. See CDC's recommendations (www.cdc.gov/coronavirus/2019-ncov/vaccines/ recommendations/immuno.html) for full details and talk to your healthcare provider to determine if getting an additional primary shot is right for you. (CDC does not recommend an additional primary shot of the COVID-19 vaccine for people with HIV who are virally suppressed or who do not have advanced HIV.)
- **Booster shots**. CDC recommends that everyone, including people with HIV, get a booster shot when they are eligible. Get information about who can get a booster shot, when to get a booster, and which booster you can get.
- **Vaccine safety**. COVID-19 vaccines are safe for people with HIV. COVID-19 vaccines meet the U.S. Food and Drug Administration's (FDA) rigorous scientific standards for safety, effectiveness, and manufacturing quality, and people with HIV were included in vaccine clinical trials.

If you have questions about getting the COVID-19 vaccine and whether it is right for you, talk to your healthcare provider.

WHAT TO KNOW ABOUT HIV AND COVID-19

People with HIV may have concerns and questions about COVID-19, including the risk of serious illness and vaccine safety. The CDC will continue to provide updated information as it becomes available.

Are People with HIV at Higher Risk for COVID-19 than Other People?

We are still learning about COVID-19 and how it affects people with HIV. Nearly half of people in the United States with diagnosed HIV are ages 50 and older. People with HIV also have higher rates of certain underlying health conditions. Older age and underlying health conditions can make people more likely to become seriously ill if they get COVID-19. This is especially true for people with advanced HIV or people with HIV who are not on treatment.

People at increased risk for severe illness, and those who live with or visit them, should take precautions (including getting vaccinated and wearing a well-fitting mask) to protect themselves and others from COVID-19.

Are COVID-19 Vaccines Safe for People with HIV?

Yes. COVID-19 vaccines are safe for people with HIV. COVID-19 vaccines meet the FDA's rigorous scientific standards for safety, effectiveness, and manufacturing quality, and people with HIV were included in vaccine clinical trials.

Authorized or approved COVID-19 vaccines will continue to undergo the most intensive safety monitoring. This includes using established and new safety monitoring systems to make sure that COVID-19 vaccines are safe.

Find a COVID-19 vaccine or booster: Search vaccines.gov, text your ZIP code to 438829, or call 800-232-0233 to find locations near you.

How Many Doses of the COVID-19 Vaccine Do People with HIV Need to Get?
COVID-19 VACCINE PRIMARY SERIES

COVID-19 vaccines are recommended for everyone who is eligible. The number of vaccine doses you need depends on the type of vaccine you receive.

ADDITIONAL PRIMARY SHOT

After completing the COVID-19 vaccine primary series, some people who have advanced HIV (including an AIDS diagnosis) or who have HIV and are not taking HIV treatment should get an additional primary shot. The additional primary shot is intended to improve a person's immune response to their two-dose COVID-19 vaccine primary series. People who are eligible for an additional primary shot should receive this dose before they get a booster shot. Talk to your healthcare provider to determine if getting an additional primary shot is right for you.

The CDC does not recommend an additional primary shot of the COVID-19 vaccine for people with HIV who are virally suppressed or who do not have advanced HIV.

BOOSTER SHOT

The CDC recommends that everyone, including people with HIV, get a booster shot when they are eligible. Learn more about who should get a booster, when to get a booster, and which booster you should get (www.cdc.gov/coronavirus/2019-ncov/vaccines/booster-shot.html).

Will COVID-19 Vaccines Interfere with HIV Medicine to Prevent or Treat HIV?

There is no evidence that COVID-19 vaccines interfere with PrEP to prevent HIV or with AR) to treat HIV. Learn more about the different COVID-19 vaccines (www.cdc.gov/coronavirus/2019-ncov/vaccines/different-vaccines.html).

What Can People with HIV Do to Protect Themselves from COVID-19?

People with HIV can protect themselves from COVID-19 by following CDC's COVID-19 prevention recommendations.

If you have HIV and are taking your HIV medicine as prescribed, it is important to continue your treatment and follow your healthcare provider's advice. This is the best way to keep your immune system healthy. People with HIV should also continue to maintain a healthy lifestyle.

Here are more steps that people with HIV can take:
- Make sure you have at least a 30-day (or longer) supply of your HIV medicine and any other medicines or

medical supplies you need for managing HIV. Ask your healthcare provider about getting your medicine by mail.

- Talk to your healthcare provider and make sure all your vaccinations are up to date, including vaccinations against seasonal influenza (flu) and bacterial pneumonia. These vaccine-preventable diseases affect people with HIV more than others.
- When possible, keep your medical appointments. Check with your healthcare provider about safety precautions for office visits and ask about telemedicine or remote clinical care options.
- People with HIV can sometimes be more likely than others to need extra help from friends, family, neighbors, community health workers, and others. If you become sick, make sure you stay in touch by phone or email with people who can help you.

What Should You Do If You Think You Might Have COVID-19?

Call your healthcare provider if you develop symptoms that could be consistent with COVID-19.

It is important to continue taking your HIV medicine as prescribed. This will help keep your immune system healthy.

Can HIV Medicine (Antiretroviral Therapy) Be Used to Treat COVID-19?

Currently, treatment for COVID-19 is limited. Evidence does not show that any medicines used to treat HIV are effective against COVID-19. People with HIV should not switch their HIV medicine in an attempt to prevent or treat COVID-19.

Some clinical trials are looking at whether HIV medicines can treat COVID-19. Other trials are looking at the effectiveness of different drugs to treat COVID-19 in people with HIV. They are also looking to better understand how people with HIV manage COVID-19.

Should People with HIV Travel at This Time?

Everyone, including people with HIV, should follow CDC's COVID-19 travel recommendations.

What Can Everyone Do to Minimize Stigma about COVID-19?

Minimizing stigma and misinformation about COVID-19 is very important. People with HIV have experience in dealing with stigma and can be allies in preventing COVID-19 stigma. Learn how you can reduce stigma and help prevent the spread of rumors about COVID-19.

COVID-19 AND TRAVEL

Do not travel if:

- You are sick
- You tested positive for COVID-19
- Do not travel until a full 10 days after your symptoms started or the date your positive test was taken if you had no symptoms
- You are waiting for the results of a COVID-19 test
- You had close contact with a person with COVID-19 and are recommended to quarantine
  - Do not travel until a full 5 days after your last close contact with the person with COVID-19. It is best to avoid travel for a full 10 days after your last exposure
  - If you must travel during days 6 through 10 after your last exposure:
    - Get tested at least 5 days after your last close contact. Make sure your test result is negative and you remain without symptoms before traveling. If you do not get tested, avoid travel until a full 10 days after your last close contact with a person with COVID-19.
    - Properly wear a well-fitting mask when you are around others for the entire duration of travel during days 6 through 10. If you are unable to wear a mask, you should not travel during days 6 through 10.

Coronavirus (COVID-19) and People with HIV

If you had close contact with a person with COVID-19 but are NOT recommended to quarantine...

- Get tested at least 5 days after your last close contact. Make sure your test result is negative and you remain without symptoms before traveling.
- If you travel during the 10 days after your last exposure, properly wear a well-fitting mask when you are around others for the entire duration of travel during the 10 days. If you are unable to wear a mask, you should not travel during the 10 days.

Part 7 | Additional Help and Information

Chapter 53 | Glossary of HIV/AIDS-Related Terms

acute HIV infection: Early stage of HIV infection that extends approximately 1–4 weeks from initial infection until the body produces enough HIV antibodies to be detected by an HIV antibody test. During acute HIV infection, HIV is highly infectious because the virus is multiplying rapidly. The rapid increase in HIV viral load can be detected before HIV antibodies are present.

adherence: Taking medications (or other treatment) exactly as instructed by a healthcare provider. The benefits of strict adherence to an HIV regimen include sustained viral suppression, reduced risk of drug resistance, improved overall health and quality of life, and decreased risk of HIV transmission.

adverse event (AE): Any undesirable experience associated with the use of a drug or other medical product.

alanine aminotransferase (ALT): A liver enzyme that plays a role in protein metabolism. Abnormally high blood levels of ALT are a sign of liver inflammation or damage from infection or drugs. A normal level is below approximately 50 IU/L.

albumin: A protein made by the liver and found in the blood. Levels of this protein may be measured as part of a liver function test.

anemia: A blood disorder caused by a reduced number or function of red blood cells. Symptoms may include shortness of breath, fatigue, and rapid heartbeat. HIV-associated causes of anemia include progression of HIV disease, opportunistic infections, and certain HIV-related drugs.

antibiotic: A drug used to kill or suppress the growth of bacteria.

This glossary contains terms excerpted from documents produced by several sources deemed reliable.

arthralgia (joint pain): A common symptom of HIV infection and may be caused by some drugs used to treat HIV and opportunistic infections.

assay: A qualitative or quantitative analysis of a substance; a test.

asymptomatic: Without symptoms or not sick. Usually, used in HIV/AIDS literature to describe a person who has a positive reaction to one of several tests for HIV antibodies, but who shows no clinical symptoms of the disease and who is not sick. Even though a person is asymptomatic, she or he may still infect another person with HIV.

baseline: An initial measurement used as the basis for future comparison. For people infected with HIV, baseline testing includes CD4 count, viral load (HIV RNA (ribonucleic acid)), and resistance testing. Baseline test results are used to guide HIV treatment choices and monitor effectiveness of antiretroviral therapy (ART).

CD4 cell count: A laboratory test that measures the number of CD4 T lymphocytes (CD4 cells) in a sample of blood. In people with HIV, the CD4 count is the most important laboratory indicator of immune function and the strongest predictor of HIV progression. The CD4 count is one of the factors used to determine when to start antiretroviral therapy (ART). The CD4 count is also used to monitor response to ART.

cervical cancer: Cancer that forms in tissues of the cervix (the organ connecting the uterus and vagina). It is usually a slow-growing cancer that may not have symptoms, but can be found with regular Papanicolaou (Pap) tests (a procedure in which cells are scraped from the cervix and looked at under a microscope). Cervical cancer is almost always caused by human papillomavirus (HPV) infection.

chemotherapy: In general, it is the use of medicines to treat any disease. It is more commonly used to describe medicines to treat cancer.

chlamydia: A sexually transmitted disease (STD) caused by *Chlamydia trachomatis* that infects the genital tract. The infection is frequently asymptomatic (i.e., shows no symptoms), but if left untreated, it can cause sterility in women.

chronic HIV infection: Also known as "asymptomatic HIV infection" or "clinical latency." The stage of HIV infection between acute HIV infection and the onset of AIDS. During chronic HIV infection, HIV levels gradually increase and the number of CD4 cells decrease. Declining CD4 cell levels indicate increasing damage to the immune system. Antiretroviral therapy

Glossary of HIV/AIDS-Related Terms

(ART) can prevent HIV from destroying the immune system and advancing to AIDS.

clinical progression: Advance of disease that can be measured by observable and diagnosable signs or symptoms. For example, HIV progression can be measured by change in CD4 count.

cluster of differentiation 4 (CD4) cell: A type of lymphocyte. CD4 T lymphocytes (CD4 cells) help coordinate the immune response by stimulating other immune cells, such as macrophages, B lymphocytes (B cells), and CD8 T lymphocytes (CD8 cells), to fight infection. HIV weakens the immune system by destroying CD4 cells.

coccidioidomycosis: An infectious fungal disease caused by the breathing in of *Coccidioides immitis*, which are carried on windblown dust particles.

coinfection: When a person has two or more infections at the same time. For example, a person infected with HIV may be coinfected with hepatitis C virus (HCV) or tuberculosis (TB) or both.

combination therapy: Two or more drugs or treatments used together to obtain the best results against HIV infection and/or AIDS. Combination drug therapy (treatment) has proven more effective than monotherapy (single-drug therapy) in controlling the growth of the virus. An example of combination therapy would be the use of two drugs such as zidovudine and lamivudine together.

computed tomography (CT) scan: A procedure that uses a computer linked to an x-ray machine to make a series of detailed pictures of areas inside the body. The pictures are taken from different angles and are used to create 3-dimensional (3-D) views of tissues and organs. A dye may be injected into a vein or swallowed to help the tissues and organs show up more clearly. A CT scan may be used to help diagnose disease, plan treatment, or find out how well treatment is working. Also called "CAT scan," "computed tomography scan," "computerized axial tomography scan," and "computerized tomography."

core biopsy: The removal of a tissue sample with a wide needle for examination under a microscope. Also called "core needle biopsy."

drug resistance: When a bacteria, virus, or other microorganism mutates (changes form) and becomes insensitive to (resistant to) a drug that was previously effective. Drug resistance can be a cause of HIV treatment failure.

false negative: A negative test result that incorrectly indicates that the condition being tested for is not present when, in fact, the condition is actually present. For example, a false negative HIV test indicates a person does not have HIV when, in fact, the person is infected with HIV.

false positive: A positive test result that incorrectly indicates that the condition being tested for is present when, in fact, the condition is actually not present. For example, a false positive HIV test indicates a person has HIV when, in fact, the person is not infected with HIV.

highly active antiretroviral therapy (HAART): The name given to treatment regimens recommended by HIV experts to aggressively decrease viral multiplication and progress of HIV disease. The usual HAART treatment combines three or more different drugs, such as two nucleoside reverse transcriptase inhibitors (NRTIs) and a protease inhibitor, two NRTIs and a nonnucleoside reverse transcriptase inhibitor (NNRTI), or other combinations. These treatment regimens have been shown to reduce the amount of virus so that it becomes undetectable in a patient's blood.

Hodgkin lymphoma: A cancer of the immune system that is marked by the presence of a type of cell called the "Reed-Sternberg cell." The two major types of Hodgkin lymphoma are classical Hodgkin lymphoma and nodular lymphocyte-predominant Hodgkin lymphoma (NLPHL). Symptoms include the painless enlargement of lymph nodes, spleen, or other immune tissue. Other symptoms include fever, weight loss, fatigue, or night sweats. Also called "Hodgkin disease."

human herpesvirus 8 (HHV-8): A type of virus that causes Kaposi sarcoma (KS) (a rare cancer in which lesions grow in the skin, lymph nodes, lining of the mouth, nose, and throat, and other tissues of the body). Human herpesvirus 8 also causes certain types of lymphoma (cancer that begins in cells of the immune system). Also called "HHV8," "Kaposi sarcoma-associated herpesvirus," and "KSHV."

human papillomavirus (HPV): A type of virus that can cause abnormal tissue growth (e.g., warts) and other changes to cells. Infection for a long time with certain types of HPV can cause cervical cancer. HPV may also play a role in some other types of cancer, such as anal, vaginal, vulvar, penile, oropharyngeal, and squamous cell skin cancers.

immune system: A complex network of cells, tissues, organs, and the substances they make that helps the body fight infections and other diseases. The immune system includes white blood cells and organs and tissues of the lymph system, such as the thymus, spleen, tonsils, lymph nodes, lymph vessels, and bone marrow.

immunocompromised: When the body is unable to produce an adequate immune response. A person may be immunocompromised because of a disease or an infection, such as HIV, or as the result of treatment with drugs or radiation.

immunosuppression: A state of the body in which the immune system is damaged and does not perform its normal functions. Immunosuppression may be induced by drugs (e.g., in chemotherapy) or result from certain disease processes, such as HIV infection.

incisional biopsy: A surgical procedure in which a portion of a lump or suspicious area is removed for diagnosis. The tissue is then examined under a microscope to check for signs of disease.

incubation period: The time between infection with a pathogen and the onset of disease symptoms.

latency: The period when an infecting organism is in the body, but is not producing any clinically noticeable ill effects or symptoms. In HIV disease, clinical latency is an asymptomatic period in the early years of HIV infection. The period of latency is characterized by near-normal cluster of differentiation 4+ (CD4+) T-cell counts.

lymphocyte: A type of immune cell that is made in the bone marrow and is found in the blood and in lymph tissue. The two main types of lymphocytes are B lymphocytes and T lymphocytes. B lymphocytes make antibodies, and T lymphocytes help kill tumor cells and help control immune responses. A lymphocyte is a type of white blood cell.

monotherapy: Using only one drug to treat an infection or disease. Monotherapy for the treatment of HIV is not recommended outside of a clinical trial. The optimal regimen for initial treatment of HIV includes three antiretroviral (ARV) drugs from at least two different HIV drug classes.

nonnucleoside reverse transcriptase inhibitor (NNRTI): Antiretroviral (ARV) HIV drug class. Nonnucleoside reverse transcriptase inhibitors (NNRTIs) bind to and block HIV reverse transcriptase (an HIV enzyme). HIV uses reverse transcriptase to convert its ribonucleic acid (RNA) into deoxyribonucleic acid (DNA) (reverse transcription). Blocking reverse transcriptase and reverse transcription prevents HIV from replicating.

nucleoside reverse transcriptase inhibitor (NRTI): Antiretroviral (ARV) HIV drug class. Nucleoside reverse transcriptase inhibitors (NRTIs) block reverse transcriptase (an HIV enzyme). HIV uses reverse transcriptase to convert its RNA into DNA (reverse transcription). Blocking reverse transcriptase and reverse transcription prevents HIV from replicating.

opportunistic infection (OI): An infection that occurs more frequently or is more severe in people with weakened immune systems, such as people with HIV or people receiving chemotherapy, than in people with healthy immune systems.

positron emission tomography (PET) scan: A procedure in which a small amount of radioactive glucose (sugar) is injected into a vein, and a scanner is used to make detailed, computerized pictures of areas inside the body where the glucose is taken up. Because cancer cells often take up more glucose than normal cells, the pictures can be used to find cancer cells in the body. Also called "PET scan."

post-exposure prophylaxis (PEP): Short-term treatment started as soon as possible after high-risk exposure to an infectious agent, such as HIV, hepatitis B virus (HBV), or hepatitis C virus (HCV). The purpose of PEP is to reduce the risk of infection. An example of a high-risk exposure is exposure to an infectious agent as the result of unprotected sex.

protease inhibitor: Antiretroviral (ARV) HIV drug class. Protease inhibitors (PIs) block protease (an HIV enzyme). By blocking protease, PIs prevent new (immature) HIV from becoming a mature virus that can infect other CD4 cells.

rapid HIV test: A screening test for detecting antibody to HIV that produces very quick results, usually in 5–30 minutes. For diagnosis of HIV infection, a positive rapid test is confirmed with a second rapid test made by a different manufacturer.

reverse transcription: The third of seven steps in the HIV life cycle. Once inside a CD4 cell, HIV releases and uses reverse transcriptase (an HIV enzyme) to convert its genetic material – HIV RNA – into HIV DNA. The conversion of HIV RNA to HIV DNA allows HIV to enter the CD4 cell nucleus and combine with the cell's genetic material – cell DNA.

serologic test: Any number of tests that are performed on the clear fluid portion of blood. Often refers to a test that determines the presence of antibodies to antigens such as viruses.

Glossary of HIV/AIDS-Related Terms

syphilis: A primarily sexually transmitted disease (STD) resulting from infection with the spirochete (a bacterium) Treponema pallidum. Syphilis can also be acquired in the uterus during pregnancy.

T cell: A type of lymphocyte. There are two major types of T lymphocytes: cytotoxic T lymphocytes (CD8 cells) and CD4 T lymphocytes (CD4 cells); both T cell types are essential for a healthy immune system. HIV infects and destroys CD4 cells, gradually destroying the immune system.

thymus: An organ of the lymph system where T lymphocytes (T cells) develop and mature. The thymus is important for normal immune system development early in life and is at its largest size at puberty.

transmitted resistance: When a person acquires a strain of HIV that is already resistant to certain antiretroviral (ARV) drugs.

treatment failure: When an antiretroviral (ARV) regimen is unable to control HIV infection. Treatment failure can be clinical failure, immunologic failure, virologic failure, or any combination of the three. Factors that can contribute to treatment failure include drug resistance, drug toxicity, or poor treatment adherence.

treatment regimen: A structured treatment plan designed to improve and maintain health. Recommended regimens for the initial treatment of HIV generally include a combination of three or more antiretroviral (ARV) drugs from at least two different HIV drug classes.

triglycerides: A type of fat in blood and adipose (fat) tissue.

undetectable viral load: When the amount of HIV in the blood is too low to be detected with a viral load (HIV RNA) test. Antiretroviral (ARV) drugs may reduce a person's viral load to an undetectable level; however, that does not mean the person is cured.

varicella zoster virus (VZV): A type of herpesvirus that causes chicken pox. After initial infection with varicella zoster virus (VZV), the inactive (latent) form of the virus can remain in the body. If the latent virus becomes active again, it can cause shingles.

viral load: The amount of HIV in a sample of blood. Viral load is reported as the number of HIV RNA copies per milliliter of blood.

viral suppression: When antiretroviral therapy (ART) reduces a person's viral load (HIV RNA) to an undetectable level. Viral suppression does not mean a person is cured; HIV still remains in the body. If ART is discontinued, the person's viral load will likely return to a detectable level.

virologic failure: A type of HIV treatment failure. Virologic failure occurs when antiretroviral therapy (ART) fails to suppress and sustain a person's viral load to less than 200 copies/mL.

white blood cell (WBC): A type of cell found in blood and lymph. White blood cells (WBCs) are key components of the immune system and help fight infection and disease. Examples of white blood cells include lymphocytes, neutrophils, eosinophils, macrophages, and mast cells.

window period: The time period from infection with HIV until the body produces enough HIV antibodies to be detected by standard HIV antibody tests. The length of the window period varies depending on the antibody test used. During the window period, a person can have a negative result on an HIV antibody test despite being infected with HIV.

Chapter 54 | Directory of Organizations for People with HIV/AIDS and Their Families and Friends

GOVERNMENT AGENCIES THAT PROVIDE INFORMATION ABOUT HIV/AIDS

Centers for Disease Control and Prevention (CDC)
1600 Clifton Rd.
Atlanta, GA 30329-4027
Toll-Free: 800-CDC-INFO
(800-232-4636)
Phone: 404-639-3311
Toll-Free TTY: 888-232-6348
Website: www.cdc.gov
E-mail: cdcinfo@cdc.gov

HIVinfo
5601 Fishers Ln.
Bldg. 5601, Fl. Rm. 2F02., MSC 9840
Rockville, MD 20892-9840
Toll-Free: 800-448-0440
Website: hivinfo.nih.gov
E-mail: ContactUs@HIVinfo.NIH.gov

Resources in this chapter were compiled from several sources deemed reliable; all contact information was verified and updated in February 2022.

Office of Minority Health (OMH)
Tower Oaks Bldg.
1101 Wootton Pkwy, Ste. 100
Rockville, MD 20852
Phone: 240-453-2882
Fax: 240-453-2883
Website: www.minorityhealth.hhs.
gov
E-mail: info@minorityhealth.hhs.
gov

National Cancer Institute (NCI)
9609 Medical Center Dr.
Rockville, MD 20850
Toll-Free: 800-4-CANCER
(800-422-6237)
Website: www.cancer.gov
E-mail: NCIinfo@nih.gov

National Institute of Allergy and Infectious Diseases (NIAID)
5601 Fishers Ln.
MSC 9806
Bethesda, MD 20892-9806
Toll-Free: 866-284-4107
Phone: 301-496-5717
Toll-Free TDD: 800-877-8339
Fax: 301-402-3573
Website: www.niaid.nih.gov
E-mail: ocpostoffice@niaid.nih.gov

National Institute on Aging (NIA)
Bldg. 31, Rm. 5C27
31 Center Dr., MSC 2292
Bethesda, MD 20892
Toll-Free: 800-222-2225
Toll-Free TTY: 800-222-4225
Website: www.nia.nih.gov
E-mail: niaic@nia.nih.gov

National Institute on Drug Abuse (NIDA)
6001 Executive Blvd.
Rm. 5213, MSC 9561
Bethesda, MD 20892
Phone: 301-443-6245
Website: nida.nih.gov

National Institutes of Health (NIH)
9000 Rockville Pike
Bethesda, MD 20892
Phone: 301-496-4000
TTY: 301-402-9612
Website: www.nih.gov

National Institutes of Mental Health (NIMH)
6001 Executive Blvd.
Rm. 6200, MSC 9663
Bethesda, MD 20892-9663
Toll-Free: 866-615-6464
Website: www.nimh.nih.gov
E-mail: nimhinfo@nih.gov

National Prevention Information Network (NPIN)
Website: npin.cdc.gov
E-mail: NPIN-info@cdc.gov

Office of AIDS Research (OAR)
5601 Fishers Ln.
Rm. 2F40
Rockville, MD 20892
Phone: 301-496-0357
Website: www.oar.nih.gov
E-mail: oarinfo@nih.gov

Office of Minority Health Resource Center (OMHRC)

1101 Wootton Pkwy.
Tower Oaks Bldg.
Rockville, MD 20852
Toll-Free: 800-444-6472
TDD: 301-251-1432
Fax: 301-251-2160
Website: minorityhealth.hhs.gov
E-mail: info@minorityhealth.hhs.gov

U.S. Department of Health and Human Services (HHS)

200 Independence Ave., S.W.
Washington, DC 20201
Toll-Free: 877-696-6775
Website: www.hhs.gov

U.S. Department of Veterans Affairs (VA)

810 Vermont Ave., N.W.
Washington, DC 20420
Toll-Free: 877-222-VETS
(877-222-8387)
Website: www.va.gov

U.S. Food and Drug Administration (FDA)

10903 New Hampshire Ave.
Silver Spring, MD 20993-0002
Toll-Free: 888-INFO-FDA
(888-463-6332)
Website: www.fda.gov

PRIVATE AGENCIES THAT PROVIDE INFORMATION ABOUT HIV/AIDS

African Aid Organization

1325 G St., N.W., Ste. 500
Washington, DC 20005
Phone: 202-449-7708
Website: afaid.org
E-mail: info@afaid.org

AID Atlanta

1605 Peachtree St., N.E.
Atlanta, GA 30309-2955
Toll-Free: 800-551-2728
Phone: 404-870-7700
Website: aidatlanta.org

AIDS Action

75 Amory St.
Boston, MA 02119
Phone: 617-437-6200
Website: aac.org

AIDS Foundation Houston

6260 Westpark Dr., Ste. 100
Houston, TX 77057
Phone: 713-623-6796
Fax: 713-623-4029
Website: afhouston.org

AIDS Healthcare Foundation (AHF)
6255 Sunset Blvd.
21st Fl.
Los Angeles, CA 90028
Phone: 323-860-5200
Website: www.aidshealth.org

AIDS InfoNet
2200 Pennsylvania Ave., N.W.
4th Fl., E.
Washington, DC 20037
Website: www.aidsinfonet.org

AIDS United
1634 Eye St., Ste. 1100
Washington, DC 20006-4003
Phone: 202-408-4848
Fax: 202-408-1818
Website: aidsunited.org
E-mail: cba@aidsunited.org

AIDS Vaccine Advocacy Coalition (AVAC)
423 W. 127th St.
4th Fl.
New York, NY 10027
Phone: 212-796-6423
Fax: 646-365-3452
Website: www.avac.org
E-mail: avac@avac.org

AIDSVu
Phone: 202-854-0480
Website: www.aidsvu.org
E-mail: info@aidsvu.org

American Academy of Family Physicians (AAFP)
11400 Tomahawk Creek Pkwy.
Leawood, KS 66211
Toll-Free: 800-274-2237
Phone: 913-906-6000
Fax: 913-906-6075
Website: www.aafp.org
E-mail: aafp@aafp.org

American Academy of HIV Medicine (AAHIVM)
1627 Eye St., N.W., Ste. 835
Washington, DC 20006
Phone: 202-659-0699
Fax: 202-659-0976
Website: www.aahivm.org

American Sexual Health Association (ASHA)
P.O. Box 13827
Research Triangle Park, NC 27709
Phone: 919-361-8400
Fax: 919-361-8425
Website: www.ashasexualhealth.org
E-mail: info@ashasexualhealth.org

Antiretroviral Pregnancy Registry (APR)
301 Government Center Dr.
Wilmington, NC 28403
Toll-Free: 800-258-4263
Toll-Free Fax: 800-800-1052
Website: www.apregistry.com
E-mail: SM_APR@INCResearch.com

Black AIDS Institute

1833 W. 8th St., Ste. 200
Los Angeles, CA 90057-4920
Website: blackaids.org
E-mail: Info@BlackAIDS.org

Black Health, Inc.

215 W. 125th St.
2nd Fl.
New York, NY 10027
Phone: 212-614-0023
Fax: 212-614-0508
Website: nblch.org
E-mail: info@nblch.org

The Body

461 5th Ave.
14th Fl.
New York, NY 10017
Phone: 212-695-2223
Fax: 212-695-2936
Website: www.thebody.com

CARE for AIDS, Inc

977 Grant Cove Pl.
Atlanta, GA 30315
Phone: 678-595-2999
Website: www.careforaids.org

Elizabeth Glaser Pediatric AIDS Foundation (EGPAF)

1140 Connecticut Ave., N.W., Ste. 200
Washington, DC 20036
Toll-Free: 888-499-HOPE
(888-499-4673)
Phone: 202-296-9165
Fax: 202-296-9185
Website: www.pedaids.org
E-mail: info@pedaids.org

Elton John AIDS Foundation (EJAF)

584 Bdwy., Ste. 906
New York, NY 10012
Phone: 212-219-0670
Website: www.
eltonjohnaidsfoundation.org
E-mail: admin@
eltonjohnaidsfoundation.org

The Foundation for AIDS Research (amfAR)

120 Wall St.
13th Fl.
New York, NY 10005-3908
Toll-Free: 800-39-amfAR
(800-392-6327)
Phone: 212-806-1600
Fax: 212-806-1601
Website: www.amfar.org
E-mail: info@amfar.org

HIV Medicine Association (HIVMA)

4040 Wilson Blvd., Ste. 300
Arlington, VA 22203
Phone: 703-299-0200
Fax: 703-299-0204
Website: www.hivma.org
E-mail: info@hivma.org

HIV Vaccine Trials Network (HVTN)

1100 Fairview Ave., N. Ste. 300
Seattle, WA 98109
Phone: 206-667-6300
Fax: 206-667-6366
Website: www.hvtn.org
E-mail: info@hvtn.org

International AIDS Vaccine Initiative (IAVI)
125 Broad St.
9th Fl.
New York, NY 10004
Phone: 212-847-1111
Fax: 212-847-1112
Website: www.iavi.org
E-mail: info@iavi.org

Lifelong
210 S. Lucile St.
Seattle, WA 98108
Toll-Free: 877-297-0576
Phone: 206-957-1600
Fax: 206-257-3300
Website: www.lifelong.org

National Clinician Consultation Center (NCCC)
1001 Potrero Ave.
Bldg. 20, Ward 2203
San Francisco, CA 94110
Toll-Free: 800-933-3413
Phone: 628-206-8700
Fax: 415-476-3454
Website: aidsetc.org/aetc-program/
national-clinician-consultation-
center

National Minority AIDS Council (NMAC)
1000 Vermont Ave., N.W., Ste. 200
Washington, DC 20005-4903
Phone: 202-815-3129
Website: www.nmac.org
E-mail: communications@nmac.
org

North American Syringe Exchange Network (NASEN)
535 Dock St., Ste. 113
Tacoma, WA 98402
Phone: 253-272-4857
Fax: 253-272-8415
Website: www.nasen.org

NYU School of Medicine
550 1st Ave.
New York, NY 10016
Website: www.med.nyu.edu

Pacific AIDS Education and Training Center (PAETC)
550 16th St.
3rd Fl., UCSF MC 0661
San Francisco, CA 94158-2549
Phone: 415-476-6153
Website: www.paetc.org

SAGE
305 7th Ave.
15th Fl.
New York, NY 10001
Phone: 212-741-2247
Fax: 212-366-1947
Website: www.sageusa.org
E-mail: info@sageusa.org

San Francisco AIDS Foundation
1035 Market St., Ste. 400
4th Fl.
San Francisco, CA 94103
Phone: 415-487-3000
Website: sfaf.org
E-mail: info@sfaf.org

Directory of Organizations

Treatment Action Group
90 Broad St., Ste. 2503
New York, NY 10004
Phone: 212-253-7922
Website: www.
treatmentactiongroup.org
E-mail: tag@treatmentactiongroup.
org

U.S. Military HIV Research Program (MHRP)
6720A Rockledge Dr., Ste. 400
Bethesda, MD 20817
Phone: 301-500-3600
Fax: 301-500-3666
Website: www.hivresearch.org
E-mail: communications@
hivresearch.org

Vivent Health
7215 Cameron Rd., Ste. B
Austin, TX 78752
Toll-Free: 833-366-6664
Phone: 512-220-7609
Toll-Free Fax: 877-770-9910
Website: viventhealth.org

The Well Project
P.O. Box 220410
Brooklyn, NY 11222
Toll-Free: 888-616-WELL
(888-616-9355)
Website: www.thewellproject.org

Whitman-Walker
1377 R St., N.W., Ste. 200
Washington, DC 20009
Phone: 202-745-7000
Fax: 202-332-1049
Website: www.whitman-walker.org

World AIDS Museum and Educational Center
1350 E. Sunrise Blvd.
Fort Lauderdale, FL 33304
Phone: 954-390-0550
Website: worldaidsmuseum.org
E-mail: info@worldaidsmuseum.
org

Melanoma Education Foundation (MEF)
P.O. Box 2023
Peabody, MA 01960
Phone: 978-535-3080
Fax: 978-535-5602
Website: www.skincheck.org
E-mail: mef@skincheck.org

Multiple Myeloma Research Foundation (MMRF)
383 Main Ave.
5th Fl.
Norwalk, CT 06851
Phone: 203-229-0464
Website: www.themmrf.org
E-mail: info@themmrf.org

National Brain Tumor Foundation (NBTF)

55 Chapel St., Ste. 200
Newton, MA 02458
Phone: 617-924-9997
Fax: 617-924-9998
Website: www.braintumor.org
E-mail: development@braintumor.org

National Lymphedema Network (NLN)

P.O. Box 1008
New York, NY 10276
Toll-Free: 800-541-3259
Website: www.lymphnet.org
E-mail: nln@lymphnet.org

Pancreatic Cancer Action Network (PanCAN)

1500 Rosecrans Ave., Ste. 200
Manhattan Beach, CA 90266
Toll-Free: 877-272-6226
Phone: 310-725-0025
Fax: 310-725-0029
Website: www.pancan.org
E-mail: info@pancan.org

The Pink Fund

P.O. Box 603
Bloomfield Hills, MI 48303
Toll-Free: 877-234-7465
Website: pinkfund.org
E-mail: info@thepinkfund.org

The Skin Cancer Foundation

205 Lexington Ave.
11th Fl.
New York, NY 10016
Phone: 212-725-5176
Fax: 212-725-5751
Website: www.skincancer.org
E-mail: research@skincancer.org

ThyCa: Thyroid Cancer Survivors' Association, Inc.

P.O. Box 1102
Olney, MD 20830-1102
Toll-Free: 877-588-7904
Fax: 630-604-6078
Website: www.thyca.org
E-mail: thyca@thyca.org

INDEX

INDEX

Page numbers followed by 'n' indicate a footnote. Page numbers in *italics* indicate a table or illustration.

Index

antiretroviral therapy (ART),
 continued
 COVID-19, 633
 drug interaction, 329
 early treatment, 401
 fungal infections, 431
 HIV/AIDS prevention, 141
 HIV infection, 9
 HIV testing, 199
 HIV treatment, 35, 249, 279
 kidney disease, 535
 long-acting HIV prevention, 190
 Mycobacterium avium complex
  (MAC), 421
 older adults, 594
 progressive multifocal
  leukoencephalopathy
  (PML), 497
 sex workers, 106
 smoking, 566
 therapeutic HIV vaccine, 349
 treatment adherence, 295
 vaccines, 175
 viral load, 115
antiretrovirals (ARVs)
 HIV treatment, 350
 myopathy, 529
 pregnancy, 167
appetite
 hepatitis B virus (HBV)
  infection, 500
 hepatotoxicity, 316
 HIV medicine, 555
 marijuana, 343
 wasting syndrome, 539
Apretude®, pre-exposure prophylaxis
 (PrEP), 184
aromatherapy, alternative
 therapies, 338
ARS. *See* acute retroviral syndrome
ART. *See* antiretroviral therapy
arthralgia (joint pain), defined, 640
ARVs. *See* antiretrovirals

Asian American
 HIV infection rate, 46
 type 2 diabetes, 314
Asians, HIV infections, 52
aspartate aminotransferase (AST),
 blood chemistry tests, 242
assay, defined, 640
asthma
 Affordable Care Act (ACA), 616
 candidiasis, 436
 HIV testing, 204
asymptomatic, defined, 640
asymptomatic HIV infection
 AIDS, 25
 Strategic Timing of AntiRetroviral
  Treatment (START)
  study, 401
atazanavir, HIV protease
 inhibitor, 334
atorvastatin, statin dose
 limitations, 333
azidothymidine (AZT), HIV
 treatment, 272

B

baseline
 antiretroviral regimens, 17
 defined, 640
 HIV clinical trials, 366
 HIV tests, 239
behavioral intervention
 HIV prevention research, 388
 HIV prevention, 56
 impact of HIV, 70
 transgender population, 105
β-D-glucan, *Pneumocystis* pneumonia
 (PCP), 463
bilirubin, blood
 chemistry, 242
binge drinking, HIV
 transmission, 119

Index

Index

Index

distal symmetric polyneuropathy
(DSP), described, 523–24
DNA. *See* deoxyribonucleic acid
drug interactions
  described, 261–62
  overview, 329–31
  substance use and HIV, 569
drug resistance
  antiretroviral therapy (ART), 250
  defined, 641
  HIV medicine and side effects, 312
  overview, 18–19
drug toxicity, pediatric HIV
  treatment, 298
drug use
  HIV stigma, 577
  opportunistic infections (OIs), 415
  organ transplantation, 137
  pre-exposure prophylaxis
    (PrEP), 58
  socioeconomic factors, 107
  syringe services programs
    (SSPs), 123
drug-drug interaction
  atorvastatin, 333
  virologic failure, 287
drug-food interaction, virologic
  failure, 289
drug-injection equipment
  HIV risk behavior, 56
  opportunistic infections (OIs), 412
drug-resistant strain, antiretroviral
  treatment, 282
dry mouth
  antiretroviral therapy (ART), 251
  candidiasis, 436
  oral health issues, 530
dual energy x-ray absorptiometry,
  osteoporosis, 323

E

e-cigarettes, described, 567

early diagnosis, clinical trials and
  research, 397
Effective Health Care Program
  publication
    Marijuana, 343n
electrodesiccation, surgery, 512
electrolyte test, blood chemistry
  tests, 242
Elizabeth Glaser Pediatric AIDS
  Foundation (EGPAF), contact, 651
Elton John AIDS Foundation (EJAF),
  contact, 651
emergency contraception, birth
  control, 589
emtricitabine, antiretroviral regimens, 16
encephalitis, herpes zoster virus, 492
encephalopathy, opportunistic
  infections (OIs), 412
Epstein-Barr virus (EBV)
  high risk cancer types, 506
  lymphoma, 519
  oral health symptoms, 532
  radiculopathies, 528
esophageal candidiasis, co-occurring
  fungal infections, 435
ethnicity
  hispanic/latinx, 56
  HIV incidence, 30
  HIV stigma, 577
  osteoporosis, 322
exercise
  lipodystrophy, 321
  myopathy, 529
  osteoporosis, 324
  overview, 557–59
  yoga, 338

F

facial palsies, described, 525
false negative
  defined, 642
  OraQuick In-Home HIV Test, 220

Index

Index

Index

opportunistic infections (OIs),
continued
  T-cell count, 240, 249
  traveling, 572
  tuberculosis (TB), 427
  wasting syndrome, 539
opt-out screening, overview 206–07
oral candidiasis, oral health issues, 530
oral contraceptive, birth control, 589
oral health
  allied healthcare professionals, 237
  candidiasis, 436
  overview, 530–32
oral sex
  alcohol use, 119
  described, 113
  herpes simplex virus type 1 (HSV-1), 485, 486, 487
  human papillomavirus (HPV), 493
  latex barrier, 591
  protection during sex, 145
  risky sex, 588
  sexual behaviors, 153
  sexually transmitted diseases (STDs), 125, 126, 127
oral ulcers, oral sex, 113
OraQuick In-Home HIV test
  overview, 219–22
  rapid self-test, 202
osteoporosis
  exercise, 558
  overview, 322–24
  treatment side effects, 313

P

Pacific AIDS Education and Training Center (PAETC), contact, 652
Pacific Islanders,
  overview, 67–70
Pancreatic Cancer Action Network (PanCAN), contact, 654

Pap test
  cancer risk, 508
  human papillomavirus (HPV), 495
PAPs. *See* Patient Assistance Programs
Patient Assistance Programs (PAPs),
  non-federal resources, 407
PCR. *See* polymerase chain reaction
PEP. *See* postexposure prophylaxis
perinatal transmission
  children and adolescents, 73
  HIV and pregnancy, 18, 77, 112, 169
  HIV medicines, 167
  overview, 169–71
  scheduled cesarean delivery, 168
peripheral neuropathy, treatment side effects, 313
peripheral/systemic lymphoma, AIDS related lymphoma, 519
personality change, progressive multifocal leukoencephalopathy (PML), 497
persons who inject drugs (PWIDs)
  described, 143
  oral daily preps, 374
pertussis, vaccines, 177
pet exposure, described, 416
PHN. *See* postherpetic neuralgia
The Pink Fund, contact, 654
PIs. *See* protease inhibitors
PML. *See* progressive multifocal leukoencephalopathy
Pneumocystis jirovecii
  fungal infections, 433
  See also Pneumocystis pneumonia (PCP)
Pneumocystis pneumonia (PCP)
  opportunistic infections (OIs), 412
  overview, 461–64

Index

S

Index

Index

triglyceride
  defined, 645
  exercise, 558
  HIV protease inhibitors, 332
  lipid profile, 243
trimethoprim/sulfamethoxazole
  (TMP/SMX), *Pneumocystis*
  pneumonia (PCP), 464
Truvada
  HIV prevention, 370
  pre-exposure prophylaxis
    (PrEP), 184
Truvada®, pre-exposure prophylaxis
  (PrEP), 184
TSpotTB, tuberculosis (TB) test, 244
tubal ligation, birth control and
  HIV, 589

U
U.S. Department of Labor (DOL)
  publications
    Family and Medical Leave
      (FMLA), 607n
    FAQs on HIPAA Portability
      and Nondiscrimination
      Requirements for
      Employers and
      Advisers, 607n
U.S. Department of Veterans Affairs
  (VA)
  contact, 649
  publications
    Alternative (Complementary)
      Therapies for HIV/
      AIDS, 337n
    Drugs, Alcohol, and HIV, 562n
    Exercise for People with
      HIV, 557n
    Frequently Asked Questions:
      How Accurate Is the Rapid
      Oral HIV Test? 213n

Getting an HIV Diagnosis –
  Your Next Steps: Entire
  Lesson, 543n
HIV Wasting Syndrome, 539n
Preventing Opportunistic
  Infections (OIs), 415n
Rapid Oral HIV Test: Patient
  Fact Sheet, 213n
Sex and Sexuality for People
  with HIV, 583n
Treatment Decisions for
  HIV, 253n
Understanding Laboratory
  Tests, 239n
U.S. Equal Employment Opportunity
  Commission (EEOC)
  publication
    Living with HIV Infection
    Your Legal Rights in the
    Workplace Under the
    ADA, 603n
U.S. Food and Drug Administration
  (FDA)
  contact, 649
  publications
    HIV or Hepatitis C Drugs
      Interactions and Muscle
      Injury, 331n
    Home Access HIV-1 Test
      System, 216n
    OraQuick In-Home HIV
      Test, 216n
U.S. Military HIV Research Program
  (MHRP), contact, 653
U.S. Social Security Administration
  (SSA)
  publication
    Social Security for People Living
      with HIV/AIDS, 613n
unapproved test, home test, 218, 221
undetectable viral load
  alcohol and drugs, 120

Index